T0263819

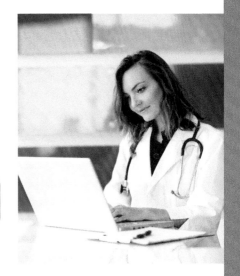
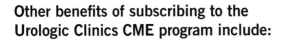

Testicular Cancer

Editor

DANIEL W. LIN

UROLOGIC CLINICS
OF NORTH AMERICA

www.urologic.theclinics.com

Consulting Editor
SAMIR S. TANEJA

August 2015 • Volume 42 • Number 3

ELSEVIER

1600 John F. Kennedy Boulevard ● Suite 1800 ● Philadelphia, Pennsylvania, 19103-2899

http://www.theclinics.com

UROLOGIC CLINICS OF NORTH AMERICA Volume 42, Number 3
August 2015 ISSN 0094-0143, ISBN-13: 978-0-323-39360-7

Editor: Kerry Holland
Developmental Editor: Susan Showalter

Urologic Clinics of North America (ISSN 0094-0143) is published quarterly by Elsevier Inc., 360 Park Avenue South, New York, NY 10010-1710. Months of issue are February, May, August, and November. Business and Editorial Offices: 1600 John F. Kennedy Blvd., Suite 1800, Philadelphia, PA 19103-2899. Periodicals postage paid at New York, NY and additional mailing offices. Subscription prices are $355.00 per year (US individuals), $602.00 per year (US institutions), $415.00 per year (Canadian individuals), $752.00 per year (Canadian institutions), $515.00 per year (foreign individuals), and $752.00 per year (foreign institutions). Foreign air speed delivery is included in all *Clinics* subscription prices. All prices are subject to change without notice. **POSTMASTER:** Send address changes to *Urologic Clinics of North America*, Elsevier Health Sciences Division, Subscription Customer Service, 3251 Riverport Lane, Maryland Heights, MO 63043. **Customer Service: 1-800-654-2452 (US). From outside the United States, call 1-314-447-8871. Fax: 1-314-447-8029. E-mail: JournalsCustomerServiceusa@elsevier.com (for print support)** and **JournalsOnlineSupport-usa@elsevier.com (for online support)**.

Reprints. For copies of 100 or more, of articles in this publication, please contact the Commercial Reprints Department, Elsevier Inc., 360 Park Avenue South, New York, New York 10010-1710. Tel.: 212-633-3874; Fax: 212-633-3820; E-mail: reprints@elsevier.com.

Urologic Clinics of North America is covered in MEDLINE/PubMed (*Index Medicus*), *Excerpta Medica, Current Contents/Clinical Medicine, Science Citation Index,* and *ISI/BIOMED*.

PROGRAM OBJECTIVE

The goal of *Urologic Clinics of North America* is to keep practicing urologists and urology residents up to date with current clinical practice in urology by providing timely articles reviewing the state of the art in patient care.

TARGET AUDIENCE

Practicing urologists, urology residents and other health care professionals practicing in the discipline of urology.

LEARNING OBJECTIVES

Upon completion of this activity, participants will be able to:
1. Review the epidemiology and diagnosis of testicular cancer.
2. Discuss the roles of surgery and chemotherapy in the management of the different stages of testicular cancer.
3. Recognize the long term outcomes and health risks associated with testicular cancer, such as infertility.

ACCREDITATION

The Elsevier Office of Continuing Medical Education (EOCME) is accredited by the Accreditation Council for Continuing Medical Education (ACCME) to provide continuing medical education for physicians.

The EOCME designates this enduring material for a maximum of 15 *AMA PRA Category 1 Credit*(s)™. Physicians should claim only the credit commensurate with the extent of their participation in the activity.

All other health care professionals requesting continuing education credit for this enduring material will be issued a certificate of participation.

DISCLOSURE OF CONFLICTS OF INTEREST

The EOCME assesses conflict of interest with its instructors, faculty, planners, and other individuals who are in a position to control the content of CME activities. All relevant conflicts of interest that are identified are thoroughly vetted by EOCME for fair balance, scientific objectivity, and patient care recommendations. EOCME is committed to providing its learners with CME activities that promote improvements or quality in healthcare and not a specific proprietary business or a commercial interest.

The planning committee, staff, authors and editors listed below have identified no financial relationships or relationships to products or devices they or their spouse/life partner have with commercial interest related to the content of this CME activity:

Brett S. Carver, MD; Clint Cary, MD, MPH; Lisly Chéry, MD; Siamak Daneshmand, MD; Atreya Dash, MD; Jasreman Dhillon, MD; Tanya Dorff, MD; Scott E. Eggener, MD; Darren R. Feldman, MD; Anjali Fortna; Sophie D. Fossa, MD, PhD; Richard S. Foster, MD; Chunkit Fung, MD, MS; Kerry Holland; Brian Hu, MD; Gino In, MD, MPH; Günter Janetschek, MD; Evan Kovac, MD CM, FRCSC; Indu Kumari; Thomas Kunit, FEBU; Stanley L. Liauw, MD; Daniel W. Lin, MD; William T. Lowrance, MD, MPH; Timothy A. Masterson, MD; James M. McKiernan, MD; Matthew J. O'Shaughnessy, MD, PhD; Kevin A. Ostrowski, MD; Shane M. Pearce, MD; Kevin R. Rice, MD; Wade J. Sexton, MD; Pranav Sharma, MD; Joel Sheinfeld, MD; Andrew J. Stephenson, MD, FRCSC, FACS; Scott M. Stevenson, MD; Megan Suermann; Lois B. Travis, MD, ScD; Thomas J. Walsh, MD; Annalynn Williams, MS; Solomon L. Woldu, MD.

The planning committee, staff, authors and editors listed below have identified financial relationships or relationships to products or devices they or their spouse/life partner have with commercial interest related to the content of this CME activity:

Samir S. Taneja, **MD** is a consultant/advisor for Bayer HealthCare AG; Eigen Pharma, LLC; GTx, Inc.; HealthTronics, Inc.; and Hitachi, Ltd.

UNAPPROVED/OFF-LABEL USE DISCLOSURE

The EOCME requires CME faculty to disclose to the participants:
1. When products or procedures being discussed are off-label, unlabelled, experimental, and/or investigational (not US Food and Drug Administration [FDA] approved); and
2. Any limitations on the information presented, such as data that are preliminary or that represent ongoing research, interim analyses, and/or unsupported opinions. Faculty may discuss information about pharmaceutical agents that is outside of FDA-approved labelling. This information is intended solely for CME and is not intended to promote off-label use of these medications. If you have any questions, contact the medical affairs department of the manufacturer for the most recent prescribing information.

TO ENROLL

To enroll in the *Urologic Clinics of North America* Continuing Medical Education program, call customer service at 1-800-654-2452 or sign up online at http://www.theclinics.com/home/cme. The CME program is available to subscribers for an additional annual fee of USD 270.

METHOD OF PARTICIPATION

In order to claim credit, participants must complete the following:

1. Complete enrolment as indicated above.
2. Read the activity.
3. Complete the CME Test and Evaluation. Participants must achieve a score of 70% on the test. All CME Tests and Evaluations must be completed online.

CME INQUIRIES/SPECIAL NEEDS

For all CME inquiries or special needs, please contact elsevierCME@elsevier.com.

Contributors

CONSULTING EDITOR

SAMIR S. TANEJA, MD
The James M. Neissa and Janet Riha Neissa
Professor of Urologic Oncology; Professor of
Urology and Radiology; Director, Division of
Urologic Oncology; Co-Director, Department
of Urology, Smilow Comprehensive Prostate
Cancer Center, NYU Langone Medical Center,
New York, New York

EDITOR

DANIEL W. LIN, MD
Professor and Chief of Urologic Oncology,
Department of Urology, Bridges Endowed
Professorship in Prostate Cancer Research,
University of Washington, Seattle, Washington

AUTHORS

BRETT S. CARVER, MD
Associate Member, Associate Attending,
Department of Surgery, Division of Urology,
Memorial Sloan Kettering Cancer Center,
New York, New York

CLINT CARY, MD, MPH
Assistant Professor of Urology, Department of
Urology, Indiana University School of
Medicine, Indianapolis, Indiana

LISLY CHÉRY, MD
Department of Urology, University of
Washington School of Medicine, Seattle,
Washington

SIAMAK DANESHMAND, MD
Associate Professor of Urology (Clinical
Scholar); Director of Urologic Oncology;
Director of Clinical Research; Urologic
Oncology Fellowship Director, Institute of
Urology, USC/Norris Comprehensive Cancer
Center, Keck School of Medicine University of
Southern California, Los Angeles, California

ATREYA DASH, MD
Department of Urology, University of
Washington School of Medicine, Seattle,
Washington

JASREMAN DHILLON, MD
Assistant Member, Department of
Genitourinary Anatomic Pathology, H. Lee
Moffitt Cancer Center, Tampa, Florida

TANYA DORFF, MD
Division of Medical Oncology, USC Keck
School of Medicine, USC Norris
Comprehensive Cancer Center, Los Angeles,
California

SCOTT E. EGGENER, MD
Section of Urology, Department of Surgery,
University of Chicago, Chicago, Illinois

DARREN R. FELDMAN, MD
Assistant Attending, Genitourinary Oncology
Service, Department of Medicine, Memorial
Sloan Kettering Cancer Center, New York,
New York

SOPHIE D. FOSSA, MD, PhD
Professor Emeritus, Departments of Clinical
Radiotherapy and Oncology, Norwegian
Radium Hospital, Oslo, Norway

RICHARD S. FOSTER, MD
Professor of Urology, Department of Urology,
Indiana University School of Medicine,
Indianapolis, Indiana

CHUNKIT FUNG, MD, MS
Assistant Professor, Division of Medical
Oncology, James P. Wilmot Cancer Institute,
University of Rochester Medical Center,
Rochester, New York

BRIAN HU, MD
Institute of Urology, USC/Norris
Comprehensive Cancer Center, Keck School
of Medicine University of Southern California,
Los Angeles, California

GINO IN, MD, MPH
Division of Medical Oncology, USC Keck
School of Medicine, USC Norris
Comprehensive Cancer Center, Los Angeles,
California

GÜNTER JANETSCHEK, MD
Professor, Department of Urology, Paracelsus
Medical University Salzburg, Salzburg, Austria

EVAN KOVAC, MD CM, FRCSC
Urologic Oncology Fellow, Glickman
Urological & Kidney Institute, Cleveland Clinic,
Cleveland, Ohio

THOMAS KUNIT, FEBU
Department of Urology, Paracelsus Medical
University Salzburg, Salzburg, Austria

STANLEY L. LIAUW, MD
Department of Radiation and Cellular
Oncology, University of Chicago, Chicago,
Illinois

WILLIAM T. LOWRANCE, MD, MPH
Assistant Professor, Department of Surgery,
Division of Urology, Huntsman Cancer
Institute, University of Utah, Salt Lake City,
Utah

TIMOTHY A. MASTERSON, MD
Associate Professor of Urology, Department of
Urology, Indiana University School of
Medicine, Indianapolis, Indiana

JAMES M. MCKIERNAN, MD
Chair and Professor, Department of Urology,
Columbia University Medical Center, New York
Presbyterian Hospital, New York, New York

MATTHEW J. O'SHAUGHNESSY, MD, PhD
Clinical Instructor, Urology Service,
Department of Surgery, Memorial Sloan
Kettering Cancer Center, New York,
New York

KEVIN A. OSTROWSKI, MD
Department of Urology, Oregon Health and
Science University, Portland, Oregon

SHANE M. PEARCE, MD
Section of Urology, Department of Surgery,
University of Chicago, Chicago, Illinois

KEVIN R. RICE, MD
Urologic Surgery, Walter Reed National Military
Medical Center, Bethesda, Maryland

WADE J. SEXTON, MD
Senior Member, Department of Genitourinary
Oncology, H. Lee Moffitt Cancer Center,
Tampa, Florida

PRANAV SHARMA, MD
GU Oncology Fellow, Department of
Genitourinary Oncology, H. Lee Moffitt Cancer
Center, Tampa, Florida

JOEL SHEINFELD, MD
Deputy Chief, Urology Service; William Cahan
Chair in Surgery, Urology Service, Department
of Surgery, Memorial Sloan Kettering Cancer
Center, New York, New York

**ANDREW J. STEPHENSON, MD, FRCSC,
FACS**
Director, Center for Urologic Oncology,
Glickman Urological & Kidney Institute,
Cleveland Clinic, Cleveland, Ohio

SCOTT M. STEVENSON, MD
Urology Resident, Division of Urology,
University of Utah School of Medicine, Salt
Lake City, Utah

LOIS B. TRAVIS, MD, ScD
Professor, Department of Radiation Oncology;
Director, Rubin Center for Cancer Survivorship,
University of Rochester Medical Center,
Rochester, New York

THOMAS J. WALSH, MD
Department of Urology, University of
Washington, Seattle, Washington

ANNALYNN WILLIAMS, MS
Graduate Student, Department of Public
Health Sciences, University of Rochester
Medical Center, University of Rochester

School of Medicine and Dentistry, Rochester,
New York

SOLOMON L. WOLDU, MD
Postdoctural Residency Fellow, Department of
Urology, Columbia University Medical Center,
New York Presbyterian Hospital, New York,
New York

Contents

Testis cancer is the most commonly diagnosed cancer in young men. Most cases represent sporadic occurrences. Most commonly it presents at an early stage (clinical stage I) and is highly curable with radical orchiectomy. Even more advanced stages of testicular cancer are curable with a multimodality treatment approach. There are no widely accepted screening strategies for germ cell tumors. This article discusses the known risk factors and epidemiology of testis cancer, the presentation, and work up for new patients, and the prognosis and cure rates based on the staging and current treatment modalities for testis cancer patients.

Intratubular germ cell neoplasia (ITGCN) is a precursor lesion for testicular germ cell tumors, most of which are early stage. ITGCN is also associated with testicular cancer or ITGCN in the contralateral testis, leading to a risk of bilateral testicular malignancy. Testicular biopsy detects most cases, and orchiectomy is the treatment of choice in patients with unilateral ITGCN. Low-dose radiation therapy is recommended in patients with bilateral ITGCN or ITGCN in the solitary testis, but the long-term risks of infertility and hypogonadism need to be discussed with the patient. Rare histologies of primary testicular cancer are also discussed.

Management of testicular seminoma has benefited from numerous advances in imaging, radiotherapy, and chemotherapy over the last 50 years leading to nearly 100% disease-specific survival for low-stage seminoma. This article examines the evaluation and management of low-stage testicular seminoma, which includes clinical stage I and IIA disease. Excellent outcomes for stage I seminoma are achieved with active surveillance, adjuvant radiotherapy, and adjuvant single-agent carboplatin. Current areas of research focus on optimizing surveillance regimens and minimizing the morbidity and long-term complications of adjuvant treatment. Radiotherapy continues to be the primary treatment option for patients with clinical stage IIa disease.

Desperation postchemotherapy retroperitoneal lymph node dissection is performed in select patients following second-line chemotherapy. Adjuvant postoperative chemotherapy is not indicated in patients following second-line chemotherapy.

The rate of diagnosis of germ cell tumors has remained fairly constant. By the International Germ Cell Cancer Consensus Classification, roughly 60% of all metastatic germ cell tumors are classified as good risk. This group of patients has an excellent prognosis, with greater than 90% expectation of cure. Treatment standards have not changed much in recent years. This article focuses on key concepts in the development of the currently accepted first-line regimens and addresses some evolving areas of interest, if not controversy.

Germ cell tumors of the testis have an overall survival rate greater than 90% as a result of a successful multidisciplinary approach to management. Late relapse affects a subset of patients however, and tends to be chemorefractory and the overall prognosis is poor. Surgery is the mainstay in management of late relapse but salvage chemotherapy can be successful. In this review, the clinical presentation and detection of late relapse, clinical outcomes, and predictors of survival in late relapse and the importance of a multidisciplinary treatment approach for successful management of late relapse are discussed.

Surgery remains an integral component of treating metastatic testicular germ cell tumors outside the retroperitoneum. Defining the role of surgery in extraretroperitoneal (ERP) disease can be challenging because metastases can vary in terms their volume, pattern, timing, and responsiveness to systemic therapy. Some of the philosophies on treating ERP disease have come from robust data on outcomes following postchemotherapy retroperitoneal lymph node dissection. The remaining knowledge is gained from retrospective series of different ERP sites from institutions with expertise in treating testis cancer. This article describes how ERP surgery should be integrated into a multidisciplinary treatment plan.

Retroperitoneal recurrences following retroperitoneal lymph node dissection (RPLND) are rare events and, with few exceptions, should be regarded as either surgical or technical failures, or a result of inappropriate modifications to the original RPLND template. Although not a substitute for an adequate initial RPLND, reoperative retroperitoneal surgery is a viable option for properly selected patients. In the hands of experienced surgeons at tertiary care centers, reoperative retroperitoneal surgery is associated with long-term survival in a significant proportion of patients, with an acceptable degree of morbidity.

Second malignant neoplasms, cardiovascular disease, neurotoxicity and ototox-icity, pulmonary complications, hypogonadism, and nephrotoxicity are potentially life-threatening long-term complications of testicular cancer and its therapy. This article describes the pathogenesis, risks, and management of these late effects experienced by long-term testicular cancer survivors, who are defined as individuals who are disease free 5 years or more after primary treatment. Testicular cancer sur-vivors should follow applicable national guidelines for cancer screening and man-agement of cardiovascular disease risk factors. In addition, health care providers should capitalize on the time of cancer diagnosis as a teachable moment to intro-duce and promote lifestyle changes.

Testicular germ cell cancer is one of the most curable cancers. Most patients are treated during their reproductive years, making infertility a significant quality of life issue after successful treatment. This focused review evaluates the factors that contribute to infertility and specific fertility risks with the various testicular can-cer treatments. Timing of patient discussions and current fertility treatments are reviewed.

UROLOGIC CLINICS OF NORTH AMERICA

THE CLINICS ARE AVAILABLE ONLINE!
Access your subscription at:
www.theclinics.com

Foreword
Testicular Cancer

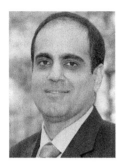

Samir S. Taneja, MD
Consulting Editor

In recent years, we have made a concerted effort to thematically devote current issues of *Urologic Clinics of North America* to areas of Urology, which best demonstrate interdisciplinary interaction and perspective in the approach to disease. In Urology, there is no better example of an interdisciplinary approach to disease than that of the evolved approach to germ cell cancers of the testis. While initially tested as a surgical disease, the advent of platinum-based chemotherapy not only improved disease outcomes but also reinvented the role of surgery in the overall management of the disease. With efficacious therapeutic modalities in hand, highly standardized, stage- and cell-type-specific treatment paradigms could be developed.

Now, those focused on the management of testicular cancer are in a luxurious position relative to those focused on other solid tumors. Given the exceedingly high cure rates demonstrated over the last 20 years, along with the accumulated body of evidence defining risk factors for progression/recurrence and predictors of response, one can easily envision the possibility of a highly individualized approach to the disease. By utilizing therapy when needed, and withholding or minimizing when possible, we can achieve the delicate balance between cure and avoidance of toxicity for which we all strive. In this way, the management of testis cancer serves as an admirable example that can be followed in other organ sites.

In this issue of *Urologic Clinics of North America*, edited by Dr Daniel Lin, the invited authors focus upon issues related to refining the craft of testis cancer management. The issue serves as a wonderful example of physicians of many disciplines offering insight on how to further improve the management of the individual patient. Practical issues, related to challenging clinical scenarios, long-term sequelae of successful therapy, and the management of recurrence, are reviewed in a systematic manner with expert opinions on the best approach. For practicing urologists, the issue serves as an update to already deeply engrained concepts. For those in training, it serves to solidify old concepts and to provoke new ideas that may challenge the existing paradigms. I am deeply indebted to Dr Lin and the many esteemed contributors to this issue for their willingness to provide such fantastic content.

Samir S. Taneja, MD
Division of Urologic Oncology
Smilow Comprehensive Prostate Cancer Center
Department of Urology
NYU Langone Medical Center
150 East 32nd Street, Suite 200
New York, NY 10016, USA

E-mail address:
samir.taneja@nyumc.org

Urol Clin N Am 42 (2015) xv
http://dx.doi.org/10.1016/j.ucl.2015.06.002
0094-0143/15/$ – see front matter © 2015 Published by Elsevier Inc.

Preface

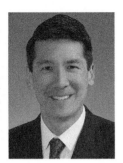

Daniel W. Lin, MD
Editor

In 2015, there will be over 8000 new cases of testicular cancer and nearly 400 deaths. For unknown reasons, the incidence of testicular cancer has been rising in both the United States and Europe, and it represents the most common malignancy in men 18 to 35 years of age. The management of testicular cancer has evolved over the past several decades, in particular with the advent of effective systemic chemotherapy over 30 years ago. The result of the multimodality approach to testicular cancer, in particular advanced testicular cancer, has resulted in remarkably high cure rates, even in the setting of distant metastatic disease. This has made testicular cancer the role-model disease in oncology, with a rich history of clinical trials and established treatment paradigms.

Although outwardly there have been few dramatic changes in treatment of testicular cancer since the last *Urologic Clinics of North America* issue in 2007, there are noteworthy evolving strategies across the disease spectrum and survivorship considerations that merit consideration. For example, we understand more about the late effects of testicular cancer therapy and how these affect survivorship issues. In addition, we are focusing efforts on individualizing therapy to minimize morbidity, preserve quality of life, and enhance recovery from therapy. All of these endeavors have been undertaken with a backdrop of maintaining the oncologic efficacy of the historic treatments, namely, preserving the high-cure rates that were obtained through years of clinical trials and established multidisciplinary approaches. This issue of *Urologic Clinics of North America* highlights key aspects of current testicular cancer management and specifically addresses practical considerations that confront all clinicians who are involved in the management of patients with testicular cancer. As a reflection of current testicular cancer multidisciplinary team approaches, this issue is authored by a wide range of distinguished urologists, medical oncologists, and pathologists.

Daniel W. Lin, MD
Department of Urology
University of Washington
1959 Northeast Pacific Street, Box 356510
Seattle, WA 98195, USA

E-mail address:
dlin@uw.edu

Urol Clin N Am 42 (2015) xvii
http://dx.doi.org/10.1016/j.ucl.2015.06.001
0094-0143/15/$ – see front matter © 2015 Published by Elsevier Inc.

Epidemiology and Diagnosis of Testis Cancer

Scott M. Stevenson, MD[a], William T. Lowrance, MD, MPH[b],*

KEYWORDS

- Testis cancer • Germ cell tumors • Seminoma • Nonseminoma • Epidemiology

KEY POINTS

- Testis cancer is the most commonly diagnosed cancer in young men.
- Although there are multiple risk factors for testis cancer, most cases represent sporadic occurrences.
- Testis cancer most commonly presents at an early stage (clinical stage I) and is highly curable with radical orchiectomy.
- Advanced stages of testis cancer are highly curable with multimodality treatment options.
- There are no widely accepted screening strategies for germ cell tumors, but disease awareness and early detection via self-examination may improve outcomes for those diagnosed.

EPIDEMIOLOGY

The objective of this article is to examine and describe the epidemiology of testicular cancer. The article will outline the general disease patterns of germ cell cancers and potential risk factors that are seen in men with testicular cancer.

An estimated 1 out of every 250 men in the United States will be diagnosed with testis cancer in their lifetime.[1,2] The rate at which testis cancer is diagnosed and found was approximately 5.6 cases per 100,000 men in the United States in 2011, and for unknown reasons this rate has been increasing over the past decades in the United States and other Western countries.[1–5] The incidence of testis cancer peaks at age 25 to 29 years, with 14.3 cases diagnosed per 100,000 men per year, although testis cancer can affect men of all ages.[1,2]

There were an estimated 227,406 testicular cancer survivors in the United States in 2011. In 2014 there was an estimated 8820 new testis cancer diagnoses.[1,2]

The therapies for testis cancer are effective in most cases, as the death rate from testis cancer is relatively low, at 0.23 deaths per 100,000 men per year. The death rate has improved over the past decades, which speaks to the effectiveness of the current multimodality treatment strategies employed for testis cancer. Despite the effectiveness of treatment, anestimated 380 men were expected to die from the disease in 2014 in the United States alone, which was less than 0.2% of all men currently surviving with a history with testicular cancer.[1,2]

Fig. 1 depicts the relationship of the changing incidence and death rates of testis cancer from 1975 to 2011.[1]

The 5-year survival rate for all stages of testis cancer is 96.6%, meaning the vast majority of patients diagnosed with testis cancer can be cured of disease. Testis cancer is one of the few malignancies that can commonly be cured even after it has metastasized. The 5-year survival for localized, regional, or distant disease is 99.2%,

Funding: None.
a Division of Urology, University of Utah School of Medicine, 30 North 1900 East, Salt Lake City, UT 84132, USA;
b Department of Surgery, Division of Urology, Huntsman Cancer Institute, University of Utah, 1950 Circle of Hope, #6405, Salt Lake City, UT 84112, USA
* Corresponding author.
E-mail address: will.lowrance@hci.utah.edu

Urol Clin N Am 42 (2015) 269–275
http://dx.doi.org/10.1016/j.ucl.2015.04.001
0094-0143/15/$ – see front matter © 2015 Elsevier Inc. All rights reserved.

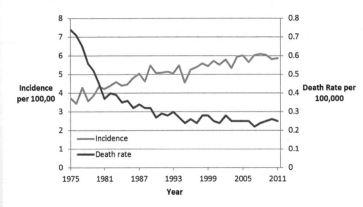

Fig. 1. Incidence and death rates of testicular cancer over time. (*Data from* SEER Cancer Statistics. 2014. Available at: seer.cancer.gov. Accessed November 22, 2014.)

96.0%, and 73.1%, respectively, highlighting the curability of even advanced germ cell tumors. In contrast, patients diagnosed with lung cancer, pancreatic cancer, or esophageal cancer only have a 5-year survival rate of 16.8%, 6.7%, and 17.5%, respectively.[1,2]

RISK FACTORS FOR TESTIS CANCER

Box 1 lists the risk factors, which incude personal history, cryptorchism, family history, intratubular germ cell neoplasia, race, geography, environmental exposures, infertility and microcalcifications.

Personal History

One of the most significant risk factors for development of testis cancer is a personal history of testis cancer. A man has a 12-fold increased risk of developing another primary tumor after his initial diagnosis of testis cancer, which occurs in approximately 2% to 3% of testis tumor survivors.[6,7] Close medical follow-up and diligent patient self-examination are key in facilitating the early detection of second primary tumors. Overall, bilateral germ cell tumors comprise 2% of all testis tumors seen on initial presentation.[8]

Cryptorchidism

History of an undescended testicle, or cryptorchidism, increases the risk of developing a testis tumor by up to eightfold if left surgically uncorrected or corrected after puberty.[9] If corrected with orchiopexy prior to puberty, the relative risk of developing testis cancer is decreased to twofold.[9,10]

Family History

There is evidence suggesting that a family history of testis cancer is a significant risk factor for development of the disease. However, this may be confounded by the result of shared environmental exposures. Some estimate that brothers and sons of men with testis cancer have as high as a 10-fold increased risk of developing testis cancer themselves.[11] There appears to be a stronger link with brothers compared with fathers as a risk factor for developing testis cancer.[12]

Intratubular Germ Cell Neoplasia

Intratubular germ cell neoplasia, also known as carcinoma in situ, is a well-established risk factor for testis cancer. It is often an associated finding with cryptorchid testicles, and contralateral testicles in men with a history of testis cancer.[11]

Race

There is wide variability in the rates of testis cancer based on race. The highest rates are among Caucasians, and the lowest rates among blacks and Asians. In the United States, the incidence of testis cancer among Caucasians is roughly 5 times higher than among blacks, 4 times higher than among Asians, and one-and-a-half times higher

---

Box 1
Risk factors for testicular cancer

- Personal history of testicular cancer in contralateral testicle
- Cryptorchidism
- Family history
- Intratubular germ cell neoplasia
- Race (highest among whites, lowest among blacks and Asians)
- Geography
- Environmental exposures
- Infertility
- Microcalcifications (association)

than among American Indians and Hispanics.[1] The exact reasons or potential genetic underpinnings for the differences in rates according to race are not known.

Geography

There is wide geographic variation in the rates of testis cancer, which correlates well with race as one might expect. Some of the highest rates are in Scandinavian countries and Germany. Some of the lowest rates are in Asian and African countries.[11] Again, there is uncertainty as to whether genetic differences, environmental exposures, or a combination of the two drive these geographic differences.

Environmental Exposures

There is a growing body of evidence implicating toxic exposures and an increased risk of testicular cancer. The main substances with a potential association with testicular cancer include organochlorines, polychlorinated biphenyls, polyvinyl chlorides, phthalates, marijuana, and tobacco.[13,14] Prenatal estrogen exposure has been implicated as a risk factor as well, but remains controversial.[15,16]

Infertility

Male factor infertility increases the risk of developing testis tumors by nearly threefold.[17] Men with primary infertility also have higher rates of testicular cancer compared with men who have undergone a vasectomy.[18] This link suggests a possible common etiology between testicular cancer and certain causes of infertility, such as testicular dysgenesis syndrome, Hiwi protein and chromosome 12 aneuploidy, DNA mismatch repair, and Y-chromosome instability.[19]

Microcalcifications

Microcalcifications are often seen on testicular ultrasonography. These are not known to be risk factors per se, but are associated with testicular cancer. Testicular tumors are more likely to be found in young men with microcalcifications compared to those without.[20] Some have reported up to an eightfold increased rate of testis tumors in those undergoing testicular ultrasound who were found to have microlithiasis compared to those without.[21]

TYPES OF GERM CELL TUMORS

Most testis cancers are germ cell tumors (roughly 95%), while the remainder are the more rare stromal tumors (eg, Leydig cell, sertoli cell, and granulosa cell tumors). Germ cell tumors can be further divided into seminoma and nonseminoma germ cell tumors, comprising 52% and 48% of total tumors, respectively.[22] The most common presentation of testis cancer is a localized seminoma.[22] Nonseminoma germ cell tumors include embryonal cell carcinomas, choriocarcinomas, yolk sac tumors, and teratomas. Pure seminomas typically peak slightly later in life (during the fourth decade) compared with other testis tumors.[3]

SCREENING

There are currently no recommended guidelines for testicular cancer screening in otherwise healthy asymptomatic men. Although earlier detection of testis cancer likely results in improved cure rates, most testis tumors are already detected at early stages of the disease, and as mentioned, have high rates of cure with current treatment paradigms. Any screening program must balance the potential to improve outcomes via early detection with the cost and negative impact of false-positive or false-negative screening results.

The United States Preventive Services Task Force currently recommends against any screening modalities for asymptomatic adolescents and adult men.[23,24] Men with symptoms, history of testicular tumors, cryptorchidism, or other high-risk factors should be given special consideration for targeted screening. Self-examination remains an important practice for those at higher risk of developing testis tumors.

There is some debate among professionals regarding the significance of microlithiasis and whether it warrants special consideration for a testicular screening program. There are no current guidelines in the United States regarding screening in the setting of microlithiasis. However, the European Society of Urogenital Radiology has proposed guidelines to perform repeat screening ultrasound in patients with microlithiasis who also have risk factors, notably either personal or family history of testis tumor or history of maldescent, orchidopexy, or testicular atrophy.[25]

PRESENTATION AND DIAGNOSIS
Initial Presentation

The classical presentation for testicular tumors is a painless testicular mass. This may be discovered on a routine physical examination, or the patient may discover the mass by self-examination and seek evaluation. Often, patients will report recent trauma to their scrotum or testicles, and while this is not a cause for tumor growth, it brings the already present testicular mass to the attention of the patient who then seeks further evaluation.

Up to 20% of patients may present with testicle pain within the mass, usually due to hemorrhage or infarction of the tumor. Sometimes patients may present with a hydrocele that obscures the mass and can make palpation of the mass challenging. Others may be mistakenly diagnosed with epididymitis, orchitis, inguinal hernia, hydrocele, or even testicular torsion.[11] If beta human chorionic gonadotropin (hCG) levels are elevated, patients may then present with gynecomastia or nipple tenderness. These symptoms may also be seen among men with Leydig cell tumors. When presenting with bulky advanced disease, patients might complain of weight loss; palpable abdominal or neck mass; flank or back pain; or pulmonary, neurologic, or gastrointestinal complaints.

History and Physical Examination

Important components of the history and physical examination parallel much of what has already been discussed regarding risk factors and presenting symptoms. Key questions to ask are timing of onset and duration of the testicular mass, pain or swelling, recent scrotal trauma, and history of fevers or recent illnesses. Sexual history may also be of value if there is suspicion for infectious etiologies. Personal and family history of testis tumors should be elicited, as well as a history of scrotal surgeries including hydrocele or hernia repairs, orchidopexy for cryptorchidism, or history of hypospadias.

During the physical examination, careful examination of both testicles should be performed and any abnormalities noted. In addition, attention should be paid to any palpable abdominal or retroperitoneal masses, inguinal or supraclavicular lymphadenopathy, or gynecomastia.

Imaging

Scrotal ultrasound is the initial primary imaging study for a suspected testicular tumor. It is nearly 100% sensitive in detecting testicular parenchymal tumors.[3] Tumors typically present as hypoechoic lesions with evidence of blood flow on Doppler imaging. In men with a testicular tumor, chest and cross-sectional imaging of the abdomen and pelvis (most commonly computed tomography [CT] imaging) are typically performed as an integral part of the staging evaluation.

Laboratory Testing

Once a suspected tumor is identified on a testicular ultrasound or physical examination, the measurement of serum tumor markers are an important next step in diagnosis and staging. Tumor markers for testis cancer include alpha fetoprotein (AFP), beta hCG, and lactate dehydrogenase (LDH). Other basic laboratories are often obtained as well (eg, compete blood count, creatinine, and liver function tests).

Depending on the results of the serum tumor markers, one can often predict certain histologic findings. By definition, pure seminomas will not have AFP elevation. Approximately 20% of pure seminomas may have beta hCG elevation. With pure choriocarcinoma, AFP is rarely elevated, and hCG will nearly always be elevated. Teratomas rarely have AFP or hCG elevation. Mixed germ cell tumors, depending on the histologic subtypes, may or may not have elevated serum tumor markers. Tumor marker elevation in relation to histologic subtype is further described in **Table 1**.

Other reasons for serum tumor marker elevation should be taken into consideration. AFP levels may also be raised in patients with hepatocellular carcinoma as well as other gastrointestinal cancers, including stomach, pancreas, biliary tract, and lung. Beta hCG levels may be elevated in men with primary hypergonadotrophic hypogonadism due to elevated levels of leutinizing hormones. In addition, marijuana use may elevate levels of hCG in men. LDH levels may be elevated in a variety of disease states. Isoenzyme 1 is the most dominant form of LDH in testis cancer.

Table 1
Testes Cancer Subtypes and Tumor Marker Production

Histologic Subtype	Tumor Markers			Lymphatic Spread	Hematogenous Spread
	AFP	hCG	LDH		
Seminoma	Never	Possible	Possible	Common	Rare
Choriocarcinoma	Rare	Usually	Possible	Common	Possible
Teratoma	Rare	Rare	Possible	Common	Rare
Embryonal	Possible	Possible	Possible	Common	Rare
Yolk sac	Possible	Possible	Possible	Common	Possible

Postorchiectomy serum tumor markers are an integral part of the staging evaluation. Serum tumor markers are usually obtained after the orchiectomy once an appropriate number of half-lives (typically 5 half-lives) have passed, therefore allowing the markers to normalize or reach their new baseline level. Beta hCG has the shortest half-life of 1 to 3 days; LDH-1 has a half-life of 4.0 to 4.5 days, and AFP has the longest half-life of 5 to 7 days. Using preorchiectomy serum tumor markers rather than postorchiectomy tumor markers is a common testis cancer staging error, and unfortunately can result in undertreatment or overtreatment of men with this disease.

STAGING

Radical inguinal orchiectomy provides both treatment as well as diagnostic and staging information. It provides definitive/curative treatment in nearly 80% of men with low stage seminomas and approximately 60% to 70% of men with low stage nonseminomas. Importantly, the histologic subtype(s) of the tumor can be determined. The pathologic T-stage of the tumor is assigned according to the presence or absence of lymphovascular invasion and depth of invasion (tunica vaginalis, spermatic cord, scrotal involvement).

Again, a complete staging evaluation for men with newly diagnosed testis cancer includes postorchiectomy serum tumor markers, chest imaging (eg, chest radiograph or chest CT scan), and cross-sectional imaging of the abdomen and pelvis (eg, CT scan or MRI).

The American Joint Committee on Cancer (AJCC) staging system for testicular cancer, which is the most commonly used staging system, can be found in the AJCC Cancer Staging Handbook, 7th edition.[26]

METASTATIC SPREAD

During human development, the gonads are formed in the abdomen and descend into the scrotum. As a result, the blood supply and lymphatic channels drain to the abdominal retroperitoneal nodes, and typically not the pelvis unless scrotal violation has occurred. Most testis tumors metastasize via predictable lymphatic channels, rather than a hematogenous route. As

Table 2
Prognostic Risk Grouping for Advanced Germ Cell Tumors

	Primary Site	Metastatis	AFP (ng/mL)	hCG (IU/L)	LDH (ULN)
Seminoma					
Good prognosis (all of the following criteria)	Any	No nonpulmonary visceral metastases	Normal	Any	Any
Intermediate prognosis (any of the following criteria)	Any	Nonpulmonary visceral metastases	Normal	Any	Any
Poor prognosis	No patients classified as poor	—	—	—	—
Nonseminoma					
Good prognosis (all of the following criteria)	Testis/ retroperitoneum	No nonpulmonary visceral metastases	<1000	<5000	<1.5×
Intermediate prognosis (all of the following criteria)	Testis/ retroperitoneum	No nonpulmonary visceral metastases	1000– 10,000 or	5000– 50,000 or	1.5–10×
Poor prognosis (any of the following criteria)	Mediastinum	Nonpulmonary visceral metastases	>10,000	>50,000	>10×

Adapted from International Germ Cell Consensus Classification: a prognostic factor-based staging system for metastatic germ cell cancers. International Germ Cell Cancer Collaborative Group. J Clin Oncol 1997;15:594–603.

a result, testicular cancer metastasis to retroperitoneal lymph nodes has been well-mapped and described for right- and left-sided primary tumors.[27,28]

Right-sided tumors typically spread to the interaortocaval lymph nodes. Left-sided tumors commonly spread to the left para-aortic lymph nodes. Spread from the right to left retroperitoneal lymph nodes is seen more commonly than spread from the left to right.[29–31]

It is not uncommon to see choriocarcinoma tumors initially spread hematogenously. Distant hematogenous spread may be seen in the lung, liver, brain, bones, kidney, adrenal gland, gastrointestinal tract, or spleen.[32]

Areas of metastatic spread are further described in **Table 1**.

PROGNOSIS

One of the important points to emphasize when counseling patients with a new diagnosis of testicular cancer is that it is generally a treatable and highly curable disease. Staging the patient appropriately is paramount in being able to assess his risk of disease progression and mortality as it relates to their overall prognosis.

For men with clinical stage I germ cell cancer, the cure rates are high with orchiectomy alone. Over 80% of men with stage I seminoma and nearly 70% with nonseminoma are cured by radical orchiectomy. Clinical stage II disease (defined as metastatic spread to the retroperitoneal lymph nodes) is also highly curable with the addition of cisplatin-based chemotherapy, retroperitoneal lymph node dissection, radiation therapy to the retroperitoneum, or some combination of these therapies to radical orchiectomy. Testis cancer is one of the few cancers wherein, long-term cure rates are still achievable even when there is distant metastatic spread (clinical stage III disease).

A prognostic staging system is used to assist and inform treatment recommendations for practitioners and patients with advanced testicular cancer. It was developed by the International Germ Cancer Collaborative Group in 1997. The system classifies patients based on histology, site of primary tumor, metastatic disease, and serum tumor markers. Patients with advanced testis cancer are categorized into either good, intermediate, or poor prognostic groups.[3,33] Chemotherapy treatment regimens and outcomes differ according to one's risk group. The descriptions of these groups, as well as the 5-year progression-free survival and 5-year overall survival rates are listed in **Tables 2** and **3**, respectively.

Table 3
Survival of Advanced Germ Cell Tumors According to Risk Group

Risk Group	5-Year Progression Free Survival	5-Year Overall Survival
Seminoma		
Good	82%	86%
Intermediate	67%	72%
Poor	No patients	No patients
Nonseminoma		
Good	89%	92%
Intermediate	75%	80%
Poor	41%	48%

Adapted from International Germ Cell Consensus Classification: a prognostic factor-based staging system for metastatic germ cell cancers. International Germ Cell Cancer Collaborative Group. J Clin Oncol 1997;15:594–603.

When comparing localized, regional, or distant disease, the 5-year overall survival rates are 99.2%, 96.0%, and 73.1%, respectively.[1,2]

SUMMARY

Testis cancer is the most commonly diagnosed cancer in young men. Although there are multiple risk factors including race, family or personal history of the disease, cryptorchidism, infertility, and others, most cases represent sporadic occurrences. Most commonly it presents at an early stage (clinical stage I) and is highly curable with radical orchiectomy. Even more advanced stages of testicular cancer are curable with a multimodality treatment approach. There are no widely accepted screening strategies for germ cell tumors, but disease awareness and early detection via self- examination may improve outcomes for the nearly 9000 men expected to be diagnosed with testis cancer this year in the United States.

REFERENCES

1. SEER Cancer Statistics. 2014. Available at: seer. cancer.gov. Accessed November 22, 2014.
2. DeSantis CE, Lin CC, Mariotto AB, et al. Cancer treatment and survivorship statistics, 2014. CA Cancer J Clin 2014;64:252–71.
3. Albers P, Albrecht W, Algaba F, et al. EAU guidelines on testicular cancer: 2011 update. Eur Urol 2011;60: 304–19.
4. Le Cornet C, Lortet-Tieulent J, Forman D, et al. Testicular cancer incidence to rise by 25% by 2025 in Europe? Model-based predictions in 40

countries using population-based registry data. Eur J Cancer 2014;50:831–9.

5. Purdue MP, Devesa SS, Sigurdson AJ, et al. International patterns and trends in testis cancer incidence. Int J Cancer 2005;115:822–7.

6. Theodore C, Terrier-Lacombe MJ, Laplanche A, et al. Bilateral germ-cell tumours: 22-year experience at the Institut Gustave Roussy. Br J Cancer 2004;90:55–9.

7. Fossa SD, Chen J, Schonfeld SJ, et al. Risk of contralateral testicular cancer: a population-based study of 29,515 U.S. men. J Natl Cancer Inst 2005; 97:1056–66.

8. Fossa SD, Aass N, Harvei S, et al. Increased mortality rates in young and middle-aged patients with malignant germ cell tumours. Br J Cancer 2004;90: 607–12.

9. Wood HM, Elder JS. Cryptorchidism and testicular cancer: separating fact from fiction. J Urol 2009; 181:452–61.

10. Pettersson A, Richiardi L, Nordenskjold A, et al. Age at surgery for undescended testis and risk of testicular cancer. N Engl J Med 2007;356:1835–41.

11. Scardino PT, Linehan M, Zelefsky M, et al. Comprehensive textbook of genitourinary oncology. 4th edition. Philadelphia: Wolters Kluwer Health/Lippincott Williams & Wilkins; 2011.

12. Hemminki K, Chen B. Familial risks in testicular cancer as aetiological clues. Int J Androl 2006; 29:205–10.

13. Meeks JJ, Sheinfeld J, Eggener SE. Environmental toxicology of testicular cancer. Urol Oncol 2012;30: 212–5.

14. Lacson JC, Bernstein L, Cortessis VK. Potential impact of age at first marijuana use on the development of nonseminomatous testicular germ cell tumors. Cancer 2013;119:1284–5.

15. Martin OV, Shialis T, Lester JN, et al. Testicular dysgenesis syndrome and the estrogen hypothesis: a quantitative meta-analysis. Environ Health Perspect 2008;116:149–57.

16. Giannandrea F, Paoli D, Figa-Talamanca I, et al. Effect of endogenous and exogenous hormones on testicular cancer: the epidemiological evidence. Int J Dev Biol 2013;57:255–63.

17. Walsh TJ, Croughan MS, Schembri M, et al. Increased risk of testicular germ cell cancer among infertile men. Arch Intern Med 2009;169:351–6.

18. Eisenberg ML, Li S, Brooks JD, et al. Increased risk of cancer in infertile men: analysis of US claims data. J Urol 2014;193:1596–601.

19. Hotaling JM, Walsh TJ. Male infertility: a risk factor for testicular cancer. Nat Rev Urol 2009;6:550–6.

20. Cooper ML, Kaefer M, Fan R, et al. Testicular microlithiasis in children and associated testicular cancer. Radiology 2014;270:857–63.

21. Heller HT, Oliff MC, Doubilet PM, et al. Testicular microlithiasis: prevalence and association with primary testicular neoplasm. J Clin Ultrasound 2014; 42:423–6.

22. Powles TB, Bhardwa J, Shamash J, et al. The changing presentation of germ cell tumours of the testis between 1983 and 2002. BJU Int 2005;95:1197–200.

23. U.S. Preventive Services Task Force. Available at: http://www.uspreventiveservicestaskforce.org/uspstf/uspstest.htm. Accessed June 20, 2014.

24. Lin K, Sharangpani R. Screening for testicular cancer: an evidence review for the U.S. Preventive Services Task Force. Ann Intern Med 2010;153:396–9.

25. Richenberg J, Belfield J, Ramchandani P, et al. Testicular microlithiasis imaging and follow-up: guidelines of the ESUR scrotal imaging subcommittee. Eur Radiol 2014;25:323–30.

26. Edge S, Greene FL, Page DL, et al. American Joint Committee on Cancer Staging manual. 7th edition. New York: Springer; 2009.

27. Whitmore WF Jr. Surgical treatment of clinical stage I nonseminomatous germ gell tumors of the testis. Cancer Treat Rep 1982;66:5–10.

28. Ray B, Hajdu SI, Whitmore WF Jr. Proceedings: distribution of retroperitoneal lymph node metastases in testicular germinal tumors. Cancer 1974;33:340–8.

29. Donohue JP, Zachary JM, Maynard BR. Distribution of nodal metastases in nonseminomatous testis cancer. J Urol 1982;128:315–20.

30. Weissbach L, Boedefeld EA. Localization of solitary and multiple metastases in stage II nonseminomatous testis tumor as basis for a modified staging lymph node dissection in stage I. J Urol 1987;138: 77–82.

31. Busch FM, Sayegh ES. Roentgenographic visualization of human testicular lymphatics: a preliminary report. J Urol 1963;89:106–10.

32. Park WW, Lees JC. Choriocarcinoma; a general review, with an analysis of 516 cases. AMA Arch Pathol 1950;49:204–41.

33. International Germ Cell Consensus Classification: a prognostic factor-based staging system for metastatic germ cell cancers. International Germ Cell Cancer Collaborative Group. J Clin Oncol 1997;15: 594–603.

Intratubular Germ Cell Neoplasia of the Testis, Bilateral Testicular Cancer, and Aberrant Histologies

Pranav Sharma, MD[a], Jasreman Dhillon, MD[b],
Wade J. Sexton, MD[a],*

KEYWORDS

- Intratubular germ cell neoplasia • Bilateral testicular cancer • Rare histologies
- Testicular germ cell tumor • Testicular biopsy • Infertility • Cryptorchidism • Microlithiasis

KEY POINTS

- ITGCN is a premalignant lesion for TGCTs.
- Risk factors for ITGCN include family history, contralateral TGCT, cryptorchidism, male factor infertility, and testicular microlithiasis.
- ITGCN is diagnosed with testicular biopsy, which is controversial in patients with contralateral ITGCN or TGCT.
- Radical inguinal orchiectomy is the accepted treatment of unilateral ITGCN, and low-dose local radiotherapy is the accepted treatment of bilateral ITGCN or ITGCN in the solitary testis to preserve Leydig cell function.
- Although non–germ cell tumors of the testis are rare, they can affect survival if not identified and treated appropriately.

INTRODUCTION

In 1972, Skakkebaek[1] in a landmark study described a possible precursor lesion for malignant testicular germ cell tumors (TGCTs) in the testes of 2 infertile men who went on to develop testicular cancer. This cluster of atypical germ cells was initially termed carcinoma in situ, but it has also been referred to as testicular intraepithelial neoplasia in the literature and is now commonly known as intratubular germ cell neoplasia, unclassified (ITGCN).

ITGCN is considered to be the premalignant lesion for most TGCTs, with the exception of pediatric germ cell tumors (yolk sac, mature teratoma) and spermatocytic seminoma.[2] Many have advocated early detection and treatment of these lesions in an effort to reduce the incidence of testicular cancer. As a result, significant advances in the understanding of ITGCN, including its pathogenesis, risk factors, diagnosis, and treatment, have been made over the last 3 decades.

Because a unilateral testicular tumor is one of the most important risk factors for the development of a contralateral testicular malignancy, bilateral TGCTs occur in 1% to 5% of cases, with metachronous onset being more common than synchronous.[3] In a recent systematic review of 50,376 patients with testicular cancer, Zequi Sde and colleagues[4] reported a prevalence of

a Department of Genitourinary Oncology, H. Lee Moffitt Cancer Center, 12902 Magnolia Drive, Tampa, FL 33612, USA; b Department of Genitourinary Anatomic Pathology, H. Lee Moffitt Cancer Center, 12902 Magnolia Drive, Tampa, FL 33612, USA
* Corresponding author.
E-mail address: wade.sexton@moffitt.org

Urol Clin N Am 42 (2015) 277–285
http://dx.doi.org/10.1016/j.ucl.2015.04.002

urologic.theclinics.com

bilateral TCGTs in 1.82% of cases. Metachronous tumors were seen in 56.6% of men with bilateral testicular masses, and synchronous tumors were seen in 43.4%. Bilateral TGCTs may also have long-term implications on fertility and risk of hypogonadism.

Although more than 95% to 98% of testicular cancers comprise TGCTs, primary non–germ cell testicular malignancies exist, including sex-cord/gonadal stromal tumors (SCGSTs) (Leydig cell, Sertoli cell, granulosa cell tumors), neuroendocrine/carcinoid tumors, leiomyosarcoma, lymphoma, signet-ring stromal tumors (SRSTs), ovarian-type surface epithelial carcinomas of the testis, squamous cell carcinoma (SCC), and testicular hemangiomas.[5] This article focuses on ITGCN and its role in bilateral TGCTs; aberrant histologies of testicular cancer are also discussed.

INTRATUBULAR GERM CELL NEOPLASIA
Risk Factors of Intratubular Germ Cell Neoplasia

The prevalence of ITGCN has been reported to be less than 1% in the normal male population, and 0.43% to 0.8% in autopsy studies, with most cases being unilateral.[6,7] Because ITGCN leads to the development of TGCT, they have similar risk factors, including familial susceptibility.[8] **Table 1** lists the various risk factors of ITGCN and its associated prevalence rate.

One of the strongest risk factors for ITGCN is a history of contralateral testicular cancer.[9] Patients who have testicular cancer with an atrophic contralateral testis who present before the age of 31 years are considered to be high risk for ITGCN.[10] Heterogeneous parenchyma of the contralateral testis on ultrasonography in a patient with testicular cancer is also suggestive of ITGCN, with a positive predictive value of 22.2% and negative predictive value of 97.6%.[11,12] Rud and colleagues[13] reported that lower sperm concentration, small contralateral testis volume, irregular ultrasonic echo pattern of the contralateral testis, and younger age can be used to predict those patients with unilateral TGCT more likely to harbor a contralateral ITGCN lesion with a prevalence rate as high as 8%. Because ITGCN is associated with poor spermatogenesis and with testicular atrophy, the National Comprehensive Cancer Network (NCCN) and European Association of Urology (EAU) guidelines recommend investigation with contralateral testicular biopsy in patients with testicular cancer with a contralateral testicular volume less than 12 mL, poor spermatogenesis, and age less than 40 years.[14,15]

Infertility is another major risk factor for the development of ITGCN. Older literature initially reported no increased risk of ITGCN in infertile men with a sperm density lower than 10 million/mL or lower than 20 million/mL associated with testicular atrophy (<15 mL).[16] However, in a subsequent study 10 years later, Olesen and colleagues[17] reported a 3-fold increased prevalence of ITGCN in men with severe oligozoospermia (sperm density ≤2.06 million/mL) compared with an age-matched cohort of normal men.

Cryptorchidism carries an increased risk of ITGCN.[18] The NCCN and the EAU, therefore, recommend biopsy of the contralateral undescended testis in a patient with unilateral TGCT. However, immunohistochemical markers have failed to detect ITGCN in prepubertal boys with cryptorchidism.[19]

ITGCN has also been noted in children with disorders of sexual differentiation. Ramani and colleagues[20] reviewed more than 100 cases of children with various intersex states and reported a 10-fold increased frequency of ITGCN in the testis. No evidence of ITGCN was seen in cases of androgen insensitivity syndrome (testicular feminization), but previous reports have shown higher prevalence rates associated with this disease.[21]

Testicular microlithiasis (TM) has not been associated with an increased prevalence of ITGCN in healthy, asymptomatic men, but in those with risk factors such as a unilateral TGCT, infertility, testicular atrophy, or sonographic heterogeneity, it can signify an increased occurrence of ITGCN.[22] Although TM is seen in approximately 5% of healthy patients, the prevalence of TM is higher in those with these significant risk factors.[23,24] It has also been suggested that bilateral TM may harbor an increased risk of ITGCN.[25] Guidelines advocate the consideration of testicular biopsy in young men with TM and at least 1 risk factor for TGCT, and self-examination is recommended for all other patients, including asymptomatic men with TM.[26]

Table 1 Risk factors and prevalence of ITGCN	
Risk Factor	**Prevalence (%)**
Contralateral TGCT[8]	5
Male factor infertility[16]	0.5–2
Cryptorchidism[17]	1.5–5
DSD[19,20]	5–10
TM[22]	<1

Abbreviations: DSD, disorders of sexual differentiation; TM, testicular microlithiasis.

Adapted from Zequi Sde C, da Costa WH, Santana TB, et al. Bilateral testicular germ cell tumours: a systematic review. BJU Int 2012;110(8):1102–9.

Pathogenesis of Intratubular Germ Cell Neoplasia

There are 2 proposed mechanisms for the development of ITGCN. The first suggests the abnormal persistence of primordial gonocytes beyond the neonatal period that fail to differentiate into spermatogonia, and the second mechanism involves the regression of spermatogonia toward a precursor germ cell phenotype.[27] These fetal gonocytes are pluripotent, with the ability to accumulate mutations and develop into various germinal and somatic tissues. Gondos and colleagues[28] noted morphologic similarities between ITGCN and germ cells at early stages of differentiation under the microscope (**Fig. 1**). This link was further reinforced by the discovery of many similar markers as well as gene expression profiles in ITGCN and fetal gonocytes.[29,30] Modulation of protein expression in ITGCN also occurs with similar mechanisms as in primordial germ cells, strengthening evidence to its origin from persistent fetal gonocytes.[31]

Diagnosis of Intratubular Germ Cell Neoplasia

ITGCN diagnosis is based on testicular biopsy. Histologically, ITGCN consists of enlarged cells with clear cystoplasm, large hyperchromatic nuclei, and prominent nucleoli (**Fig. 2**).[32] Tubular basement membranes are thickened, and ITGCN is often interspersed among normal Sertoli cells and seminiferous tubules showing intact spermatogenesis.[33] Immunohistochemical staining also distinguishes ITGCN from nonneoplastic spermatogenic cells, because markers for placentallike alkaline phosphatase and octamer-binding

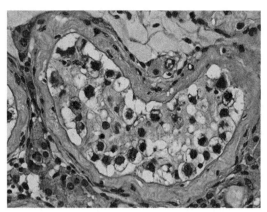

Fig. 2. ITGCN is identified on microscopic examination by germ cells with enlarged hyperchromatic nuclei, prominent nucleoli, and clear cytoplasm. These cells are typically arranged along the basement membrane of the seminiferous tubule with frequent mitotic figures. H&E stain, 60×.

transcription factor 3/4 show high sensitivity and specificity rates on biopsy specimens.[34,35]

Testicular biopsy has an approximately 0.5% false-negative rate for ITGCN.[36] This finding is secondary to the focal nature of the disease, with a certain degree of sampling error. Two-site biopsies have further improved the sensitivity of detection, but subsequent TGCTs in patients with 1 or 2 previous negative biopsies have been described.[37–39]

Controversy still exists with regards to the type of patient who would benefit from testicular biopsy. Although most of the academic world recommends testicular biopsy in patients with unilateral TGCT and a risk factor for contralateral disease, certain centers in Germany and Denmark perform routine contralateral testicular biopsies on all patients with TGCT at the time of orchiectomy. Proponents of routine biopsies argue that early detection allows treatment with radiation therapy (XRT) and preserves testicular hormone production in contrast to future orchiectomy, whereas opponents claim that many cases of recurrence exist even after XRT, with reports of hypogonadism in these patients as high as 40%.[40,41]

Prognosis of Intratubular Germ Cell Neoplasia

The relationship between ITGCN and the development of TGCTs is well established, and the malignant potential of ITGCN does not occur until after the hormonal changes of puberty.[42] Longitudinal studies have reported that when ITGCN is present on testicular biopsy, 40% of patients develop a TGCT within 3 years and 50% within 5 years.[43] Loss of PTEN and p18 expression and gain of

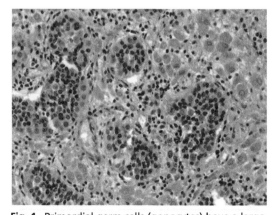

Fig. 1. Primordial germ cells (gonocytes) have a large, round central nucleus with absent or inconspicuous nucleoli and scant cytoplasm. Their persistence on microscopy has been associated with the development of ITGCN. Hematoxylin and eosin stain (H&E stain), 40×.

chromosome 12p have all been associated with progression of ITGCN to TGCT.[44–46] This process also seems to occur independent of Sertoli cell interaction.[47]

Treatment of Intratubular Germ Cell Neoplasia

Treatment of ITGCN includes surveillance, orchiectomy, or low-dose external beam radiation (XRT) to the affected testis. Chemotherapy for TGCT is not effective in controlling ITGCN in the contralateral testicle.[48]

For patients with unilateral ITGCN and a normal contralateral testis, orchiectomy is the preferred treatment option. Orchiectomy may also be considered in patients with ITGCN in an atrophic, poorly functioning testis or in patients with ITGCN associated with oligospermia who are pursuing assisted reproductive techniques. ITGCN in the solitary testicle is more controversial, with some advocating surveillance with testicular self-examination and others recommending early low-dose XRT to the affected testis. Treatment of ITGCN should be weighed against the consequences of resultant infertility and possible hypogonadism with reliance on long-term testosterone supplementation.

ITGCN responds to XRT most effectively at doses of 18 to 20 Gy. Giwercman and colleagues[49] reported resolution of ITGCN in patients treated with 20 Gy of XRT with up to 2 years follow-up, but 25% of patients required hormone supplementation because of Leydig cell dysfunction. In addition, patients who undergo XRT to a solitary testicle are rendered infertile as a result of destruction of normal spermatogonia. Lower doses ranging from 14 to 16 Gy have been used with varying degrees of success, but an increased risk of recurrence has been reported.[41]

Surveillance remains an option for patients who wish to preserve fertility and endocrine function. However, patients need to be compliant with follow-up and regular testicular self-examination.

BILATERAL TESTICULAR GERM CELL TUMOR

The prevalence of bilateral TGCTs ranges from 0.5% to 5.0% based on several large single-institutional series.[50,51] Patients with bilateral ITGCN or contralateral ITGCN in the presence of a unilateral TGCT are typically affected. Certain genetic mutations in phosphodiesterase 11A have been implicated in bilateral and familial TGCTs.[52] Men with bilateral TGCTs are also significantly more likely to have brothers with testis cancer than those with unilateral disease.[53]

Table 2 shows the clinical and pathologic features of metachronous versus synchronous bilateral TGCTs based on a meta-analysis of 916 patients.[4] Synchronous patients were on average 3 years older than metachronous patients, as a result of a higher incidence of seminoma. However, metachronous patients had better cancer-specific survival and overall survival (OS) associated with a lower incidence of clinical stage II and III disease compared with synchronous patients. The time interval between tumors also influenced the histology of the second tumor in the

Table 2
Metachronous versus synchronous bilateral TGCTs

Characteristic	Metachronous	Synchronous
Number (%)	341 (56.6)	261 (43.4)
Mean age (y)	30.90	33.54
Histology, no. (%)		
Bilateral seminoma	102 (29.9)	155 (59.4)
Bilateral nonseminoma	107 (31.3)	22 (8.4)
Discordant histology	132 (38.7)	84 (32.2)
Clinical stage, no. (%)		
I	250 (73.3)	130 (49.8)
II	74 (21.7)	75 (28.7)
III	17 (5.0)	56 (21.5)
5-year CSS (%)	95	89
5-year OS (%)	95	88

Abbreviations: CSS, cancer-specific survival; OS, overall survival.

Adapted from Zequi Sde C, da Costa WH, Santana TB, et al. Bilateral testicular germ cell tumours: a systematic review. BJU Int 2012;110(8):1104; with permission.

metachronous group. When the time interval was less than 60 months, there was a higher incidence of seminoma, but when the interval between primary tumors was greater than 60 months, the incidence of seminoma was less resulting in inferior cancer-related outcomes because of a higher incidence of nonseminoma.

Partial orchiectomy has been used in patients with bilateral testicular masses, with favorable outcomes in terms of survival, preserved endocrine function, and preserved fertility.[54] It is typically indicated for organ confined tumors less than 3 cm in clinical diameter with use of biopsies of the tumor bed to rule out adjacent ITGCN and assess margin status.[55] Adjuvant XRT can also reduce local recurrence rates, although this can affect long-term fertility. OS rates are comparable with those with unilateral disease, and long-term testosterone production was preserved in 90% of patients at 7-year follow-up.[56] Half of patients who postponed local XRT also successfully fathered a child.

ABERRANT TESTICULAR HISTOLOGIES

SCGSTs are the most common non–germ cell tumors, accounting for 5% to 6% of all testicular tumors.[57] They consist of Leydig cell, Sertoli cell, and granulosa cell tumors.

Leydig cell tumors are capable of testosterone or estrogen production, and endocrine manifestations such as gynecomastia, loss of libido, erectile dysfunction, or precocious puberty in children are seen in 20% to 30% of cases.[58,59] Sertoli cell tumors are classified as sclerosing or large cell calcifying type (**Fig. 3**). Unlike Leydig cell tumors, virilization is rarely seen, yet, signs of hyperestrogenism such as gynecomastia are present in 20% to 30% of cases.[60] Granulosa cell tumors are divided into adult and juvenile types. Adult granulosa cell tumors have been associated with gynecomastia, and the juvenile type has been associated with ambiguous genitalia and ipsilateral cryptorchidism.[61]

Most SCGSTs are benign, treated with orchiectomy or partial orchiectomy, but 10% to 20% can metastasize and lead to death within 2 years.[62,63] Kim and colleagues[64] established 5 histopathologic high-risk criteria predictive of the metastatic potential of all SCGSTs including tumor size greater than 5 cm, necrosis, moderate or severe nuclear atypia, angiolymphatic invasion, infiltrating margins, and greater than 5 mitotic features per 10 high power fields. In a recent review of 48 patients with testicular SCGST, Silberstein and colleagues[65] advocated that patients with 2 or more high-risk criteria or patients with evidence of retroperitoneal disease on cross-sectional imaging (at least clinical stage IIA disease) may benefit from early retroperitoneal lymph node dissection to prevent future disease relapse and improve cancer-related outcomes.

Primary testicular neuroendocrine tumors (ie, carcinoid tumors) are characterized by the presence of nests of small round cells with uniform nuclei forming sheets (**Fig. 4**).[66] Tumor cells stain positive for neuroendocrine markers like chromogranin and synaptophysin. Vasoactive products produced by the tumor can cause carcinoid syndrome, characterized by sweating, flushing, wheezing, diarrhea, and abdominal pain.[67] Orchiectomy is the treatment of choice, but adjuvant

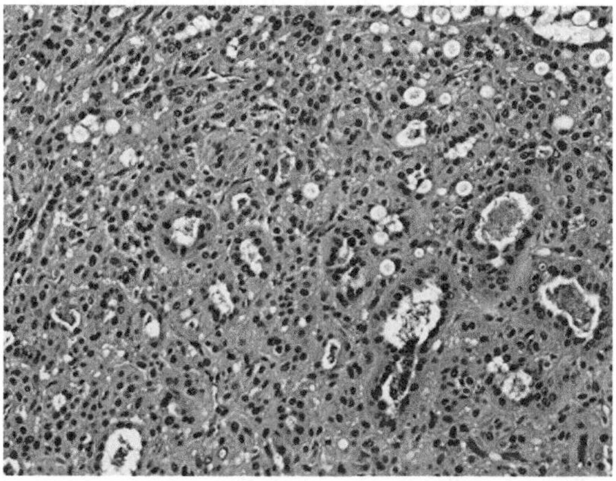

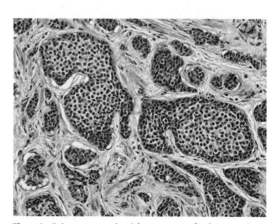

Fig. 3. Sertoli cell tumors are composed of tubules, sheets, nests, or cords containing Sertoli cells, which are present in a myxoid or fibrous stroma. Cystoplasmic lipid-containing vacuoles and dystrophic calcifications, including psammomatous calcifications, can also be present. H&E stain, 20×.

Fig. 4. Primary carcinoid tumor of the testis is composed of islands of monomorphic cells arranged in a nested trabecular pattern forming sheets. The tumor cells have granular chromatin and scarce mitotic figures. H&E stain, 20×.

treatment with an octreotide analog can stabilize the tumor and improve any carcinoid-related symptoms.[68,69] Regimens of chemotherapy have not been established, and XRT has little effect.[70]

Intratesticular leiomyosarcoma is a malignant soft tissue tumor arising from the contractile cells of seminiferous tubules, smooth muscle of blood vessels, and tunica albuginea.[71] Risk factors include previous XRT, high doses of anabolic steroids, and chronic inflammation.[72] Most cases are clinical stage I with slow-growing local disease, which can be adequately treated with radical orchiectomy followed by surveillance. Prognosis is typically good, with rare occurrences of metastasis. This situation is in contrast to paratesticular leiomyosarcoma, which is more aggressive, mandating wide local resection to obtain a negative margin status, with some evidence supporting the use of adjuvant radiotherapy because of an increased risk of locoregional recurrence, ranging from 30% to 50%.[73]

Primary testicular lymphoma consists of 1% to 2% of non-Hodgkin lymphoma and is most commonly diffuse large B-cell lymphoma (69%–75%) (**Fig. 5**).[74] The age of presentation is usually beyond the sixth decade of life, and it has a high predilection for the contralateral testicle and distant sites such as the skin, lungs, and central nervous system (CNS).[75] Typical treatment of unilateral stage I-II disease includes a multimodal approach involving orchiectomy, anthracycline-based combination chemotherapy with rituximab, contralateral prophylactic scrotal XRT, and prophylactic intrathecal chemotherapy (methotrexate) or cranial XRT, because of the high risk of CNS

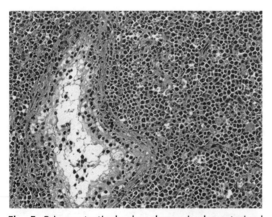

Fig. 5. Primary testicular lymphoma is characterized by a distinctive intertubular growth pattern with splaying of the seminiferous tubules by solid sheets of neoplastic cells. Lymphoma cells show brisk mitotic activity and have ill-defined cell membranes, pleomorphic, twisted nuclei, and small nucleoli. H&E stain, 20×.

relapse.[76] Five-year OS is estimated around 85% with poor ECOG (Eastern Cooperative Oncology Group) performance status, infiltration of adjacent tissues, and bulky disease denoted as poor prognostic features.[77]

Ovarian-type surface epithelial carcinomas of the testis (such as mucinous adenocarcinoma) are rare, with fewer than 25 cases reported to date.[78] Orchiectomy is the standard treatment of localized disease, and most reported cases have not shown metastases with a good prognosis.[79] Adjuvant chemotherapy with paclitaxel and carboplatin might have potential efficacy in advanced disease, but solid evidence is lacking.[80]

Michal and colleagues[81] first described SRST of the testis in 2005. Like Leydig and Sertoli cell tumors, SRSTs are rarely malignant and easily treatable with orchiectomy or partial orchiectomy. Some argue that it is a specific variant of Sertoli cell tumors and should be grouped under the category of SCGSTs, but controversy remains in part because of its rare occurrence.

Primary testicular SCC is extremely rare, and metastasis from other sites should be excluded first. Reports have associated primary testicular SCC with malignant transformation of an epidermal cyst, a teratoma, or a hydrocele.[82,83] It may be related to chronic scrotal irritation or an inflammatory process with subsequent squamous metaplasia, but this relationship is difficult to examine because of its low incidence.[84]

Primary testicular hemangiomas have also been described, with 43 individual cases reported over the last 55 years.[85] Cavernous, capillary, cellular capillary, epithelioid, and juvenile subtypes have been noted with a common infiltrative growth pattern and entrapment of adjacent benign seminiferous tubules that are atrophic, sclerotic, and lack spermatogenesis. Although their histologic appearance can sometimes be concerning with the presence of prominent vascularity, no recurrences have been noted after orchiectomy or partial orchiectomy.

SUMMARY

ITGCN is an important precursor to TGCTs. The risk of bilateral TGCTs in patients with unilateral disease is small but not negligible. Although there is still debate in regards to screening, effective treatment options are available. Appropriate counseling of patients regarding the consequence of treatment is essential. In addition, non–germ cell tumors of the testicle do exist. Although rare, they can still cause significant patient morbidity and mortality if not recognized and treated appropriately.

REFERENCES

1. Skakkebaek NE. Possible carcinoma-in-situ of the testis. Lancet 1972;2(7776):516–7.
2. Klein FA, Melamed MR, Whitmore WF Jr. Intratubular malignant germ cells (carcinoma in situ) accompanying invasive testicular germ cell tumors. J Urol 1985;133(3):413–5.
3. Fossa SD, Chen J, Schonfeld SJ, et al. Risk of contralateral testicular cancer: a population-based study of 29,515 US men. J Natl Cancer Inst 2005;97(14):1056–66.
4. Zequi Sde C, da Costa WH, Santana TB, et al. Bilateral testicular germ cell tumours: a systematic review. BJU Int 2012;110(8):1102–9.
5. Trabert B, Chen J, Devesa SS, et al. International patterns and trends in testicular cancer incidence, overall and by histologic subtype, 1973-2007. Andrology 2014;3:4–12.
6. Giwercman A, Muller J, Skakkebaek NE. Prevalence of carcinoma in situ and other histopathological abnormalities in testes from 399 men who died suddenly and unexpectedly. J Urol 1991;145(1):77–80.
7. Linke J, Loy V, Dieckmann KP. Prevalence of testicular intraepithelial neoplasia in healthy males. J Urol 2005;173(5):1577–9.
8. Greene MH, Mai PL, Loud JT, et al. Familial testicular germ cell tumors (FTGCT)–overview of a multidisciplinary etiologic study. Andrology 2014;3:47–58.
9. Ruf CG, Gnoss A, Hartmann M, et al. Contralateral biopsies in patients with testicular germ cell tumours: patterns of care in Germany and recent data regarding prevalence and treatment of testicular intra-epithelial neoplasia. Andrology 2014;3:92–8.
10. Harland SJ, Cook PA, Fossa SD, et al. Intratubular germ cell neoplasia of the contralateral testis in testicular cancer: defining a high risk group. J Urol 1998;160(4):1353–7.
11. Giwercman A, Lenz S, Skakkebaek NE. Carcinoma in situ in atrophic testis: biopsy based on abnormal ultrasound pattern. Br J Urol 1993;72(1):118–20.
12. Lenz S, Skakkebaek NE, Hertel NT. Abnormal ultrasonic pattern in contralateral testes in patients with unilateral testicular cancer. World J Urol 1996;14(Suppl 1):S55–8.
13. Rud CN, Daugaard G, Rajpert-De Meyts E, et al. Sperm concentration, testicular volume and age predict risk of carcinoma in situ in contralateral testis of men with testicular germ cell cancer. J Urol 2013;190(6):2074–80.
14. Albers P, Albrecht W, Algaba F, et al. EAU guidelines on testicular cancer: 2011 update. European Association of Urology. Actas Urol Esp 2012;36(3):127–45 [in Spanish].
15. Motzer RJ, Agarwal N, Beard C, et al. NCCN clinical practice guidelines in oncology: testicular cancer. J Natl Compr Canc Netw 2009;7(6):672–93.
16. Giwercman A, Thomsen JK, Hertz J, et al. Prevalence of carcinoma in situ of the testis in 207 oligozoospermic men from infertile couples: prospective study of testicular biopsies. BMJ 1997;315(7114):989–91.
17. Olesen IA, Hoei-Hansen CE, Skakkebaek NE, et al. Testicular carcinoma in situ in subfertile Danish men. Int J Androl 2007;30(4):406–11 [discussion: 412].
18. Giwercman A, Bruun E, Frimodt-Moller C, et al. Prevalence of carcinoma in situ and other histopathological abnormalities in testes of men with a history of cryptorchidism. J Urol 1989;142(4):998–1001 [discussion: 1001–2].
19. Kvist K, Clasen-Linde E, Cortes D, et al. Adult immunohistochemical markers fail to detect intratubular germ cell neoplasia in prepubertal boys with cryptorchidism. J Urol 2014;191(4):1084–9.
20. Ramani P, Yeung CK, Habeebu SS. Testicular intratubular germ cell neoplasia in children and adolescents with intersex. Am J Surg Pathol 1993;17(11):1124–33.
21. Cassio A, Cacciari E, D'Errico A, et al. Incidence of intratubular germ cell neoplasia in androgen insensitivity syndrome. Acta Endocrinol (Copenh) 1990;123(4):416–22.
22. Tan IB, Ang KK, Ching BC, et al. Testicular microlithiasis predicts concurrent testicular germ cell tumors and intratubular germ cell neoplasia of unclassified type in adults: a meta-analysis and systematic review. Cancer 2010;116(19):4520–32.
23. Elzinga-Tinke JE, Sirre ME, Looijenga LH, et al. The predictive value of testicular ultrasound abnormalities for carcinoma in situ of the testis in men at risk for testicular cancer. Int J Androl 2010;33(4):597–603.
24. Peterson AC, Bauman JM, Light DE, et al. The prevalence of testicular microlithiasis in an asymptomatic population of men 18 to 35 years old. J Urol 2001;166(6):2061–4.
25. de Gouveia Brazao CA, Pierik FH, Oosterhuis JW, et al. Bilateral testicular microlithiasis predicts the presence of the precursor of testicular germ cell tumors in subfertile men. J Urol 2004;171(1):158–60.
26. van Casteren NJ, Looijenga LH, Dohle GR. Testicular microlithiasis and carcinoma in situ overview and proposed clinical guideline. Int J Androl 2009;32(4):279–87.
27. Rajpert-De Meyts E. Developmental model for the pathogenesis of testicular carcinoma in situ: genetic and environmental aspects. Hum Reprod Update 2006;12(3):303–23.
28. Gondos B, Berthelsen JG, Skakkebaek NE. Intratubular germ cell neoplasia (carcinoma in situ): a preinvasive lesion of the testis. Ann Clin Lab Sci 1983;13(3):185–92.
29. Honecker F, Stoop H, de Krijger RR, et al. Pathobiological implications of the expression of markers of

testicular carcinoma in situ by fetal germ cells. J Pathol 2004;203(3):849–57.

30. Sonne SB, Almstrup K, Dalgaard M, et al. Analysis of gene expression profiles of microdissected cell populations indicates that testicular carcinoma in situ is an arrested gonocyte. Cancer Res 2009;69(12): 5241–50.

31. Eckert D, Biermann K, Nettersheim D, et al. Expression of BLIMP1/PRMT5 and concurrent histone H2A/H4 arginine 3 dimethylation in fetal germ cells, CIS/IGCNU and germ cell tumors. BMC Dev Biol 2008;8:106.

32. Gondos B, Migliozzi JA. Intratubular germ cell neoplasia. Semin Diagn Pathol 1987;4(4):292–303.

33. van Casteren NJ, de Jong J, Stoop H, et al. Evaluation of testicular biopsies for carcinoma in situ: immunohistochemistry is mandatory. Int J Androl 2009;32(6):666–74.

34. Jacobsen GK, Norgaard-Pedersen B. Placental alkaline phosphatase in testicular germ cell tumours and in carcinoma-in-situ of the testis. An immunohistochemical study. Acta Pathol Microbiol Immunol Scand A 1984;92(5):323–9.

35. van Casteren NJ, Stoop H, Dohle GR, et al. Noninvasive detection of testicular carcinoma in situ in semen using OCT3/4. Eur Urol 2008;54(1):153–8.

36. Dieckmann KP, Loy V. False-negative biopsies for the diagnosis of testicular intraepithelial neoplasia (TIN)–an update. Eur Urol 2003;43(5):516–21.

37. Cappelen T, Fossa SD, Stenwig AE, et al. False-negative biopsy for testicular intraepithelial neoplasia and high-risk features for testicular cancer. Acta Oncol 2000;39(1):105–9.

38. Dieckmann KP, Kulejewski M, Pichlmeier U, et al. Diagnosis of contralateral testicular intraepithelial neoplasia (TIN) in patients with testicular germ cell cancer: systematic two-site biopsies are more sensitive than a single random biopsy. Eur Urol 2007; 51(1):175–83 [discussion: 183–5].

39. Souchon R, Gertenbach U, Dieckmann KP, et al. Contralateral testicular cancer in spite of TIN-negative double biopsies and interval cisplatin chemotherapy. Strahlenther Onkol 2006;182(5): 289–92.

40. Dieckmann KP, Lauke H, Michl U, et al. Testicular germ cell cancer despite previous local radiotherapy to the testis. Eur Urol 2002;41(6):643–9 [discussion: 649–50].

41. Petersen PM, Giwercman A, Daugaard G, et al. Effect of graded testicular doses of radiotherapy in patients treated for carcinoma-in-situ in the testis. J Clin Oncol 2002;20(6):1537–43.

42. Skakkebaek NE. Carcinoma in situ of the testis: frequency and relationship to invasive germ cell tumours in infertile men. Histopathology 1978;2(3): 157–70.

43. von der Maase H, Rorth M, Walbom-Jorgensen S, et al. Carcinoma in situ of contralateral testis in patients with testicular germ cell cancer: study of 27 cases in 500 patients. Br Med J 1986; 293(6559):1398–401.

44. Bartkova J, Thullberg M, Rajpert-De Meyts E, et al. Cell cycle regulators in testicular cancer: loss of p18INK4C marks progression from carcinoma in situ to invasive germ cell tumours. Int J Cancer 2000;85(3):370–5.

45. Di Vizio D, Cito L, Boccia A, et al. Loss of the tumor suppressor gene PTEN marks the transition from intratubular germ cell neoplasias (ITGCN) to invasive germ cell tumors. Oncogene 2005;24(11): 1882–94.

46. Looijenga LH, Zafarana G, Grygalewicz B, et al. Role of gain of 12p in germ cell tumour development. APMIS 2003;111(1):161–71 [discussion: 172–3].

47. Summersgill B, Osin P, Lu YJ, et al. Chromosomal imbalances associated with carcinoma in situ and associated testicular germ cell tumours of adolescents and adults. Br J Cancer 2001;85(2):213–20.

48. Kleinschmidt K, Dieckmann KP, Georgiew A, et al. Chemotherapy is of limited efficacy in the control of contralateral testicular intraepithelial neoplasia in patients with testicular germ cell cancer. Oncology 2009;77(1):33–9.

49. Giwercman A, von der Maase H, Berthelsen JG, et al. Localized irradiation of testes with carcinoma in situ: effects on Leydig cell function and eradication of malignant germ cells in 20 patients. J Clin Endocrinol Metab 1991;73(3):596–603.

50. Che M, Tamboli P, Ro JY, et al. Bilateral testicular germ cell tumors: twenty-year experience at M. D. Anderson Cancer Center. Cancer 2002;95(6): 1228–33.

51. Holzbeierlein JM, Sogani PC, Sheinfeld J. Histology and clinical outcomes in patients with bilateral testicular germ cell tumors: the Memorial Sloan Kettering Cancer Center experience 1950 to 2001. J Urol 2003;169(6):2122–5.

52. Horvath A, Korde L, Greene MH, et al. Functional phosphodiesterase 11A mutations may modify the risk of familial and bilateral testicular germ cell tumors. Cancer Res 2009;69(13):5301–6.

53. Harland SJ, Rapley EA, Nicholson PW. Do all patients with bilateral testis cancer have a hereditary predisposition? Int J Androl 2007;30(4):251–5 [discussion: 255].

54. Bojanic N, Bumbasirevic U, Vukovic I, et al. Testis sparing surgery in the treatment of bilateral testicular germ cell tumors and solitary testicle tumors: a single institution experience. J Surg Oncol 2014; 111:226–30.

55. Steiner H, Holtl L, Maneschg C, et al. Frozen section analysis-guided organ-sparing approach in testicular tumors: technique, feasibility, and long-term results. Urology 2003;62(3):508–13.

56. Heidenreich A, Weissbach L, Holtl W, et al. Organ sparing surgery for malignant germ cell tumor of the testis. J Urol 2001;166(6):2161–5.

57. Dilworth JP, Farrow GM, Oesterling JE. Non-germ cell tumors of testis. Urology 1991;37(5):399–417.

58. Al-Agha OM, Axiotis CA. An in-depth look at Leydig cell tumor of the testis. Arch Pathol Lab Med 2007; 131(2):311–7.

59. Gabrilove JL, Nicolis GL, Mitty HA, et al. Feminizing interstitial cell tumor of the testis: personal observations and a review of the literature. Cancer 1975; 35(4):1184–202.

60. Halat SK, Ponsky LE, MacLennan GT. Large cell calcifying Sertoli cell tumor of testis. J Urol 2007; 177(6):2338.

61. Arzola J, Hutton RL, Baughman SM, et al. Adult-type testicular granulosa cell tumor: case report and review of the literature. Urology 2006;68(5):1121. e13–6.

62. Bozzini G, Picozzi S, Gadda F, et al. Long-term follow-up using testicle-sparing surgery for Leydig cell tumor. Clin Genitourin Cancer 2013;11(3):321–4.

63. Grem JL, Robins HI, Wilson KS, et al. Metastatic Leydig cell tumor of the testis. Report of three cases and review of the literature. Cancer 1986;58(9): 2116–9.

64. Kim I, Young RH, Scully RE. Leydig cell tumors of the testis. A clinicopathological analysis of 40 cases and review of the literature. Am J Surg Pathol 1985;9(3): 177–92.

65. Silberstein JL, Bazzi WM, Vertosick E, et al. Clinical outcomes of local and metastatic testicular sex cord-stromal tumors. J Urol 2014;192(2):415–9.

66. Wang WP, Guo C, Berney DM, et al. Primary carcinoid tumors of the testis: a clinicopathologic study of 29 cases. Am J Surg Pathol 2010;34(4):519–24.

67. Soga J, Yakuwa Y, Osaka M. Carcinoid syndrome: a statistical evaluation of 748 reported cases. J Exp Clin Cancer Res 1999;18(2):133–41.

68. Hayashi T, Iida S, Taguchi J, et al. Primary carcinoid of the testis associated with carcinoid syndrome. Int J Urol 2001;8(9):522–4.

69. Stroosma OB, Delaere KP. Carcinoid tumours of the testis. BJU Int 2008;101(9):1101–5.

70. Zuetenhorst JM, Taal BG. Metastatic carcinoid tumors: a clinical review. Oncologist 2005;10(2): 123–31.

71. Yachia D, Auslaender L. Primary leiomyosarcoma of the testis. J Urol 1989;141(4):955–6.

72. Yoshimine S, Kono H, Nakagawa K, et al. Primary intratesticular leiomyosarcoma. Can Urol Assoc J 2009;3(6):E74–6.

73. Haran S, Balakrishan V, Neerhut G. A rare case of paratesticular leiomyosarcoma. Case Rep Urol 2014;2014:715395.

74. Miedler JD, MacLennan GT. Primary testicular lymphoma. J Urol 2007;178(6):2645.

75. Fonseca R, Habermann TM, Colgan JP, et al. Testicular lymphoma is associated with a high incidence of extranodal recurrence. Cancer 2000; 88(1):154–61.

76. Vitolo U, Chiappella A, Ferreri AJ, et al. First-line treatment for primary testicular diffuse large B-cell lymphoma with rituximab-CHOP, CNS prophylaxis, and contralateral testis irradiation: final results of an international phase II trial. J Clin Oncol 2011; 29(20):2766–72.

77. Wang Y, Li ZM, Huang JJ, et al. Three prognostic factors influence clinical outcomes of primary testicular lymphoma. Tumour Biol 2013;34(1):55–63.

78. Azuma T, Matayoshi Y, Nagase Y. Primary mucinous adenocarcinoma of the testis. Case Rep Med 2012; 2012:685946.

79. Ulbright TM, Young RH. Primary mucinous tumors of the testis and paratestis: a report of nine cases. Am J Surg Pathol 2003;27(9):1221–8.

80. Vaughn DJ, Rizzo TA, Malkowicz SB. Chemosensitivity of malignant ovarian-type surface epithelial tumor of testis. Urology 2005;66(3):658.

81. Michal M, Hes O, Kazakov DV. Primary signet-ring stromal tumor of the testis. Virchows Arch 2005; 447(1):107–10.

82. Bryan RL, Liu S, Newman J, et al. Squamous cell carcinoma arising in a chronic hydrocoele. Histopathology 1990;17(2):178–80.

83. Shah KH, Maxted WC, Chun B. Epidermoid cysts of the testis: a report of three cases and an analysis of 141 cases from the world literature. Cancer 1981; 47(3):577–82.

84. Shih DF, Wang JS, Tseng HH. Primary squamous cell carcinoma of the testis. J Urol 1996;156(5):1772.

85. Kryvenko ON, Epstein JI. Testicular hemangioma: a series of 8 cases. Am J Surg Pathol 2013;37(6): 860–6.

Management of Low-Stage Testicular Seminoma

Shane M. Pearce, MD[a],*, Stanley L. Liauw, MD[b],
Scott E. Eggener, MD[a]

KEYWORDS

- Seminoma • Stage I • Stage II • Surveillance • Chemotherapy • Radiotherapy

KEY POINTS

- Initial staging evaluation of seminoma after orchiectomy with serum tumor markers and imaging of chest, abdomen, and pelvis is critical.
- Disease-specific survival approaching 100% achieved for low-stage seminoma with active surveillance, adjuvant radiotherapy, or adjuvant single-agent carboplatin.
- Patient selection depends on specific patient and cancer characteristics.
- Risk of unnecessary treatment and sequelae of adjuvant therapy must be weighed against pitfalls of active surveillance such as poor compliance.
- Further research is needed to guide patient selection for adjuvant therapy and to optimize active surveillance protocols.

INTRODUCTION

Epidemiology

Although testicular cancer is the most commonly diagnosed cancer among men aged 14 to 44 years worldwide, it is a rare disease accounting for only 1% to 2% of malignancies.[1,2] Over the last 40 years, for unknown reasons, the global incidence of testicular cancer has doubled. In the United States, there will be an estimated 8820 new cases of testicular cancer in 2014, accounting for 380 deaths.[3] Testicular cancers are classified as seminomatous or nonseminomatous, with a nearly 1:1 incidence ratio. Among testicular cancer diagnoses, seminoma accounts for 46% to 60%.[4]

Histologic Subtypes

Classic or typical seminoma accounts for 95% of seminomas. Gross pathology reveals a white or tan tumor with lobulations. Microscopic examination demonstrates large uniform cells in a sheetlike distribution with a characteristic "fried egg" appearance. Syncytiotrophoblasts may be present, which accounts for the 10% to 15% of seminomas that produce abnormally high levels of human chorionic gonadotropin (hCG).[5] Immunohistochemistry plays a limited role in the diagnosis of seminoma, but nearly all seminomas stain strongly positive for placental alkaline phosphatase (87%–100% of cases). However, placental alkaline phosphatase staining is not specific for seminoma.[5]

Histologic variants of seminoma include tubular seminoma, which histologically mimics Sertoli cell tumor, and anaplastic seminoma.[6] Anaplastic seminoma is a subtype of historical significance referring to seminomas with high mitotic activity. Both tubular and anaplastic seminomas have a

No relevant disclosures to report.
[a] Section of Urology, Department of Surgery, University of Chicago, 5841 South Maryland Avenue, MC 6038, Chicago, IL 60637, USA; [b] Department of Radiation and Cellular Oncology, University of Chicago; 5841 South Maryland Avenue, MC 6038, Chicago, IL 60637, USA
* Corresponding author. The University of Chicago Medicine & Biological Sciences, 5841 South Maryland Avenue, MC 6038, Chicago, IL 60637.
E-mail address: pearce.shane@gmail.com

urologic.theclinics.com

similar prognosis and clinical management strategy as classic seminoma.[5,7]

Spermatocytic seminoma is rare (<1% of germ cell tumors [GCTs]), originates from more mature germ cells compared with classic seminoma, and has entirely different genetic and morphologic signatures.[8,9] These tumors are also unique because cryptorchidism is not a risk factor and they typically present in older men (mean age at diagnosis, 54 years).[10] Microscopy shows 3 distinct cell types (small, medium, and large) with round nuclei and no placental alkaline phosphatase expression.[11] Spermatocytic seminomas have very low malignant potential and are usually cured with radical orchiectomy followed by surveillance, with the exception of rare cases containing sarcomatous differentiation.[12]

Patterns of Spread

Classic seminoma metastasizes via lymphatic spread to the retroperitoneum if lymphatic flow has not been altered, such as after previous inguinal or scrotal surgery. The primary landing zone for right-sided tumors is the interaortocaval retroperitoneal nodes, compared with left-sided tumors, which typically spread initially to the left paraaortic (PA) nodes. Lymphatic spread within the retroperitoneum tends to be from right to left. Although rare, advanced seminoma presents with supradiaphragmatic lymphadenopathy or visceral metastases in the lung, liver, brain, and other sites. Even advanced seminoma has a relatively favorable prognosis and only liver and brain metastasis have been associated with an adverse prognosis.[13]

CLINICAL EVALUATION
Presentation and Initial Evaluation

Seminoma incidence peaks between 34 and 45 years, approximately 10 years later than other GCTs.[14] Most patients with testicular cancer will present with a painless mass. If present, pain may be owing to rapid growth of the tumor, hemorrhage, or infarction. Symptoms are observed more commonly with nonseminomatous GCTs compared with seminomas, because seminomas tend to have a more indolent disease course. Gynecomastia and infertility can rarely be presenting symptoms. Additionally, a small percentage of cases present with symptoms of metastatic disease, such as abdominal or flank pain, back pain, palpable mass of the abdomen or neck, lower extremity swelling, or a unilateral right-sided varicocele.[15,16] There is a well-recognized diagnostic delay between the onset of symptoms

and diagnosis of seminoma, with a mean delay of 4.9 months.[17]

Clinicians should assess for GCT risk factors when taking a history from patients with a testicular mass. A history of undescended testicle is the most significant risk factor for testicular GCT with a relative risk of between 2.7 and 8. Prepubertal orchiopexy seems to result in a significant reduction in the relative risk of testicular GCTs.[18] Orchiopexy seems to reduce specifically the risk of seminoma, evidenced by a 74% incidence of seminoma among malignant tumors arising from uncorrected cryptorchid testicles compared with a 29% incidence of seminoma among GCTs arising after orchiopexy.[18,19] Other established risk factors that should be assessed include a family history of testicular cancer, personal history of testicular cancer, presence of intratubular germ cell neoplasia, or a history of other urogenital abnormalities such as hypospadias.[20,21]

The initial evaluation of a patient presenting with a testicular mass should routinely involve scrotal ultrasonography as an extension of the physical examination. Both testes should be examined. Ultrasonography will usually reveal a solitary, hypoechoic lesion. Seminomas tend to have a more homogenous appearance compared with nonseminomatous GCTs. They can also seem to be lobulated or multinodular with cystic spaces.[22,23]

Serum Tumor Markers

Before radical orchiectomy, serum tumor markers such as α-fetoprotein (AFP), hCG, and lactate dehydrogenase should be obtained. The presence of syncytiotrophoblastic elements in approximately 10% to 15% of classical seminomas account for the increased hCG level in this subset of seminomatous GCTs.[24,25] When hCG is increased, it is typically less than 500 IU/mL. Although increased tumor markers do play a role in the staging of testis cancer (**Table 1**), patients with hCG-producing seminomas do not have a worse prognosis compared with nonsecretors.[26] In contrast with nonseminomatous GCTs, tumor markers are not utilized in the International Germ Cell Cancer Collaborative Group risk stratification schema (**Table 2**) for seminomas.[27] Detection of lactate dehydrogenase does not aid in the differential diagnosis of seminomatous or nonseminomatous GCTs, although levels may reflect overall disease burden.[28] Pure seminoma never secretes AFP; therefore, an increased AFP level indicates a nonseminomatous component or the presence of liver metastases, even when the primary tumor is pure seminoma on final histology.[29] Several recent

Table 1
AJCC/UICC serum tumor marker based staging

Stage	AFP (μg/L)	hCG (IU/L)	LDH
S0	Normal	Normal	Normal
S1	<1000	<5000	<1.5 × NL[a]
S2	1000–10,000	5000–50,000	1.5–10 × NL[a]
S3	>10,000	>50,000	>10 × NL[a]

Abbreviations: AFP, α-fetoprotein; AJCC, American Joint Committee on Cancer; hCG, human chorionic gonadotropin; LDH, lactate dehydrogenase; UICC, International Union Against Cancer.
[a] NL indicates upper limit of normal for LDH assay.

studies have investigated the role of serum microRNAs as a novel class of tumor markers for the management of testicular GCTs, but further prospective evaluation is needed.[30,31]

As stated, serum tumor markers should be measured before radical orchiectomy, after radical orchiectomy, and later as part of surveillance protocols or during treatment of metastatic disease. Declining serum tumor markers at a rate consistent with the marker's well-established half-life is expected after radical orchiectomy. Persistent markers or a decline slower than expected typically indicates the presence of metastatic disease.

Orchiectomy

After scrotal ultrasonography and serum tumor markers, the next step in management of a solid testicular mass usually involves a radical inguinal orchiectomy. Important surgical principles include high ligation of the spermatic cord using nonabsorbable suture to allow future identification if

Table 2
TNM staging groups and risk stratification of seminoma testicular cancer

Stage and Risk Category	Primary Tumor	N Stage	Clinical M Stage	Post-Orchiectomy Tumor Markers
IA	pT1 (no involvement of tunica vaginalis or spermatic cord, no LVI)	N0	M0	S0
IB	pT2 (involvement of tunica vaginalis or spermatic cord, +LVI)	N0	M0	S0
IS	Any pT stage	N0	M0	S1 or greater
IIA	Any pT stage	N1 (<5 retroperitoneal nodes and each ≤ 2 cm)	M0	S1
IIB	Any pT stage	N2 (>5 retroperitoneal nodes or ≥1 node 2–5 cm)	M0	S1
IIC	Any pT stage	N3 (retroperitoneal lymph node > 5 cm)	M0	S1
IIIA	Any pT stage	Any N stage	M1a (distant lymph nodes or lungs)	S0 or S1
IIIB	Any pT stage	Any N stage	M0 or M1a	S2
IIIC	Any pT stage	Any N stage	M0 or M1a	S3
	Any pT stage	Any N stage	M1b (N on pulmonary visceral) metastases)	Any S
Low risk	Any primary site	Any N stage	No nonpulmonary visceral metastases	Any S (normal AFP required)
Intermediate risk	Any primary site	Any N stage	Nonpulmonary visceral metastases	Any S (normal AFP required)

Abbreviations: AFP, α-fetoprotein; LVI, lymphovascular Invasion; TNM, tumor node metastasis.

retroperitoneal lymph node dissection is required subsequently. Testis-sparing surgery has been used as a treatment option for patients with bilateral tumors or a testicular mass in a solitary testicle. A number of studies have demonstrated acceptable oncologic outcomes and preservation of hormonal function and fertility with this approach, although local recurrence rates may be as high as 27% if adjuvant radiation therapy (RT) to the testicle is not used.[32–34]

Radical orchiectomy provides excellent local oncologic control in addition to establishing the histologic type, grade, and stage of the primary tumor. Pathologic review by an experienced genitourinary pathologist is strongly encouraged because tumors can be reclassified—for example, from seminoma to nonseminoma—in approximately 4% of cases and discrepancies in staging of the primary based on the presence or absence of lymphovascular invasion occur in 10% of cases.[35] Distinguishing the exact histologic type and stage of the primary tumor is critical for finalizing management options for low-stage testicular cancer.

Imaging

Complete diagnostic and staging evaluations of testicular cancer involve imaging of the retroperitoneum and lungs. Imaging of the lungs can include a CT scan or plain chest radiograph, depending on the level of suspicion. Contrast-enhanced CT of the abdomen and pelvis remains the imaging modality of choice for evaluating the retroperitoneum. Using a size criterion of 8 mm or larger in the maximum axial dimension achieves 100% specificity but only 47% sensitivity for detection of retroperitoneal lymph node metastases.[36] Other studies have shown that 25% to 30% of patients harbor occult metastases that cannot be detected on CT.[37,38] Efforts to improve the accuracy of clinical staging have examined other imaging modalities, including MRI and fluorodeoxyglucose PET. Fluorodeoxyglucose PET has demonstrated clinical utility in differentiating benign inflammation and granulation tissue from recurrent disease in retroperitoneal masses, but does not improve staging in clinical stage I disease compared with CT.[39,40] Although MRI offers the advantage of avoiding radiation, it is time consuming and costly. The use of lymphotrophic, nanoparticle-based contrast agents with MRI showed promising early results, with improved sensitivity and specificity for detection of nodal metastases compared with MRI alone; however, additional larger, prospective evaluation is needed.[41]

Staging and Risk Stratification

Patients are assigned a stage based on the primary tumor's final pathology, nodal and metastatic stage from imaging studies, and postorchiectomy serum tumor marker status (see **Table 2**).[27,42] Approximately 80% of seminoma patients are clinical stage I and 15% clinical stage II, with the majority being stage IIA or IIB.[43] Patients with advanced disease can be further categorized as either "good risk" or "intermediate risk" based on the International Germ Cell Cancer Collaborative Group (IGCCCG) prognostic factor based staging system (see **Table 2**).[27,42] Notably, in contrast with nonseminoma, there is no "poor risk" advanced seminoma.

MANAGEMENT OF CLINICAL STAGE I SEMINOMA

Men presenting with clinical stage I seminoma, who represent 80% of incident cases, can achieve long-term cure rates approaching 100%, regardless of management approach.[44–47] The primary options include adjuvant radiotherapy, chemotherapy or surveillance (**Table 3**). Owing to the exquisite radiosensitivity and chemosensitivity of seminoma, even relapse after adjuvant treatment is highly curable. In recent years, research has focused on minimizing unnecessary treatment and reducing treatment-related morbidity, while maintaining uniform cure rates.[48,49] Consideration must also be given to the cost of various treatment strategies.

Surveillance

Active surveillance has been extensively validated in numerous large institutional and population-based studies and now represents the preferred management approach in most guidelines for clinical stage I seminoma.[42,50–52] The most recent National Comprehensive Cancer Network (NCCN) guidelines for CS IA and IB seminoma (see **Table 2**) support active surveillance as the preferred management strategy for patients with a horseshoe/pelvic kidney, inflammatory bowel disease, or a prior history of radiation. Surveillance is also an appropriate option for the remainder of CS IA/IB patients. According to data from the National Cancer Database, active surveillance is now the most common treatment modality for clinical stage I seminoma in the United States, with utilization increasing from 25% in 1998% to 56% in 2011.[53]

Outcomes
Disease-specific survival for active surveillance has consistently approached 100% in multiple

Table 3
Post-orchiectomy management options for clinical stage 1 seminoma

Management	Frequency of Use	Risks	Benefits
Surveillance	55%	Relapse Compliance Radiation exposure Cost	Only treat the minority of patients who recur Treatment of relapse is almost always curative
Radiotherapy	28%	Acute toxicity Secondary malignancy Cardiovascular morbidity Unnecessary in 80%–85% of patients	Disease-specific survival near 100% Low overall recurrence rate (3%–5%) Lower cost vs surveillance
Adjuvant carboplatin	17%	Acute toxicity Long-term risk unknown Unnecessary treatment	Disease-specific survival near 100% Low overall recurrence rate (4%–7%)

Data from Jeldres C, Nichols CR, Pham K, et al. United States trends in patterns of care in clinical stage I testicular cancer: results from the National Cancer Database (1998–2011). J Clin Oncol 2014;32(Suppl 4). Abstract 369.

trials.[54–57] Relapse rates for patients with stage I seminoma managed with surveillance are between 13% and 19%.[54,56] A recent, large, multiinstitutional study of active surveillance in 1344 patients with clinical stage I seminoma showed that 99% of relapses exhibit good-risk features.[54] All of these relapses were cured with standard chemotherapy.[58]

Surveillance protocols

Typical active surveillance protocols for seminoma involve periodic physical examination, serum tumor markers (AFP and hCG, with or without lactate dehydrogenase), chest radiographs, and abdominal imaging with CT or MRI (**Table 4** for examples of surveillance protocols). Despite the widespread use of active surveillance, there are few data regarding the optimum extent and timing of diagnostic testing. More than 90% of relapses occur during the first 3 years of active surveillance; therefore, most schedules concentrate diagnostic testing during that time period. Relapses are detected on abdominal CT and tumor markers 87%

Table 4
Proposed active surveillance schedule for stage 1 seminoma after orchiectomy

Guideline	Years of Follow-Up				
	1	2	3	4	5
Kollmannsberger et al[54]					
Physical examination	Every 2 mo	Every 3 mo	Every 6 mo	Every 6 mo	Every 6 mo
Tumor markers	Every 2 mo	Every 3 mo	Every 6 mo	Every 6 mo	Every 6 mo
Chest x-ray	Every 4 mo	18 and 24 mo	—	—	—
CT/MRI[a] abdomen	Every 4 mo	18 and 24 mo	36 mo	—	60 mo
NCCN guidelines[b]					
Physical examination[c]	Every 3–6 mo	Every 6–12 mo	Every 6–12 mo	Annually	Annually
Tumor markers	Optional	Optional	Optional	Optional	Optional
Chest x-ray	As clinically indicated; consider chest CT in symptomatic patients				
CT abdomen and pelvis	At 3,6, and 12 mo	Every 6–12 mo	Every 6–12 mo	Every 12–24 mo	

[a] MRI only at experienced centers.
[b] NCCN Clinical Practice Guidelines: Testicular Cancer. V1.2015.
[c] Obtain scrotal ultrasound for equivocal examination.

Referenced with permission from the NCCN Clinical Practice Guidelines in Oncology (NCCN Guidelines®) for Testicular Cancer V.1.2015 © National Comprehensive Cancer Network, Inc 2014. All rights reserved. Accessed January 20, 2015. To view the most recent and complete version of the guideline, go online to NCCN.org. NATIONAL COMPREHENSIVE CANCER NETWORK®, NCCN®, NCCN GUIDELINES®, and all other NCCN Content are trademarks owned by the National Comprehensive Cancer Network, Inc.

and 3% of cases, respectively.[54] The added value of the physical examination and chest x-ray is very limited, and future guidelines may further reduce the number of chest x-rays.[54] The natural history of relapses after active surveillance was recently used to propose an evidence-based surveillance protocol for stage I seminoma.[54] **Table 4** compares this evidence-based surveillance protocol with current NCCN guidelines.[59]

Radiation exposure with surveillance

Radiation exposure associated with imaging is a concern with active surveillance. The average CT of the abdomen and pelvis exposes a patient to 10 to 20 mSv, with the potential for a cumulative exposure of up to 420 mSv if older surveillance protocols are followed.[43] Data from atomic bomb survivors in Japan has been used to estimate radiation exposure from CT scans is responsible for 0.6% to 2.0% of all cancers in the United States.[60] The use of MRI as an alternative imaging modality to limit radiation exposure is currently being investigated, but for now, its use should be restricted to experienced centers.[48,54] Other avenues of investigation include low-dose CTs, MR lymphography, and alternative imaging schedules to minimize the number of scans.

Patient adherence

Lack of adherence to the prescribed regimen is a major concern during active surveillance. The patient's ability to follow-up regularly, particularly during the first 3 years of surveillance, is critical for the success of this management strategy. Follow-up may be simple for some patients, with easy access to a cancer facility experienced in the management of testicular cancer. Only a minority of patients and their physicians are compliant with surveillance imaging and serum tumor marker testing.[61–64] Evaluation of a large, private insurance claims database found compliance with surveillance recommendations is poor and declines over time, with nearly 30% of patients on surveillance for stage I testis cancer receiving no abdominal imaging, chest imaging, or tumor marker tests within the first year of diagnosis.[61]

Radiotherapy

Adjuvant RT to the retroperitoneal lymph nodes has been historically the mainstay for treatment of men with stage I or IIA seminoma. The traditional approach involves a total dose of 30 Gy divided in 15 fractions administered to the PA and ipsilateral pelvic nodes (dogleg field), achieving disease-specific survival rates of nearly 100%.[65–69] The known toxicities of this approach includes acute (60%) and chronic gastrointestinal side effects (5%), risks of secondary malignancy, fertility concerns, and cardiac toxicity.[45,70,71] Toxicity concerns led to investigation of modified fields and reduced radiation dose in an attempt to minimize radiation exposure.

Evolution of radiation therapy

The UK Medical Research Council (MRC) TE10 trial randomized 478 men with stage I seminoma and undisturbed lymphatic drainage to PA strip (**Fig. 1**) or dogleg field radiation (30 Gy/15 fractions; **Fig. 2**).[72] Adjuvant radiation to the PA strip was associated with diminished hematologic, gastrointestinal, and gonadal toxicities. Although there were more pelvic recurrences in the PA strip cohort, overall recurrence rates for both approaches were equivalent at 4%, supporting PA adjuvant radiotherapy for patients with undisturbed lymphatic drainage. A second MRC

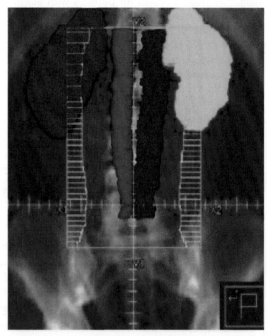

Fig. 1. Paraaortic (PA) field for adjuvant radiotherapy in stage I seminoma. Three-dimensional conformal radiation therapy planning technique utilizing vascular structures to establish lateral borders of targeted Field (*red*, aorta; *blue*, inferior vena cava). (*Referenced with permission* from the NCCN Clinical Practice Guidelines in Oncology (NCCN Guidelines®) for Testicular Cancer V.1.2015 © National Comprehensive Cancer Network, Inc 2014. All rights reserved. Accessed January 20, 2015. To view the most recent and complete version of the guideline, go online to NCCN.org. NATIONAL COMPREHENSIVE CANCER NETWORK®, NCCN®, NCCN GUIDELINES®, and all other NCCN Content are trademarks owned by the National Comprehensive Cancer Network, Inc.)

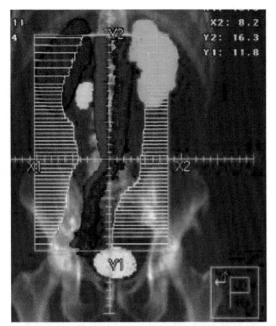

Fig. 2. Dog-leg field for adjuvant radiotherapy for right-sided primary tumor, clinical stage IIA seminoma. Three-dimensional conformal radiation therapy planning technique using vascular structures to establish lateral borders of targeted field (*red*, aorta and iliac artery; *blue*, inferior vena cava and iliac vein). (*Referenced with permission* from the NCCN Clinical Practice Guidelines in Oncology (NCCN Guidelines®) for Testicular Cancer V.1.2015 © National Comprehensive Cancer Network, Inc 2014. All rights reserved. Accessed January 20, 2015. To view the most recent and complete version of the guideline, go online to NCCN.org. NATIONAL COMPREHENSIVE CANCER NETWORK®, NCCN®, NCCN GUIDELINES®, and all other NCCN Content are trademarks owned by the National Comprehensive Cancer Network, Inc.)

prospective trial, TE18, randomly assigned 625 patients to 30 Gy/15 fractions versus 20 Gy/10 fractions to the PA field.[73] This trial demonstrated reduced morbidity in the 20 Gy arm with noninferior relapse rates. Based on these studies, current NCCN guidelines support administration of 20 Gy in 10 fractions to the PA field for patients with no history of pelvic or scrotal surgery.[59]

General radiotherapy considerations
Unnecessary radiation to the kidney, liver, and bowel can be further reduced with CT-based anteroposterior–posteroanterior 3-dimensional conformal RT compared with intensity-modulated RT; therefore, intensity-modulated RT is not recommended.[74] Clinicians are advised to consider alternative management approaches in patients with a history of ipsilateral pelvic surgery owing to the large volume of tissue that would be irradiated

with inclusion of the iliac and inguinal lymph nodes in the radiation field.[59] There is no evidence that extension of the radiation field reduces recurrences even in patients with a history of scrotal violation.[75,76]

Toxicity
It is important to recognize potential long-term toxicity secondary to RT, such as secondary malignancy and cardiovascular disease. Analysis of a pooled registry of 40,576 testicular cancer patients found RT independently increased the risk of nontesticular secondary solid malignancies, such as gastric cancers (relative risk [RR], 4.1) and sarcomas (RR, 5.1).[77] MD Anderson reported an experience of 477 patients with stage I or II seminoma treated with radiation, finding a 61% increased risk of cardiac-specific mortality.[71] The effect was limited to patients with at least 15 years of follow-up, and interestingly the increased risk of cardiovascular mortality was persistent even with exclusion of patients receiving mediastinal RT. Registry data from the United Kingdom (n = 992) found a greater than 2-fold risk of cardiovascular events (RR, 2.4) after radiotherapy for testicular cancer.[78] However, data from the Dutch testicular cancer registry (n = 2512) found the increased risk of cardiovascular morbidity was limited to patients receiving mediastinal radiation (RR, 2.5), with no increased risk after infradiaphragmatic RT alone. Overall, the data support the long-term carcinogenic potential of RT; however, there is conflicting evidence regarding the risk of cardiovascular morbidity associated with infradiaphragmatic RT.

Adjuvant Single-Agent Carboplatin

Owing to the potential toxicity associated with RT and the chemosensitive nature of seminoma, chemotherapy has been investigated as an option for stage I seminoma.

Outcomes
Adjuvant chemotherapy with single-dose carboplatin (400 mg/m^2 or an area under the curve of 7) has demonstrated very low relapse rates, ranging from 1.8% to 8.6% in numerous retrospective and prospective single-arm trials.[12] Adjuvant carboplatin therapy is now an accepted alternative to RT and surveillance for stage I seminoma. The MRC TE19 trial randomized 1477 men with stage I seminoma to RT or a single cycle of carboplatin using an area under the curve of 7.[79] This trial demonstrated noninferiority for adjuvant carboplatin with a 5-year relapse rate of 5.3%, compared with a 4% rate after RT. Adjuvant chemotherapy achieved a disease-specific survival rate of 99.9% and the 5-year rate of contralateral GCTs was lower in the carboplatin

arm (0.2% vs 1.2%). Chemotherapy also had the advantage of less missed work and decreased lethargy compared with RT.

Toxicity

Acute toxicities of carboplatin include nausea, vomiting, and myelosuppression. The long-term toxicity associated with single-agent adjuvant carboplatin is not well-characterized. A singly study of 199 patients treated with adjuvant carboplatin for stage I seminoma found no increased risk of cardiovascular disease or secondary malignancy compared with the general population with a mean follow-up of 9 years.[80] These results must be interpreted with caution because accurate long-term risk assessment for cardiovascular disease and secondary malignancy will require a markedly greater number of patients with at least 15 to 20 years of follow-up.

Cost Considerations

The financial implications of active surveillance for stage I seminoma are difficult to estimate given the variety of surveillance protocols and local–regional cost variations. Two North American studies have found surveillance is associated with $2600 to $5000 increased cost compared with adjuvant RT.[81,82] To our knowledge, no studies have examined the cost effectiveness of adjuvant single-agent carboplatin for stage I seminoma.

Patterns of Failure

Active surveillance, adjuvant radiotherapy, and adjuvant chemotherapy all achieve excellent outcomes in the management of patients with stage I seminoma, but the pattern of relapse can vary depending on the initial choice of treatment. The estimated rates of relapse vary: active surveillance (13%–19%), radiotherapy (3%–5%), and chemotherapy (4%–7%). With active surveillance, 92% of relapses occur within 3 years of diagnosis compared with greater than 99% of relapses within 3 years after adjuvant treatment.[83] The median time to recurrence on active surveillance (14 months) is comparable with the time to recurrence after adjuvant radiotherapy (12–15 months) and adjuvant chemotherapy (18 months).[54,84,85] Pooled data from the TE10, TE18, and TRE19 trials reveal that patients treated with adjuvant PA radiotherapy commonly recur in the mediastinum, neck, or pelvis, in contrast with the majority of retroperitoneal recurrences seen after active surveillance and adjuvant chemotherapy.[83] Relapses after adjuvant RT are typically treated with cisplatin-based chemotherapy (bleomycin + etoposide + cisplatin [BEP] for 3 cycles or etoposide + cisplatin [EP] for 4 cycles) with

excellent cure rates. Relapse after adjuvant carboplatin may be treated with either salvage radiotherapy or salvage cisplatin-based induction chemotherapy regimens.

Risk-Adapted Management

Although all 3 strategies yield disease-specific survival rates approaching 100%, no consensus exists regarding optimal management. Much attention is now devoted to minimizing morbidity related to unnecessary treatment and 1 potential strategy is risk-adapted management. Attempts to identify a prognostic model to guide risk-adapted management of clinical stage I seminoma have produced mixed results. In 2002, a retrospective pooled analysis of 638 patients with stage I seminoma managed with surveillance identified tumor size of greater than 4 cm and rete testis involvement as independent predictors of relapse. The presence of both adverse prognostic factors was associated with a 32% relapse rate compared with 16% for 1 risk factor and 12% for no risk factors. A recent attempt to validate these findings independently in 687 men confirmed primary tumor size as an important prognostic factor, but did not validate rete testis invasion as a significant predictor of relapse.[86] This study identified a 2% to 3% incremental increased risk of relapse for every 1 cm increase in tumor size, starting at 9% for a 1-cm seminoma to 26% for an 8-cm mass.

Nonetheless, 2 prospective studies have achieved disease-specific survival of 100% using risk-adjusted treatment guidelines with tumor size of greater than 4 cm and rete testis invasion as risk factors.[87,88] Risk-adapted management of stage I seminoma remains experimental in consensus guidelines and the most recent NCCN guidelines discouraged the use of a tumor size of greater than 4 cm and rete testis invasion for risk stratification.[59,89,90]

MANAGEMENT OF CLINICAL STAGE IIA SEMINOMA
Radiotherapy

Clinical stage II seminoma accounts for 15% to 20% of presenting cases, with most substaged as either IIA or IIB (see **Table 2**). Current NCCN guidelines for clinical stage IIA seminoma recommend RT using a modified dogleg field with a dose of 30 Gy.[59] This approach achieved a recurrence-free survival rate of 95% in a prospective trial of 66 men with stage IIA seminoma.[91] The most important factor predicting the likelihood of cure with RT alone was volume of nodal involvement, with a 91% 5-year relapse-free survival rate for patients with nodal disease less than

Table 5
National Comprehensive Cancer Network (NCCN) proposed follow-up schedule after adjuvant treatment of early stage seminoma

	Years of Follow-Up				
	1	2	3	4	5
Clinical stage I					
Physical examination[a]	Every 6–12 mo	Every 6–12 mo	Annually	Annually	Annually
Abdominal/pelvic CT	Annually	Annually	Annually	—	—
Chest x-ray	As clinically indicated, consider chest CT in symptomatic patients				
Clinical stage IIA and nonbulky IIB					
Physical examination[a]	Every 3 mo	Every 6 mo	Every 6 mo	Every 6 mo	Every 6 mo
Abdominal/pelvic CT	At 3 mo, then at 3–12 mo	Annually	Annually	As clinically indicated	
Chest x-ray	Every 6 mo	Every 6 mo	—	—	—

NCCN Clinical Practice Guidelines in Oncology I NCCN Guidelines for Testicular Cancer V.1.2015.

[a] Serum tumor markers optional, obtain scrotal utrasound for equivocal examination.

Referenced with permission from the NCCN Clinical Practice Guidelines in Oncology (NCCN Guidelines®) for Testicular Cancer V.1.2015 © National Comprehensive Cancer Network, Inc 2014. All rights reserved. Accessed January 20, 2015. To view the most recent and complete version of the guideline, go online to NCCN.org. NATIONAL COMPREHENSIVE CANCER NETWORK®, NCCN®, NCCN GUIDELINES®, and all other NCCN Content are trademarks owned by the National Comprehensive Cancer Network, Inc.

5 cm in maximal diameter, compared with 44% if greater than 5 cm.[92]

Chemotherapy

A prospective German study (n = 108) evaluated adjuvant carboplatin for stage II seminoma.[93] This study examined single-agent carboplatin for 3 cycles if clinical stage IIA and 4 cycles if clinical stage IIB. The study was terminated at interim analysis based on an increased relapse rate (18% vs 10% expected with RT), with all failures at the initial site of retroperitoneal disease. Based on this result, and the excellent outcomes achieved with radiotherapy, adjuvant RT to PA nodes and upper pelvis is the standard of care for clinical stage IIA seminoma. Multiagent chemotherapy with EP ×4 or BEP ×3 has been evaluated prospectively (n = 72) in men with clinical stage IIA and IIB seminoma.[94] The estimated 5-year progression-free survival rates were 100% for clinical stage IIA and 87% for clinical stage IIB. Multiagent chemotherapy is considered as an alternative to RT for patients with clinical stage IIA seminoma, particularly among patients with contraindications to RT such as a horseshoe kidney or prior radiation.

FOLLOW-UP REGIMENS

Men with low-stage seminoma treated with radiotherapy or chemotherapy require long-term follow-up to identify potential relapses, monitor the contralateral testicle, and evaluate for late sequelae of treatment, including secondary malignancy and cardiovascular disease. Current NCCN guidelines advise more frequent clinical evaluation and imaging of CS IIA compared with CS I seminoma after adjuvant treatment (**Table 5**).[59]

REFERENCES

1. Shanmugalingam T, Soultati A, Chowdhury S, et al. Global incidence and outcome of testicular cancer. Clin Epidemiol 2013;5:417–27.
2. Nigam M, Aschebrook-Kilfoy B, Shikanov S, et al. Increasing incidence of testicular cancer in the United States and Europe between 1992 and 2009. World J Urol 2015;33(5):623–31.
3. Siegel R, Ma J, Zou Z, et al. Cancer statistics, 2014. CA Cancer J Clin 2014;64:9–29.
4. Bray F, Ferlay J, Devesa SS, et al. Interpreting the international trends in testicular seminoma and nonseminoma incidence. Nat Clin Pract Urol 2006;3:532–43.
5. Cheville JC. Classification and pathology of testicular germ cell and sex cord-stromal tumors. Urol Clin North Am 1999;26:595–609.
6. Zavala-Pompa A, Ro JY, el-Naggar AK, et al. Tubular seminoma. An immunohistochemical and DNA flow-cytometric study of four cases. Am J Clin Pathol 1994;102:397–401.
7. Zuckman MH, Williams G, Levin HS. Mitosis counting in seminoma: an exercise of questionable significance. Hum Pathol 1988;19:329–35.

8. Verdorfer I, Rogatsch H, Tzankov A, et al. Molecular cytogenetic analysis of human spermatocytic seminomas. J Pathol 2004;204:277–81.

9. Looijenga LHJ, Hersmus R, Gillis AJM, et al. Genomic and expression profiling of human spermatocytic seminomas: primary spermatocyte as tumorigenic precursor and DMRT1 as candidate chromosome 9 gene. Cancer Res 2006;66:290–302.

10. Eble JN. Spermatocytic seminoma. Hum Pathol 1994;25:1035–42.

11. Aggarwal N, Parwani AV. Spermatocytic seminoma. Arch Pathol Lab Med 2009;133:1985–8.

12. Chung P, Mayhew LA, Warde P, et al. Management of stage I seminomatous testicular cancer: a systematic review. Clin Oncol (R Coll Radiol) 2010;22: 6–16.

13. Gholam D, Fizazi K, Terrier-Lacombe MJ, et al. Advanced seminoma–treatment results and prognostic factors for survival after first-line, cisplatin-based chemotherapy and for patients with recurrent disease: a single-institution experience in 145 patients. Cancer 2003;98:745–52.

14. Krag Jacobsen G, Barlebo H, Olsen J, et al. Testicular germ cell tumours in Denmark 1976-1980. Pathology of 1058 consecutive cases. Acta Radiol Oncol 1984;23:239–47.

15. Bahrami A, Ro JY, Ayala AG. An overview of testicular germ cell tumors. Arch Pathol Lab Med 2007; 131:1267–80.

16. Wein AJ, Kavoussi LR, Novick AC, et al. Campbell-Walsh Urology e-dition. JAMA 2007;298:2201–2.

17. Huyghe E, Muller A, Mieusset R, et al. Impact of diagnostic delay in testis cancer: results of a large population-based study. Eur Urol 2007;52: 1710–6.

18. Wood HM, Elder JS. Cryptorchidism and testicular cancer: separating fact from fiction. J Urol 2009; 181:452–61.

19. Batata MA, Whitmore WF, Chu FC, et al. Cryptorchidism and testicular cancer. J Urol 1980;124:382–7.

20. Tollerud DJ, Blattner WA, Fraser MC, et al. Familial testicular cancer and urogenital developmental anomalies. Cancer 1985;55:1849–54.

21. Prener A, Engholm G, Jensen OM. Genital anomalies and risk for testicular cancer in Danish men. Epidemiology 1996;7:14–9.

22. Dogra VS, Gottlieb RH, Oka M, et al. Sonography of the scrotum. Radiology 2003;227:18–36.

23. Mirochnik B, Bhargava P, Dighe MK, et al. Ultrasound evaluation of scrotal pathology. Radiol Clin North Am 2012;50:317–32, vi.

24. Barlow LJ, Badalato GM, McKiernan JM. Serum tumor markers in the evaluation of male germ cell tumors. Nat Rev Urol 2010;7:610–7.

25. Javadpour N, McIntire KR, Waldmann TA. Human chorionic gonadotropin (HCG) and alpha-fetoprotein (AFP) in sera and tumor cells of patients with testicular seminoma: a prospective study. Cancer 1978;42:2768–72.

26. Boujelbene N, Ozsahin M, Ugurluer G, et al. Management of chorionic gonadotropin-producing seminoma. Prog Urol 2011;21:308–13.

27. Anonymous. International germ cell consensus classification: a prognostic factor-based staging system for metastatic germ cell cancers. International Germ Cell Cancer Collaborative Group. J Clin Oncol 1997; 15:594–603.

28. Stanton GF, Bosl GJ, Whitmore WF, et al. VAB-6 as initial treatment of patients with advanced seminoma. J Clin Oncol 1985;3:336–9.

29. Javadpour N. Significance of elevated serum alphafetoprotein (AFP) in seminoma. Cancer 1980;45:2166–8.

30. Syring I, Bartels J, Holdenrieder S, et al. Circulating serum miRNA (miR-367-3p, miR-371a-3p, miR-372-3p and miR-373-3p) as biomarkers in patients with testicular germ cell cancer. J Urol 2015;193:331–7.

31. Belge G, Dieckmann KP, Spiekermann M, et al. Serum levels of microRNAs miR-371-3: a novel class of serum biomarkers for testicular germ cell tumors? Eur Urol 2012;61:1068–9.

32. Steiner H, Höltl L, Maneschg C, et al. Frozen section analysis-guided organ-sparing approach in testicular tumors: technique, feasibility, and long-term results. Urology 2003;62:508–13.

33. Bojanic N, Bumbasirevic U, Vukovic I, et al. Testis sparing surgery in the treatment of bilateral testicular germ cell tumors and solitary testicle tumors: a single institution experience. J Surg Oncol 2015; 111(2):226–30.

34. Lawrentschuk N, Zuniga A, Grabowksi AC, et al. Partial orchiectomy for presumed malignancy in patients with a solitary testis due to a prior germ cell tumor: a large North American experience. J Urol 2011;185:508–13.

35. Delaney RJ, Sayers CD, Walker MA, et al. The continued value of central histopathological review of testicular tumours. Histopathology 2005;47: 166–9.

36. Hilton S, Herr HW, Teitcher JB, et al. CT detection of retroperitoneal lymph node metastases in patients with clinical stage I testicular nonseminomatous germ cell cancer: assessment of size and distribution criteria. AJR Am J Roentgenol 1997;169:521–5.

37. Read G, Stenning SP, Cullen MH, et al. Medical Research Council prospective study of surveillance for stage I testicular teratoma. Medical Research Council Testicular Tumors Working Party. J Clin Oncol 1992;10:1762–8.

38. Peckham MJ, Barrett A, Husband JE, et al. Orchidectomy alone in testicular stage I non-seminomatous germ-cell tumours. Lancet 1982;2:678–80.

39. De Santis M, Pont J. The role of positron emission tomography in germ cell cancer. World J Urol 2004;22: 41–6.

40. Spermon JR, De Geus-Oei LF, Kiemeney LA, et al. The role of (18)fluoro-2-deoxyglucose positron emission tomography in initial staging and re-staging after chemotherapy for testicular germ cell tumours. BJU Int 2002;89:549–56.

41. Harisinghani MG, Saksena M, Ross RW, et al. A pilot study of lymphotrophic nanoparticle-enhanced magnetic resonance imaging technique in early stage testicular cancer: a new method for noninvasive lymph node evaluation. Urology 2005;66: 1066–71.

42. Motzer RJ, Agarwal N, Beard C, et al. NCCN clinical practice guidelines in oncology: testicular cancer. J Natl Compr Cancer Netw 2009;7:672–93.

43. Chung P, Warde P. Contemporary management of stage I and II seminoma. Curr Urol Rep 2013;14: 525–33.

44. Jones G, Arthurs B, Kaya H, et al. Overall survival analysis of adjuvant radiation versus observation in stage I testicular seminoma: a surveillance, epidemiology, and end results (SEER) analysis. Am J Clin Oncol 2013;36:500–4.

45. Fosså SD, Aass N, Kaalhus O. Radiotherapy for testicular seminoma stage I: treatment results and long-term post-irradiation morbidity in 365 patients. Int J Radiat Oncol Biol Phys 1989;16:383–8.

46. Dosmann MA, Zagars GK. Post-orchiectomy radiotherapy for stages I and II testicular seminoma. Int J Radiat Oncol Biol Phys 1993;26:381–90.

47. Warde P, Gospodarowicz MK, Panzarella T, et al. Stage I testicular seminoma: results of adjuvant irradiation and surveillance. J Clin Oncol 1995;13:2255–62.

48. Tandstad T, Dahl O, Cohn-Cedermark G, et al. Risk-adapted treatment in clinical stage I nonseminomatous germ cell testicular cancer: the SWENOTECA management program. J Clin Oncol 2009;27: 2122–8.

49. Kollmannsberger C, Moore C, Chi KN, et al. Non-risk-adapted surveillance for patients with stage I nonseminomatous testicular germ-cell tumors: diminishing treatment-related morbidity while maintaining efficacy. Ann Oncol 2010;21:1296–301.

50. Albers P, Albrecht W, Algaba F, et al. EAU guidelines on testicular cancer: 2011 update. Eur Urol 2011;60: 304–19.

51. Wood L, Kollmannsberger C, Jewett M, et al. Canadian Consensus Guidelines for the management of testicular germ cell cancer. Can Urol Assoc J 2010;4:e19–38.

52. Krege S, Beyer J, Souchon R, et al. European Consensus Conference on Diagnosis and Treatment of Germ Cell Cancer: a report of the second meeting of the European Germ Cell Cancer Consensus Group (EGCCCG): part II. Eur Urol 2008;53:497–513.

53. Jeldres C, Nichols CR, Pham K, et al. United States trends in patterns of care in clinical stage I testicular cancer: results from the National Cancer Database (1998-2011). J Clin Oncol 2014;32(Suppl 4). Abstract 369.

54. Kollmannsberger C, Tandstad T, Bedard PL, et al. Patterns of relapse in patients with clinical stage I testicular cancer managed with active surveillance. J Clin Oncol 2015;33:51–7.

55. Cummins S, Yau T, Huddart R, et al. Surveillance in stage I seminoma patients: a long-term assessment. Eur Urol 2010;57:673–8.

56. Von der Maase H, Specht L, Jacobsen GK, et al. Surveillance following orchidectomy for stage I seminoma of the testis. Eur J Cancer 1993;29A: 1931–4.

57. Choo R, Thomas G, Woo T, et al. Long-term outcome of postorchiectomy surveillance for stage I testicular seminoma. Int J Radiat Oncol Biol Phys 2005;61: 736–40.

58. Sharp DS, Carver BS, Eggener SE, et al. Clinical outcome and predictors of survival in late relapse of germ cell tumor. J Clin Oncol 2008;26:5524–9.

59. Motzer RJ, Agarwal N, Beard C, et al. NCCN clinical practice guidelines in oncology: testicular cancer. J Natl Compr Cancer Netw 2009;7:672–93.

60. Brenner DJ, Hall EJ. Computed tomography–an increasing source of radiation exposure. N Engl J Med 2007;357:2277–84.

61. Yu H, Madison RA, Setodji CM, et al. Quality of surveillance for stage I testis cancer in the community. J Clin Oncol 2009;27:4327–32.

62. Alomary I, Samant R, Gallant V. Treatment of stage I seminoma: a 15-year review. Urol Oncol 2006;24: 180–3.

63. De Wit R, Bosl GJ. Optimal management of clinical stage I testis cancer: one size does not fit all. J Clin Oncol 2013;31:3477–9.

64. Hao D, Seidel J, Brant R, et al. Compliance of clinical stage I nonseminomatous germ cell tumor patients with surveillance. J Urol 1998;160:768–71.

65. Dosoretz DE, Shipley WU, Blitzer PH, et al. Megavoltage irradiation for pure testicular seminoma: results and patterns of failure. Cancer 1981;48: 2184–90.

66. Giacchetti S, Raoul Y, Wibault P, et al. Treatment of stage I testis seminoma by radiotherapy: long-term results–a 30-year experience. Int J Radiat Oncol Biol Phys 1993;27:3–9.

67. Lai PP, Bernstein MJ, Kim H, et al. Radiation therapy for stage I and IIA testicular seminoma. Int J Radiat Oncol Biol Phys 1994;28:373–9.

68. Willan BD, McGowan DG. Seminoma of the testis: a 22-year experience with radiation therapy. Int J Radiat Oncol Biol Phys 1985;11:1769–75.

69. Zagars GK, Babaian RJ. Stage I testicular seminoma: rationale for postorchiectomy radiation therapy. Int J Radiat Oncol Biol Phys 1987;13:155–62.

70. Aass N, Fosså SD, Høst H. Acute and subacute side effects due to infra-diaphragmatic radiotherapy for

testicular cancer: a prospective study. Int J Radiat Oncol Biol Phys 1992;22:1057–64.

71. Zagars GK, Ballo MT, Lee AK, et al. Mortality after cure of testicular seminoma. J Clin Oncol 2004;22: 640–7.

72. Fosså SD, Horwich A, Russell JM, et al. Optimal planning target volume for stage I testicular semi-noma: a medical research council randomized trial. medical research council testicular tumor working group. J Clin Oncol 1999;17:1146.

73. Jones WG, Fossa SD, Mead GM, et al. Randomized trial of 30 versus 20 Gy in the adjuvant treatment of stage I Testicular Seminoma: a report on Medical Research Council Trial TE18, European Organisation for the Research and Treatment of Cancer Trial 30942 (ISRCTN18525328). J Clin Oncol 2005;23: 1200–8.

74. Hall EJ, Wuu CS. Radiation-induced second can-cers: the impact of 3D-CRT and IMRT. Int J Radiat Oncol Biol Phys 2003;56:83–8.

75. Capelouto CC, Clark PE, Ransil BJ, et al. A review of scrotal violation in testicular cancer: is adjuvant local therapy necessary? J Urol 1995;153:981–5.

76. Krege S, Beyer J, Souchon R, et al. European Consensus Conference on Diagnosis and Treatment of Germ Cell Cancer: a report of the second meeting of the European Germ Cell Cancer Consensus group (EGCCCG): part I. Eur Urol 2008;53:478–96.

77. Travis LB, Fosså SD, Schonfeld SJ, et al. Second cancers among 40,576 testicular cancer patients: focus on long-term survivors. J Natl Cancer Inst 2005;97:1354–65.

78. Huddart RA, Norman A, Shahidi M, et al. Cardiovas-cular disease as a long-term complication of treat-ment for testicular cancer. J Clin Oncol 2003;21: 1513–23.

79. Oliver RTD, Mead GM, Rustin GJS, et al. Random-ized trial of carboplatin versus radiotherapy for stage I seminoma: mature results on relapse and contralateral testis cancer rates in MRC TE19/EORTC 30982 study (ISRCTN27163214). J Clin On-col 2011;29:957–62.

80. Powles T, Robinson D, Shamash J, et al. The long-term risks of adjuvant carboplatin treatment for stage I seminoma of the testis. Ann Oncol 2008;19: 443–7.

81. Warde P, Gospodarowicz MK, Panzarella T, et al. Long term outcome and cost in the management of stage I testicular seminoma. Can J Urol 2000;7: 967–72 [discussion: 973].

82. Sharda NN, Kinsella TJ, Ritter MA. Adjuvant radia-tion versus observation: a cost analysis of alternate management schemes in early-stage testicular seminoma. J Clin Oncol 1996;14:2933–9.

83. Mead GM, Fossa SD, Oliver RTD, et al. Randomized trials in 2466 patients with stage I seminoma: pat-terns of relapse and follow-up. J Natl Cancer Inst 2011;103:241–9.

84. Leung E, Warde P, Jewett M, et al. Treatment burden in stage I seminoma: a comparison of surveillance and adjuvant radiation therapy. BJU Int 2013;112: 1088–95.

85. Livsey JE, Taylor B, Mobarek N, et al. Patterns of relapse following radiotherapy for stage I seminoma of the testis: implications for follow-up. Clin Oncol (R Coll Radiol) 2001;13:296–300.

86. Chung P, Daugaard G, Tyldesley S, et al. Evaluation of a prognostic model for risk of relapse in stage I seminoma surveillance. Cancer Med 2015;4(1): 155–60.

87. Aparicio J, Germà JR, García del Muro X, et al. Risk-adapted management for patients with clinical stage I seminoma: the second Spanish Germ Cell Cancer Cooperative Group study. J Clin Oncol 2005;23: 8717–23.

88. Aparicio J, Maroto P, del Muro XG, et al. Risk-adapt-ed treatment in clinical stage I testicular seminoma: the third Spanish Germ Cell Cancer Group study. J Clin Oncol 2011;29:4677–81.

89. Beyer J, Albers P, Altena R, et al. Maintaining suc-cess, reducing treatment burden, focusing on survi-vorship: highlights from the third European consensus conference on diagnosis and treatment of germ-cell cancer. Ann Oncol 2013;24:878–88.

90. Oldenburg J, Fosså SD, Nuver J, et al. Testicular seminoma and non-seminoma: ESMO Clinical Prac-tice Guidelines for diagnosis, treatment and follow-up. Ann Oncol 2013;24(Suppl 6):vi125–32.

91. Classen J, Schmidberger H, Meisner C, et al. Radio-therapy for stages IIA/B testicular seminoma: final report of a prospective multicenter clinical trial. J Clin Oncol 2003;21:1101–6.

92. Chung PWM, Gospodarowicz MK, Panzarella T, et al. Stage II testicular seminoma: patterns of recur-rence and outcome of treatment. Eur Urol 2004;45: 754–9 [discussion: 759–60].

93. Krege S, Boergermann C, Baschek R, et al. Single agent carboplatin for CS IIA/B testicular semi-noma. A phase II study of the German Testicular Cancer Study Group (GTCSG). Ann Oncol 2006; 17:276–80.

94. Garcia-del-Muro X, Maroto P, Gumà J, et al. Chemo-therapy as an alternative to radiotherapy in the treat-ment of stage IIA and IIB testicular seminoma: a Spanish Germ Cell Cancer Group Study. J Clin On-col 2008;26:5416–21.

Management of Stage I Nonseminomatous Germ Cell Tumors

Evan Kovac, MD CM, FRCSC[a],
Andrew J. Stephenson, MD, FRCSC[b],*

KEYWORDS

- Testicular neoplasms • Neoplasms • Germ cell and embryonal • Chemotherapy • Retroperitoneum
- Lymph node excision • Neoplasm staging • Surveillance

KEY POINTS

- Clinical stage I (CSI) nonseminomatous germ cell tumor (NSGCT) is defined as a nonseminoma that is localized to the orchiectomy specimen and without clinical/radiographic evidence of metastases or increased serum tumor markers.
- Postorchiectomy options for CSI NSGCT include surveillance, retroperitoneal lymph node dissection, or primary chemotherapy.
- Regardless of the chosen treatment avenue, cure rates of up to 100% are achieved.
- There is equipoise among experts in testis cancer as to the preferred treatment strategy for CSI NSGCT.
- An individualized approach, based on clinical and histopathologic features, is recommended, and patients with CSI NSGCT should be presented with each option, along with a detailed explanation of their respective risks and benefits.

EPIDEMIOLOGY AND PRESENTATION

Clinical stage I (CSI) nonseminomatous germ cell tumor (NSGCT) is defined as disease confined to the orchiectomy specimen in the absence of increased serum tumor markers (STMs) and without clinical or radiographic evidence of metastatic disease.[1–4] Age at presentation varies between seminoma and NSGCT. Although the incidence of seminomas peaks in the 35–39 year age range, NSGCTs typically present at a younger age, peaking in the 20–24 year age range.[5] In addition, there has been a significant and favorable stage migration at initial presentation, possibly as a result of increased awareness and improved diagnostic tools. In 1973, 55% of all diagnosed germ cell tumors (GCTs) were localized to the testis, with that number increasing to 73% in 2001.[5]

Approximately 70% to 80% of patients with CSI NSGCTs have cancer pathologically localized to the testis and are cured by orchiectomy alone, whereas the other 20% to 30% have occult retroperitoneal or distant metastases. With chemotherapy, surgery, or a combination of both, cure rates approaching 100% are achieved. However, if adjuvant treatments are applied to all patients with stage I NSGCT, up to 70% of patients

Disclosures: none.
[a] Glickman Urological & Kidney Institute, Cleveland Clinic, Mail Code Q10-1, 9500 Euclid Avenue, Cleveland Clinic, Cleveland, OH 44195, USA; [b] Center for Urologic Oncology, Glickman Urological & Kidney Institute, Cleveland Clinic, Cleveland Clinic Main Campus, Mail Code Q10-1, 9500 Euclid Avenue, Cleveland, OH 44195, USA
* Corresponding author.
E-mail address: stephea2@ccf.org

urologic.theclinics.com

undergo otherwise unnecessary and morbid therapies. Proper selection of patients for adjuvant treatment versus observation based on the probability of subclinical metastatic disease is paramount for the optimal treatment of these patients.

RETROPERITONEAL WORKUP AND RISK STRATIFICATION
Imaging

The primary landing site for right-sided tumors is the interaortocaval region, whereas left-sided tumors typically land in the para-aortic region. Although no absolute size cutoff exists to define clinical stage II disease (lymphatic metastases to the retroperitoneum), a 1-cm cut point to identify suspicious lymph nodes lacks sensitivity, because clinical understaging may occur in up to 80% of patients.[6–8] Evidence suggests that a lower size threshold should be used for lymph nodes in the primary landing zone, and we view lymph nodes 6 mm or larger with a high degree of suspicion, particularly when present in the context of other risk factors. In NSGCT, otherwise healthy and young men rarely have significant retroperitoneal adenopathy at baseline. Therefore, patients presenting with visually detectable lymph nodes within the primary landing zone on abdominal computed tomography (CT), even when smaller than 1.0 cm, should be treated with a high degree of suspicion for metastatic disease. Several investigators have shown that using a cutoff of 4 mm in the primary landing zone and 10 mm outside the primary landing zone was associated with a sensitivity and specificity of pathologic stage (PS) II disease of 91% to 93% and 50% to 58%, respectively.[6,7]

Nevertheless, accurate clinical staging is an imperfect science, as exemplified by the fact that even with the latest imaging technology and risk-stratification techniques, patients with a pristine CT scan of the abdomen and pelvis are understaged up to 20% to 30% of the time and are at risk for relapse.[9] In an attempt to improve rates of understaging, fluorodeoxyglucose (FDG) positron emission tomography (PET) has been investigated as a primary staging tool in patients with newly diagnosed, low-stage (I-II) NSGCT. Although the positive predictive value exceeds 90%, the negative predictive value of FDG-PET is similar to CT, at 67% to 78%. Because teratoma is not FDG-avid, a negative PET result fares no better than CT at ruling out occult retroperitoneal metastatic disease, even when considering malignant GCT elements such as embryonal carcinoma (EC), yolk sac tumor, and choriocarcinoma.[10] Therefore, FDG-PET cannot be recommended as a staging tool for NSGCT.

Histopathologic Risk Factors

Previous work has focused on histopathologic risk factors associated with the presence of occult retroperitoneal disease. Two histologic features in the primary tumor have consistently been shown to confer a greater risk of occult metastatic disease:

1. Lymphovascular invasion (LVI)[11–26]
2. Percentage of EC[11,13,14,16–18,21,22,24,27]

Other, less reliable predictors of occult metastases include high (T3/T4) histopathologic stage of the primary tumor[28] and MIB-1 staining.[4]

Impressively, 1 series[24] showed that patients with LVI in the primary tumor carry a 48% chance of relapse, whereas those without LVI have a 14% to 22% chance of relapsing. In a series of 267 patients with CSI-IIA NSGCT and who underwent retroperitoneal lymph node dissection (RPLND),[29] the presence of EC predominance and LVI in the primary tumor was associated with a higher rate of PSII disease (54% vs 37%, $P = .009$).

Therefore, previous consensus meetings have recommended the use of LVI in the primary specimen to risk stratify patients.[4] Meanwhile, the definition of EC predominance is not clearly defined, ranging from 45% to 90%. In addition, presence of occult metastases in patients with CSI NSGCT with LVI and EC predominance varies widely, from 45% to 90% and 30% to 80%, respectively,[4] and underscores the lack of reliability of these characteristics in accurately predicting patients at higher risk of retroperitoneal relapse.

Although contemporary studies have confirmed the prognostic significance of LVI for occult metastatic disease in CSI NSGCT, the rate of metastases in these studies seems to be substantially lower ($\leq$30%–50% relative decrease) compared with the early studies from the 1980s and 1990s analyzing LVI. For example, in a population-based study of patients with LVI on surveillance in the SWENOTECA (Swedish and Norwegian Testicular Cancer Group) study, Tandstad and colleagues[30] reported a probability of relapse of 45%. Likewise, in a study of unselected surveillance patients from Princess Margaret Hospital, Sturgeon and colleagues[31] reported a 49% relapse rate for those with pure EC and LVI. The reason for the lower than expected relapse rate for these patients may be related to stage migration, improved clinical staging, or differences in the pathologic assessment of LVI over time. Thus, when counseling patients about treatment options for CSI NSGCT, urologists should endeavor to counsel patients about the probability of occult disease rather than simply identifying patients as high or low risk from LVI or EC predominance.

MANAGEMENT OF STAGE I NONSEMINOMATOUS GERM CELL TUMOR

As previously stated, stage I NSGCT, clinically, is defined by the excision of a localized testicular nonseminoma, without increased postorchiectomy markers, and an otherwise normal metastatic workup (ie, normal CT chest and abdomen). Although many patients are cured by orchiectomy alone, up to 20% to 30% of patients with CSI disease (in both low-risk and high-risk groups) are clinically understaged and have occult metastases, most commonly in the retroperitoneal lymph nodes. Therefore, options for these patients include:

1. Active surveillance
2. RPLND
3. Primary chemotherapy

The ideal postorchiectomy treatment avenue for each individual patient is controversial. Here, we discuss the postorchiectomy options for stage I NSGCT, their relative risks and benefits, and the clinical factors that influence both the patient and urologist when choosing a postorchiectomy strategy.

Active Surveillance

Data accumulated over many decades have revealed that surveillance for CSI NSGCT achieves long-term survival outcomes that are comparable with adjuvant chemotherapy and RPLND. Although identifying patients at high risk of relapse remains challenging, overall surveillance relapse rates have been consistently reported in the 20% to 30% range.[24,25,32–36] Although most relapses typically occur within 2 years, late relapses beyond 5 years have been documented in approximately 1% to 5% of cases.[25,37,38]

Table 1 summarizes the largest trials of active surveillance (AS) to date.

The rationale for surveillance is based on the fact that 70% to 80% of patients are cured by orchiectomy, whereas adjuvant chemotherapy and RPLND are both associated with defined rates of important short-term and long-term toxicity. However, the series presented in **Table 1** represent cohorts of mainly low-risk patients. As discussed previously, relapse rates in patients with high-risk features typically exceed 30%, and it is in this subset of patients in whom the rationale for surveillance is less robust. Nevertheless, both low-risk

Table 1
Largest AS trials

Study	No. Patients	Relapses (%)	Median Follow-Up (mo)	Median Time to Relapse (mo)	% Systemic Relapse*	GCT Deaths (%)
Read et al,[24] 1992	373	100 (27)	60	3 (1.5–20)	39	5 (1.3)
Daugaard et al,[37] 2003	301	86 (29)	60	5 (1–171)	66	0
Freedman et al,[34] 1987	259	70 (32)	30	NR	61	3 (1.2)
Colls et al,[32] 1999	248	70 (28)	53	NR	73	4 (1.6)
Francis et al,[33] 2000	183	52 (28)	70	6 (1–12)	54	2 (1)
Gels et al,[35] 1995	154	42 (27)	72	4 (2–24)	71	2 (1)
Sharir et al,[36] 1999	170	48 (28)	76	7 (2–21)	79	1 (0.5)
Sogani et al,[25] 1998	105	27 (26)	136	5 (2–24)	37	3 (3)
Duran et al,[39] 2007	305	77 (25)	NR	7	26	2 (0.7)
Tandstad et al,[30] 2009	350	44 (13)	56	8	27	0
Kollmannsberger et al,[38] 2010	223	59 (26)	52	NR	NR	0
Kollmannsberger et al,[9] 2015	1139	221 (19)	62	6 (4–8)	NR	3 (<1)

* Systemic relapse defined as relapse with elevated serum tumor markers and/or relapse in tissue other than retroperitoneal lymph nodes.
Data from Refs.[9,24,25,30,32–39]

and high-risk patients who relapse on surveillance are cured of their disease in most cases. Thus, surveillance reserves treatments (and potential treatment-related morbidity) to those who need it. Therefore, AS for CSI NSGCT is an attractive strategy and we believe that it should be considered the standard of care in this patient population, regardless of risk factors.

Although there is no validated method of performing surveillance, most protocols involve frequent monitoring in years 1 to 2 with clinical assessment, STM (β human chorionic gonadotropin, α-fetoprotein, and lactate dehydrogenase) determinations, chest imaging, and transaxial abdominal-pelvic imaging. Beyond 2 years, the frequency of these tests is lessened. The low (0.5%–1.0%) but defined risk of relapse beyond 5 years mandates long-term surveillance.[40,41] For patients with CSIA testicular cancer enrolled in AS, the National Comprehensive Cancer Network (NCCN) guidelines recommend a history, physical examination, and STMs every 2 months in the first year, every 3 months in year 2, every 4 to 6 months in year 3, every 6 months in year 4, and annually thereafter. Abdominal/pelvic CT imaging should be performed every 4 to 6 months in the first year, every 6 to 12 months in year 2, and annually thereafter. Chest radiographs should be performed at months 4 and 12, and annually thereafter. For CSIB patients, the NCCN guidelines recommend a similar surveillance strategy to stage IA, except with an increased frequency of abdominal/pelvic CT imaging and chest radiographs: abdominal/pelvic CT every 4 months in the first year, every 4 to 6 months in year 2, every 6 months in year 3, and annually thereafter, and chest radiographs every 2 months in the first year, every 3 months in year 2, every 4 to 6 months in year 3, every 6 months in year 4, and annually thereafter.[42]

In addition to the NCCN guidelines, other published data on surveillance imaging protocols call for up to 4 to 7 CT scans within the first 2 years after enrollment.[27,33,43] Accordingly, the frequent use of CT imaging on surveillance has come under scrutiny because of the association of secondary malignancies with numerous abdominopelvic CT scans and the associated cumulative radiation exposure; the safety threshold seems to be crossed when an individual has received 7 lifetime CT scans.[44] A recent randomized trial of 2 versus 5 CT scans in years 1 to 2 among CSI NSGCT patients on surveillance reported no differences in the relapse rate, the IGCCCG (International Germ Cell Cancer Collaborative Group) risk group at relapse, or treatment required for relapsing patients, with no differences in survival between the 2 arms.[45]

Although there were relatively few patients with LVI randomized in this trial, it seems that 2 CT scans in years 1 to 2 on surveillance is safe and effective for a low-risk cohort of patients. With improving technology, low-dose, single-phase CT scanners are becoming increasingly used and show acceptable diagnostic accuracy.[46] Although there is no absolute safe radiation threshold, low-dose scanners may allow for a greater number of abdominopelvic CT scans in high-risk patients and do not necessarily increase the long-term risk of radiation-induced secondary malignancies.

The surveillance protocol used at our institution has been previously reported.[27] Clinical assessment, chest radiograph, and STM measurements are performed every 3 months during the first year, every 4 months in year 2, every 6 months in year 3 to 5, and annually thereafter. We perform low-dose, single-phase CT abdominal-pelvis imaging at 3, 12, 24, and 60 months in otherwise asymptomatic patients with normal STMs. Other investigators have also shown the safety and reliability of low-dose, noncontrast CT imaging and magnetic resonance imaging to survey the retroperitoneum when read by experienced radiologists and clinicians.[46]

Many urologists stipulate that a reliable patient is a prerequisite for AS, and reports of nonadherence to follow-up have been reported.[47] Although it is true that frequent physician visits, along with serum markers, chest radiographs, and abdominopelvic CT imaging are the cornerstones of a surveillance protocol, patients who are lost to follow-up typically present to hospital once symptomatic relapse occurs. In these rare cases, reports of sustainable remission with either chemotherapy or RPLND have been achieved.[48] Thus, although anticipated compliance should be considered when choosing/recommending treatments, anticipated noncompliance should not be the principal reason to deny a patient surveillance. Despite high rates of noncompliance with surveillance protocols, long-term cure rates approach 100%, suggesting that available treatments are able to salvage even those patients who are noncompliant with surveillance and who relapse with advanced disease. Thus, little rationale exists for excluding these patients from surveillance.

In general, remote location or inability to access physicians/hospitals with expertise in GCT management is a relative contraindication to surveillance, and these patients may best be served by either chemotherapy or RPLND.

The emotional stress and anxiety accompanying the chance of relapse while on surveillance must be balanced against the physical stress and morbidity of either chemotherapy or RPLND. Quality-adjusted survival models have been developed in an attempt to comprehend the patient's decision-making process when considering cancer outcomes, morbidity, and patient preferences for AS, chemotherapy, and RPLND, and have found that in all scenarios, patients prefer AS to chemotherapy or RPLND, except when the risk of recurrence is greater than 33% to 37%.[49] The predominance of an aversion to the emotional stress associated with AS in a high-risk group may sway the patient toward chemotherapy or RPLND.

For those who relapse on surveillance, the standard approach has been to administer risk-appropriate chemotherapy to all patients regardless of clinical stage and marker status at relapse. In these instances, long-term cure rates approach 100%. We and others have advocated that similar treatments should be offered to similarly staged patients with metastatic NSGCT at diagnosis. Although chemotherapy is the preferred salvage treatment of those who relapse with increased markers or CSIIC-III, select patients with normal STMs and nonbulky retroperitoneal disease (<3 cm) may also be considered for RPLND as the primary intervention. In general, relapses treated with chemotherapy should be risk adapted according to IGCCCG risk group.

Retroperitoneal Lymph Node Dissection

Subclinical metastatic disease in CSI NSGCT is the principal cause of early relapse and is present in approximately 20% to 30% of patients with this clinical stage. In those with occult metastases, malignant GCTs (which may later transform into teratomatous elements at metastatic sites) are usually located in the retroperitoneum ± systemic sites. Metastatic GCT that bypasses the retroperitoneum is an uncommon event,[8] whereas teratoma, when present, is virtually always localized to the retroperitoneum. Therefore, an adjuvant treatment that effectively removes occult metastases (including teratoma) in the retroperitoneum is an ideal choice for those patients in whom surveillance is not the preferred route.

RPLND for CSI NSGCT should be considered for the following reasons:

1. Systemic disease is rare.
2. Teratoma is chemoresistant and is identified in 15% to 25% of patients with occult PSII disease.
3. After full, bilateral template RPLND, the risk of abdominopelvic relapse is as low as 2%, thus obviating routine surveillance transaxial imaging of the retroperitoneum, postoperatively.
4. Patients who relapse after RPLND can be effectively salvaged with chemotherapy.

5. In patients with pN1 disease, cure rates after RPLND exceed 75%.[50]
6. In patients with pN2 disease and greater, adjuvant chemotherapy cures virtually 100% of patients.
7. RPLND is a safe, well-tolerated surgery, with minimal short-term and long-term morbidity, when performed by experienced surgeons at high-volume centers.
8. RPLND offers the most complete and accurate staging method for the retroperitoneum.
9. Given the low relapse rates after RPLND alone for patients with PSI (pN0, <5%–10%) and pN1 (<10%–20%), RPLND is associated with the lowest use of chemotherapy (and its associated short-term and long-term toxicity) among the 3 treatment options.

Long-term recurrence after primary RPLND is exceedingly rare, ranging from 1% to 2% beyond 2 years. Predictors of occult metastatic disease and early recurrence are less robust predictors of late recurrence.[51]

In addition to removal of the ipsilateral spermatic cord, a full, bilateral template dissection involves removal of all lymphatic tissue between the boundaries of the renal arteries at the cephalad extent, the ureters laterally, and the crossing of the ureters over the common iliac arteries at the caudal extent, including removal of all lymphatic tissue in the retroaortic and retrocaval locations. Without preservation of the sympathetic trunks, the postganglionic nerves from T10 to L2, and the hypogastric plexus, virtually all patients have ejaculatory dysfunction. To minimize this risk, several modified templates have been proposed to limit contralateral dissection lateral to either the aorta (right-sided templates) or inferior vena cava (left-sided templates) to spare these nerves. When modified templates are used, ejaculation rates up to 75% have been reported. With the development of nerve-sparing techniques that endeavor to dissect the postganglionic sympathetic fibers and hypogastric plexus from the surrounding lymphatic tissue, ejaculation rates of 95% or greater have been reported. Thus, nerve-sparing techniques have obviated modified templates and many centers routinely perform a full, bilateral, nerve-sparing dissection on all patients. If modified templates are performed, they should exclude contralateral dissection only below the inferior mesenteric artery, because lesser templates risk leaving malignant GCT or teratoma behind in up to 25% of patients.[52] Although primary, bilateral template RPLND obviates frequent follow-up abdominopelvic imaging, the risk of recurrence with a modified template RPLND is sufficiently high to require follow-up CT imaging, thus negating one of the principle benefits of RPLND over surveillance. Experts agree that a full, bilateral template, nerve-sparing RPLND is the optimal approach when a surgical avenue is chosen over chemotherapy or surveillance.[53,54]

Table 2 summarizes the largest reported series of primary RPLND to date.

Long-term complications of nerve-sparing RPLND are minimal and include an approximate 1% risk of bowel obstruction,[50,53] a 0.4% risk of lymphocele or chylous ascites[60] and a midline scar.

Both laparoscopic and robotic platforms have been used to perform RPLND.[61–64] Although technically feasible, these procedures should adhere to well-honed surgical principles, which should not be compromised in the interest of expediency.

Surgeon experience in RPLND, whether approached laparoscopically or open, is a prerequisite to effective surgery and lasting recurrence-free survival. Experts in the procedure agree that RPLND should not be performed in low-volume hospitals. Yet, a recent analysis reported that 75% of urologists performing RPLND in the United States have logged only a single RPLND, whereas urologists who logged 2 RPLNDs in a year were in the top 25% of performers.[65] In a randomized trial comparing RPLND with a single cycle of bleomycin, etoposide, and cisplatinum (BEP) chemotherapy for the management of CSI NSGCT,[58] relapse rates were significantly higher in the RPLND cohort. Yet, the study was conducted across 61 centers in Germany, with participating urologists performing a range of modified templates in low-volume centers. The importance of having an RPLND performed at high-volume, experienced centers in this procedure cannot be understated.

Primary RPLND is a safe, efficacious, and viable option for patients presenting with CSI NSGCT. The procedure offers the most accurate method for staging the retroperitoneum and is of excellent therapeutic value in patients with PSII disease. The procedure effectively controls the most common site of occult metastases and drastically reduces the need for long-term radiographic follow-up and its associated radiation exposure. With refined, nerve-sparing techniques performed by experienced surgeons, ejaculatory function is restored in 95% of cases, with otherwise few and rare long-term adverse sequelae. Patients with CSI NSGCT should be offered RPLND as one of 3 standard adjuvant therapies with a comprehensive discussion regarding its risks and benefits.

Table 2
Largest reported series of primary RPLND

	No. Patients	PSII (%)	% Teratoma in Retroperitoneum	% Relapse, PSI	% Relapse, PSII	% Adjuvant Chemotherapy	GCT Deaths (%)
Donohue et al,[55] 1993	378	113 (30)	15	12	34	13	3 (0.8)
Hermans et al,[56] 2000	292	67 (23)	NR	10	22	12	1 (0.3)
Nicolai et al,[51] 2010	322	61 (19)	NR	12	32	NR	5 (1.6)
Stephenson et al,[8] 2005	297	83 (28)	15	6	19	15	0
Williams et al,[57] 2009	76	37 (49)	NR	5	11	NR	0
Albers et al,[58] 2008	173	31 (19)	NR	9	NR	19	0
Richie et al,[59] 1990	99	35 (35)	NR	6	15	15	0

Abbreviation: NR, not reported.
Data from Refs.[8,51,55–59]

Primary Chemotherapy

Many patients with PSII disease (especially PSIIB and IIC) receive chemotherapy after RPLND. In the setting of node-positive disease, 3 cycles of BEP is standard. However, for CSI disease, 2 cycles of BEP is recommended. The rationale for 2 cycles is based on the low relapse rates after 2 cycles of adjuvant chemotherapy for pN1-N3 disease after RPLND.[66] In addition to the 30% relapse rate for CSI NSGCT, there are several rationales for chemotherapy in this setting:

1. Reduced short-term and long-term morbidity from 2, rather than 3 cycles of BEP.
2. High cure rate, low relapse rate, and a high likelihood of avoiding RPLND

Chemotherapy offers the highest chance of cure with any single modality for CSI disease. However, there are several disadvantages of primary chemotherapy:

1. Up to 70% to 80% of patients who receive primary chemotherapy are never destined to relapse and are thus unnecessarily exposed to its associated toxicities.
2. Chemotherapy is ineffective against retroperitoneal teratoma.
3. Follow-up CT imaging of the abdomen and pelvis is still required after primary chemotherapy.
4. Early and late toxicities of chemotherapy.
5. Relapse after primary chemotherapy poses a challenge, because they may be resistant to conventional chemotherapy.

Despite the lack of large-scale, phase 3 trials, several case series and phase 2 trials have evaluated the efficacy of primary chemotherapy for CSI NSGCT. Several groups stratified their patients by Medical Research Council risk group, depending on the presence of 1 or several of the following risk factors within the primary tumor[67]:

1. Predominance of EC
2. Absence of yolk sac elements
3. LVI

Most patients in these studies received 2 cycles of BEP.[15,22,23,67–69] However, other platinum-based regimens have been described.[70–72] Overall, relapse rates after primary, platinum-based chemotherapy are in the range of 2.5%, whereas the risk of death from testicular cancer ranges between 0% and 1.8%. Most relapses occurred within 2 years, with a median time to relapse of 22 months. Although long-term data for primary chemotherapy are lacking, late relapses have been described.[15]

Other groups have endeavored to determine the long-term efficacy of a single cycle of BEP, albeit in smaller series. Westermann and colleagues[73] evaluated 40 patients who received 1 cycle of BEP for high-risk, CSI NSGCT. After a median follow-up of 99 months, 35 of 40 (87.5%) were relapse-free. Those who relapsed were salvaged by additional cycles of chemotherapy, or surgery. In a phase 2 clinical trial, Vidal and colleagues[74] evaluated 40 patients for the long-term results of a single cycle of BEP for high-risk CSI NSGCT. At a median follow-up of 186 months, 1 patient (2.5%) developed pulmonary metastases at 13 months after treatment, and 3 patients (7.5%) developed metachronous tumors in the contralateral testicle. In the larger, prospective, SWENOTECA study, Tandstad and colleagues[30] offered surveillance or 1 cycle of BEP to patients diagnosed with LVI-negative CSI NSGCT, or 1 to 2 cycles of BEP to patients diagnosed with LVI-positive stage I disease. At a median follow-up of 4.7 years, 41.7% of LVI-positive patients on surveillance relapsed, versus only 13.2% of LVI-negative patients. Strikingly, in patients who received 1 cycle of BEP, 3.2% of LVI-positive patients relapsed, whereas 1.3% of LVI-negative patients relapsed, showing a 90% reduction in relapse for both LVI-positive and LVI-negative patients with CSI nonseminoma.

Albers and colleagues[58] randomized 382 patients with CSI NSGCT to receive either RPLND or a single cycle of BEP after orchiectomy. After a median follow-up of 4.7 years, a significantly lower number of recurrences were noted in the chemotherapy group (2 vs 15), with RPLND showing a hazard ratio of 7.9 compared with chemotherapy. However, no GCT deaths were noted in either arm. In addition, patients with histologically negative nodes experienced a recurrence rate of 11%, a significantly higher recurrence rate than pathologically stage-matched patients treated at high-volume centers. Patients randomized to RPLND in this trial were treated at 1 of 61 centers in Germany and were not uniformly offered full, bilateral templates. The relative inexperience of surgeons, combined with the performance of a substantial number of unilateral templates likely contributed to these poor results.

The short-term and long-term adverse effects of 3 cycles of BEP are well documented and include[75]:

1. Raynaud phenomenon (30%)
2. Sensory peripheral neuropathy (20%)
3. Pulmonary toxicity
4. Ototoxicity (20%)
5. Chronic kidney disease (20% reduction in creatinine clearance, persisting hypomagnesemia, or hypophosphatemia)

6. Infertility
7. Coronary artery disease and late cardiac events
8. Secondary malignancy

In a 20-year follow-up study,[76] long-term survivors of testicular cancer who received BEP were 5.7 times more likely to develop coronary artery disease and 3.1 times more likely to experience a myocardial infarction when compared with patients who underwent surgery alone.

Data collected on the adverse effects of 2 cycles of BEP are less robust. Neurotoxicity or ototoxicity has been reported in 8% to 19% of long-term survivors,[71,72,77] whereas glomerular filtration rate is decreased by 9%.[71] The effect on fertility from 2 cycles of BEP seems to be minimal, but high-quality data are lacking.[71]

Intuitively, the side effect profile of 1 cycle of BEP should be more favorable than 2 or 3 cycles. In the small cohorts reported earlier, long-term adverse effects of a single cycle of BEP were minimal and included reports of intermittent grades I-II tinnitus and grade II peripheral neuropathy.[73,74]

A major concern for long-term survivors of testicular cancer who receive chemotherapy is the risk of secondary malignancies. In one of the largest follow-up cohorts, Fung and colleagues[78] retrospectively analyzed secondary malignancy rates in men treated with cisplatin-based chemotherapy. Patients who received chemotherapy were 40% likelier to develop solid cancers with a median latency of 12.5 years. Three-fold to 7-fold risk increases were seen for renal, thyroid, and soft tissue cancers. Others have reported on the risk of leukemia with the use of high-dose etoposide.[79] However, modern BEP regimens remain lower than the reported threshold of more than 2 to 8 g/m^2, thus greatly reducing the risk of leukemia.

Although primary chemotherapy reduces the chance of recurrence in CSI NSGCT more than any other single modality, its early and late side effect profile, along with the risk of secondary malignancy, has limited its use in North America. Single-cycle chemotherapy for CSI nonseminoma should be considered investigatory, and until long-term phase 2 and 3 trials are available, 2 cycles of cisplatin-based chemotherapy should be considered the standard regimen for stage I disease.

SUMMARY

CSI NSGCT is a highly curable disease, regardless of treatment strategy. Surveillance, primary chemotherapy with 2 cycles of BEP, and RPLND all offer cure rates that approach 100%. Each follow-up approach is accompanied by its own set of strengths and drawbacks. Surveillance allows the patient to avoid potentially morbid adjuvant treatments approximately 70% of the time, but the importance of patient adherence to follow-up, the risk of multiple CT scans over the first 2 to 3 years, and the anxiety associated with surveillance must be discussed.

RPLND is a safe, well-tolerated procedure that effectively rids the retroperitoneum of the primary sites of metastatic disease. With modern nerve-sparing techniques, short-term and long-term morbidity from the procedure is minimized, with most patients able to achieve postoperative antegrade ejaculation. In addition, recurrence after RPLND is cured with cisplatin-based chemotherapy in up to 100% of cases. Occasional CT scans may be performed when following patients after RPLND, but overall radiation exposure from CT imaging is greatly reduced compared with surveillance or chemotherapy strategies. Long-term morbidity from RPLND includes a midline scar and a 1% risk of bowel obstruction and a small risk of lymphocele and chylous ascites. A major limitation to RPLND is the fact that 15% to 30% of patients undergoing the procedure receive adjuvant chemotherapy and are thus exposed to the morbidities of both surgery and chemotherapy in many cases.

As monotherapy, primary, cisplatin-based chemotherapy is associated with the lowest risk of relapse among the 3 treatment options. However, it may be associated with important short-term and long-term side effects, including, but not limited to, Raynaud phenomenon, sensory peripheral neuropathy, pulmonary toxicity, ototoxicity, chronic kidney disease, infertility, coronary artery disease, and the risk of secondary malignancies. Nonetheless, many of these adverse effects are seen after 3 cycles of BEP, whereas robust data evaluating the long-term effects of using 2 cycles or 1 cycle are lacking, although it seems there is no safe lower limit.

Multiple series have shown an increased risk of recurrence in patients harboring primarily embryonal components and LVI. Patients with primary tumors showing one or both of these characteristics should be counseled accordingly, because their risk of recurrence is higher. Nonetheless, even high-risk patients have a high likelihood of never experiencing recurrence.

No single approach can be considered superior in the setting of CSI NSGCT. Therefore, patients presenting at this stage should be informed of all 3 options. Surveillance is likely most appropriate for patients at low risk of recurrence. RPLND is associated with high cure rate and minimal long-term morbidity. Chemotherapy is likely most appropriate for patients refusing surveillance and surgery, where no experienced surgeon in RPLND is available, or who are likely to be lost to follow-up.

We conducted a decision analysis of treatment options for CSI NSGCT, which considered evidence-based estimates of treatment outcomes and short-term and long-term complications for chemotherapy, RPLND, and surveillance and utilities (preferences) for these outcomes based on expert clinical opinion from testicular cancer physicians and surgeons at our institution. For patients with a risk of relapse less than 35%, surveillance was the preferred treatment approach, because it was associated with the highest quality-adjusted life-years. Based on the method used to assess preferences, either RPLND or chemotherapy was recommended when the risk of relapse exceeded 35% to 40%.[49] Utilities for these outcomes varied widely among expert clinicians who frequently manage this disease. This finding underscores the importance of taking an individualized approach when counseling patients about treatment options for CSI NSGCT that takes into account patient preferences and individual clinician/institutional expertise.

REFERENCES

1. de Wit R, Bosl GJ. Optimal management of clinical stage I testis cancer: one size does not fit all. J Clin Oncol 2013;31(28):3477–9.
2. Nichols CR, Roth B, Albers P, et al. Active surveillance is the preferred approach to clinical stage I testicular cancer. J Clin Oncol 2013;31(28):3490–3.
3. Oldenburg J, Cullen M, Tandstad T. Primum non nocere: do we harm stage I testicular cancer patients less by applying adjuvant chemotherapy than by failing to present this option? Ann Oncol 2015; 26(2):255–6.
4. Stephenson AJ, Aprikian AG, Gilligan TD, et al. Management of low-stage nonseminomatous germ cell tumors of testis: SIU/ICUD Consensus Meeting on Germ Cell Tumors (GCT), Shanghai 2009. Urology 2011;78(4 Suppl):S444–55.
5. McGlynn KA, Devesa SS, Graubard BI, et al. Increasing incidence of testicular germ cell tumors among black men in the United States. J Clin Oncol 2005;23(24):5757–61.
6. Hilton S, Herr HW, Teitcher JB, et al. CT detection of retroperitoneal lymph node metastases in patients with clinical stage I testicular nonseminomatous germ cell cancer: assessment of size and distribution criteria. AJR Am J Roentgenol 1997;169(2): 521–5.
7. Leibovitch L, Foster RS, Kopecky KK, et al. Improved accuracy of computerized tomography based clinical staging in low stage nonseminomatous germ cell cancer using size criteria of retroperitoneal lymph nodes. J Urol 1995;154(5):1759–63.
8. Stephenson AJ, Bosl GJ, Motzer RJ, et al. Retroperitoneal lymph node dissection for nonseminomatous germ cell testicular cancer: impact of patient selection factors on outcome. J Clin Oncol 2005;23(12):2781–8.
9. Kollmannsberger C, Tandstad T, Bedard PL, et al. Patterns of relapse in patients with clinical stage I testicular cancer managed with active surveillance. J Clin Oncol 2015;33(1):51–7.
10. de Wit M, Brenner W, Hartmann M, et al. [18F]-FDG-PET in clinical stage I/II non-seminomatous germ cell tumours: results of the German multicentre trial. Ann Oncol 2008;19(9):1619–23.
11. Albers P, Bierhoff E, Neu D, et al. MIB-1 immunohistochemistry in clinical stage I nonseminomatous testicular germ cell tumors predicts patients at low risk for metastasis. Cancer 1997;79(9):1710–6.
12. Albers P, Siener R, Kliesch S, et al. Risk factors for relapse in clinical stage I nonseminomatous testicular germ cell tumors: results of the German Testicular Cancer Study Group Trial. J Clin Oncol 2003; 21(8):1505–12.
13. Albers P, Ulbright TM, Albers J, et al. Tumor proliferative activity is predictive of pathological stage in clinical stage A nonseminomatous testicular germ cell tumors. J Urol 1996;155(2):579–86.
14. Alexandre J, Fizazi K, Mahe C, et al. Stage I nonseminomatous germ-cell tumours of the testis: identification of a subgroup of patients with a very low risk of relapse. Eur J Cancer 2001;37(5):576–82.
15. Bohlen D, Borner M, Sonntag RW, et al. Long-term results following adjuvant chemotherapy in patients with clinical stage I testicular nonseminomatous malignant germ cell tumors with high risk factors. J Urol 1999;161(4):1148–52.
16. de Riese WT, Albers P, Walker EB, et al. Predictive parameters of biologic behavior of early stage nonseminomatous testicular germ cell tumors. Cancer 1994;74(4):1335–41.
17. Heidenreich A, Schenkmann NS, Sesterhenn IA, et al. Immunohistochemical expression of Ki-67 to predict lymph node involvement in clinical stage I nonseminomatous germ cell tumors. J Urol 1997; 158(2):620–5.
18. Heidenreich A, Sesterhenn IA, Mostofi FK, et al. Prognostic risk factors that identify patients with clinical stage I nonseminomatous germ cell tumors at low risk and high risk for metastasis. Cancer 1998; 83(5):1002–11.
19. Klepp O, Dahl O, Flodgren P, et al. Risk-adapted treatment of clinical stage 1 non-seminoma testis cancer. Eur J Cancer 1997;33(7):1038–44.
20. Madej G, Pawinski A. Risk-related adjuvant chemotherapy for stage I non-seminoma of the testis. Clin Oncol 1991;3(5):270–2.

21. Moul JW, McCarthy WF, Fernandez EB, et al. Percentage of embryonal carcinoma and of vascular invasion predicts pathological stage in clinical stage I nonseminomatous testicular cancer. Cancer Res 1994;54(2):362–4.

22. Ondrus D, Matoska J, Belan V, et al. Prognostic factors in clinical stage I nonseminomatous germ cell testicular tumors: rationale for different risk-adapted treatment. Eur Urol 1998;33(6):562–6.

23. Pont J, Holtl W, Kosak D, et al. Risk-adapted treatment choice in stage I nonseminomatous testicular germ cell cancer by regarding vascular invasion in the primary tumor: a prospective trial. J Clin Oncol 1990;8(1):16–20.

24. Read G, Stenning SP, Cullen MH, et al. Medical Research Council prospective study of surveillance for stage I testicular teratoma. Medical Research Council Testicular Tumors Working Party. J Clin Oncol 1992;10(11):1762–8.

25. Sogani PC, Perrotti M, Herr HW, et al. Clinical stage I testis cancer: long-term outcome of patients on surveillance. J Urol 1998;159(3):855–8.

26. White PM, Howard GC, Best JJ, et al. The role of computed tomographic examination of the pelvis in the management of testicular germ cell tumours. Clin Radiol 1997;52(2):124–9.

27. Choueiri TK, Stephenson AJ, Gilligan T, et al. Management of clinical stage I nonseminomatous germ cell testicular cancer. Urol Clin North Am 2007; 34(2):137–48 [abstract: viii].

28. Vergouwe Y, Steyerberg EW, Eijkemans MJ, et al. Predictors of occult metastasis in clinical stage I nonseminoma: a systematic review. J Clin Oncol 2003;21(22):4092–9.

29. Stephenson AJ, Bosl GJ, Bajorin DF, et al. Retroperitoneal lymph node dissection in patients with low stage testicular cancer with embryonal carcinoma predominance and/or lymphovascular invasion. J Urol 2005;174(2):557–60 [discussion: 560].

30. Tandstad T, Dahl O, Cohn-Cedermark G, et al. Risk-adapted treatment in clinical stage I nonseminomatous germ cell testicular cancer: the SWENOTECA management program. J Clin Oncol 2009;27(13): 2122–8.

31. Sturgeon JF, Moore MJ, Kakiashvili DM, et al. Non-risk-adapted surveillance in clinical stage I nonseminomatous germ cell tumors: the Princess Margaret Hospital's experience. Eur Urol 2011;59(4):556–62.

32. Colls BM, Harvey VJ, Skelton L, et al. Late results of surveillance of clinical stage I nonseminoma germ cell testicular tumours: 17 years' experience in a national study in New Zealand. BJU Int 1999; 83(1):76–82.

33. Francis R, Bower M, Brunstrom G, et al. Surveillance for stage I testicular germ cell tumours: results and cost benefit analysis of management options. Eur J Cancer 2000;36(15):1925–32.

34. Freedman LS, Parkinson MC, Jones WG, et al. Histopathology in the prediction of relapse of patients with stage I testicular teratoma treated by orchidectomy alone. Lancet 1987;2(8554):294–8.

35. Gels ME, Hoekstra HJ, Sleijfer DT, et al. Detection of recurrence in patients with clinical stage I nonseminomatous testicular germ cell tumors and consequences for further follow-up: a single-center 10-year experience. J Clin Oncol 1995;13(5):1188–94.

36. Sharir S, Jewett MA, Sturgeon JF, et al. Progression detection of stage I nonseminomatous testis cancer on surveillance: implications for the followup protocol. J Urol 1999;161(2):472–5 [discussion: 475–6].

37. Daugaard G, Petersen PM, Rorth M. Surveillance in stage I testicular cancer. APMIS 2003;111(1):76–83 [discussion: 83–5].

38. Kollmannsberger C, Moore C, Chi KN, et al. Non-risk-adapted surveillance for patients with stage I nonseminomatous testicular germ-cell tumors: diminishing treatment-related morbidity while maintaining efficacy. Ann Oncol 2010;21(6):1296–301.

39. Duran I, Sturgeon JF, Jewett MA, et al. Initial versus recent outcomes with a non-risk adapted surveillance policy in stage I non-seminomatous germ cell tumors (NSGCT). J Clin Oncol 2007; 25(18S):5021.

40. Daugaard G, Gundgaard MG, Mortensen MS, et al. Surveillance for stage I nonseminoma testicular cancer: outcomes and long-term follow-up in a population-based cohort. J Clin Oncol 2014;32(34): 3817–23.

41. Ernst DS, Brasher P, Venner PM, et al. Compliance and outcome of patients with stage 1 nonseminomatous germ cell tumors (NSGCT) managed with surveillance programs in seven Canadian centres. Can J Urol 2005;12(2):2575–80.

42. Motzer RJ, Agarwal N, Beard C, et al. Testicular cancer. J Natl Compr Canc Netw 2012;10(4):502–35.

43. Segal R, Lukka H, Klotz LH, et al. Surveillance programs for early stage non-seminomatous testicular cancer: a practice guideline. Can J Urol 2001;8(1): 1184–92.

44. Tarin TV, Sonn G, Shinghal R. Estimating the risk of cancer associated with imaging related radiation during surveillance for stage I testicular cancer using computerized tomography. J Urol 2009;181(2): 627–32 [discussion: 632–33].

45. Rustin GJ, Mead GM, Stenning SP, et al. Randomized trial of two or five computed tomography scans in the surveillance of patients with stage I nonseminomatous germ cell tumors of the testis: Medical Research Council Trial TE08, ISRCTN56475197–the National Cancer Research Institute Testis Cancer Clinical Studies Group. J Clin Oncol 2007;25(11): 1310–5.

46. O'Malley ME, Chung P, Haider M, et al. Comparison of low dose with standard dose abdominal/pelvic

multidetector CT in patients with stage 1 testicular cancer under surveillance. Eur Radiol 2010;20(7): 1624–30.

47. Hao D, Seidel J, Brant R, et al. Compliance of clinical stage I nonseminomatous germ cell tumor patients with surveillance. J Urol 1998;160(3 Pt 1): 768–71.

48. Hentrich MU, Brack NG, Schmid P, et al. Testicular germ cell tumors in patients with human immunodeficiency virus infection. Cancer 1996;77(10):2109–16.

49. Nguyen CT, Fu AZ, Gilligan TD, et al. Defining the optimal treatment for clinical stage I nonseminomatous germ cell testicular cancer using decision analysis. J Clin Oncol 2010;28(1):119–25.

50. Foster RS, Donohue JP. Retroperitoneal lymph node dissection for the management of clinical stage I nonseminoma. J Urol 2000;163(6):1788–92.

51. Nicolai N, Miceli R, Necchi A, et al. Retroperitoneal lymph node dissection with no adjuvant chemotherapy in clinical stage I nonseminomatous germ cell tumours: long-term outcome and analysis of risk factors of recurrence. Eur Urol 2010; 58(6):912–8.

52. Eggener SE, Carver BS, Sharp DS, et al. Incidence of disease outside modified retroperitoneal lymph node dissection templates in clinical stage I or IIA nonseminomatous germ cell testicular cancer. J Urol 2007;177(3):937–42 [discussion: 942–3].

53. Heidenreich A, Pfister D, Witthuhn R, et al. Postchemotherapy retroperitoneal lymph node dissection in advanced testicular cancer: radical or modified template resection. Eur Urol 2009;55(1):217–24.

54. Large MC, Sheinfeld J, Eggener SE. Retroperitoneal lymph node dissection: reassessment of modified templates. BJU Int 2009;104(9 Pt B):1369–75.

55. Donohue JP, Thornhill JA, Foster RS, et al. Retroperitoneal lymphadenectomy for clinical stage A testis cancer (1965 to 1989): modifications of technique and impact on ejaculation. J Urol 1993; 149(2):237–43.

56. Hermans BP, Sweeney CJ, Foster RS, et al. Risk of systemic metastases in clinical stage I nonseminoma germ cell testis tumor managed by retroperitoneal lymph node dissection. J Urol 2000;163(6): 1721–4.

57. Williams SB, McDermott DW, Dock W, et al. Retroperitoneal lymph node dissection in patients with high risk testicular cancer. J Urol 2009;181(5): 2097–101 [discussion: 2101–2].

58. Albers P, Siener R, Krege S, et al. Randomized phase III trial comparing retroperitoneal lymph node dissection with one course of bleomycin and etoposide plus cisplatin chemotherapy in the adjuvant treatment of clinical stage I nonseminomatous testicular germ cell tumors: AUO trial AH 01/94 by the German Testicular Cancer Study Group. J Clin Oncol 2008;26(18):2966–72.

59. Richie JP. Clinical stage 1 testicular cancer: the role of modified retroperitoneal lymphadenectomy. J Urol 1990;144(5):1160–3.

60. Baniel J, Foster RS, Rowland RG, et al. Complications of primary retroperitoneal lymph node dissection. J Urol 1994;152(2 Pt 1):424–7.

61. Cheney SM, Andrews PE, Leibovich BC, et al. Robot-assisted retroperitoneal lymph node dissection: technique and initial case series of 18 patients. BJU Int 2015;115(1):114–20.

62. Gardner MW, Roytman TM, Chen C, et al. Laparoscopic retroperitoneal lymph node dissection for low-stage cancer: a Washington University update. J Endourol 2011;25(11):1753–7.

63. Guzzo TJ, Gonzalgo ML, Allaf ME. Laparoscopic retroperitoneal lymph node dissection with therapeutic intent in men with clinical stage I nonseminomatous germ cell tumors. J Endourol 2010; 24(11):1759–63.

64. Nielsen ME, Lima G, Schaeffer EM, et al. Oncologic efficacy of laparoscopic RPLND in treatment of clinical stage I nonseminomatous germ cell testicular cancer. Urology 2007;70(6):1168–72.

65. Flum AS, Bachrach L, Jovanovic BD, et al. Patterns of performance of retroperitoneal lymph node dissections by American urologists: most retroperitoneal lymph node dissections in the United States are performed by low-volume surgeons. Urology 2014;84(6):1325–8.

66. Behnia M, Foster R, Einhorn LH, et al. Adjuvant bleomycin, etoposide and cisplatin in pathological stage II non-seminomatous testicular cancer. the Indiana University experience. Eur J Cancer 2000;36(4): 472–5.

67. Cullen M, James N. Adjuvant therapy for stage I testicular cancer. Cancer Treat Rev 1996;22(4): 253–64.

68. Abratt RP, Pontin AR, Barnes RD, et al. Adjuvant chemotherapy for stage I non-seminomatous testicular cancer. S Afr Med J 1994;84(9):605–7.

69. Chevreau C, Mazerolles C, Soulie M, et al. Long-term efficacy of two cycles of BEP regimen in high-risk stage I nonseminomatous testicular germ cell tumors with embryonal carcinoma and/or vascular invasion. Eur Urol 2004;46(2):209–14 [discussion: 214–15].

70. Amato RJ, Ro JY, Ayala AG, et al. Risk-adapted treatment for patients with clinical stage I nonseminomatous germ cell tumor of the testis. Urology 2004;63(1):144–8 [discussion: 148–9].

71. Dearnaley DP, Fossa SD, Kaye SB, et al. Adjuvant bleomycin, vincristine and cisplatin (BOP) for high-risk stage I non-seminomatous germ cell tumours: a prospective trial (MRC TE17). Br J Cancer 2005; 92(12):2107–13.

72. Oliver RT, Ong J, Shamash J, et al. Long-term follow-up of Anglian Germ Cell Cancer Group surveillance

versus patients with stage 1 nonseminoma treated with adjuvant chemotherapy. Urology 2004;63(3): 556–61.

73. Westermann DH, Schefer H, Thalmann GN, et al. Long-term followup results of 1 cycle of adjuvant bleomycin, etoposide and cisplatin chemotherapy for high risk clinical stage I nonseminomatous germ cell tumors of the testis. J Urol 2008;179(1): 163–6.

74. Vidal AD, Thalmann GN, Karamitopoulou-Diamantis E, et al. Long-term outcome of patients with clinical stage I high-risk nonseminomatous germ-cell tumors 15 years after one adjuvant cycle of bleomycin, etoposide, and cisplatin chemotherapy. Ann Oncol 2015;26(2):374–7.

75. Kollmannsberger C, Kuzcyk M, Mayer F, et al. Late toxicity following curative treatment of testicular cancer. Semin Surg Oncol 1999;17(4):275–81.

76. Haugnes HS, Wethal T, Aass N, et al. Cardiovascular risk factors and morbidity in long-term survivors of testicular cancer: a 20-year follow-up study. J Clin Oncol 2010;28(30):4649–57.

77. Kondagunta GV, Sheinfeld J, Mazumdar M, et al. Relapse-free and overall survival in patients with pathologic stage II nonseminomatous germ cell cancer treated with etoposide and cisplatin adjuvant chemotherapy. J Clin Oncol 2004;22(3):464–7.

78. Fung C, Fossa SD, Milano MT, et al. Solid tumors after chemotherapy or surgery for testicular nonseminoma: a population-based study. J Clin Oncol 2013;31(30):3807–14.

79. Wierecky J, Kollmannsberger C, Boehlke I, et al. Secondary leukemia after first-line high-dose chemotherapy for patients with advanced germ cell cancer. J Cancer Res Clin Oncol 2005;131(4): 255–60.

The Evolution and Technique of Nerve-Sparing Retroperitoneal Lymphadenectomy

 CrossMark

Timothy A. Masterson, MD[a,*], Clint Cary, MD, MPH[a], Kevin R. Rice, MD[b], Richard S. Foster, MD[a]

KEYWORDS

- Antegrade ejaculation • Fertility • Nerve-sparing retroperitoneal lymph node dissection
- Nonseminomatous germ cell tumor • Testicular cancer

KEY POINTS

- Through a better understanding of lymphatic dissemination in testicular germ cell tumors, modifications in the boundaries of dissection have improved the long-term morbidity of retroperitoneal lymphadenectomy (RPLND) without compromising oncologic outcomes.
- Through the use of modified unilateral templates and nerve-sparing techniques, preservation of antegrade ejaculation can be expected in nearly all patients undergoing primary RPLND.
- Nerve-sparing primary RPLND offers the most accurate way to identify micrometastatic disease that is present in 26% to 30% of early-stage nonseminoma patients, while proving therapeutic in 80% to 90% of men and avoiding any long-term morbidity.
- Similar success rates for ejaculatory preservation are possible after postchemotherapy RPLND when it is feasible to incorporate either or both of these techniques.
- Nerve-sparing postchemotherapy RPLND offers the potential to reduce the morbidity of necessary surgery in a patient population in which limited therapeutic options exist for residual disease after chemotherapy.

INTRODUCTION

During the past 40 years, there has been a dramatic improvement in survival rates for men diagnosed with testicular cancer. Most important among these improvements are the incorporation of cisplatin-based chemotherapy, better cross-sectional imaging and serologic markers for diagnosis and staging, and a better understanding of the nodal distribution with tailoring of surgical templates. With these improvements in survival, the focus has been directed at minimizing the morbidity of therapy in men who have anticipated life expectancies of 30 to 50 years beyond curative treatment. In the setting of advanced or metastatic disease, many of the associated toxicities and side effects of systemic chemotherapy and surgery are necessary and unavoidable. However, in early-stage disease, the associated efficacy and side-effect profiles of the 3 primary options of surgery,

The authors have no disclosures of any commercial or financial conflicts of interest; no funding was used to support this article.
[a] Department of Urology, Indiana University School of Medicine, 535 North Barnhill Drive, Suite 420, Indianapolis, IN 46202, USA; [b] Urologic Surgery, Walter Reed National Military Medical Center, 8901 Rockville Road, Bethesda, MD 20889, USA
* Corresponding author.
E-mail address: tamaster@iupui.edu

Urol Clin N Am 42 (2015) 311–320
http://dx.doi.org/10.1016/j.ucl.2015.04.005
0094-0143/15/$ – see front matter © 2015 Elsevier Inc. All rights reserved.

chemotherapy, and surveillance can be scrutinized and compared with each other.

Historically, surgical intervention served as the best opportunity for a durable cure in the absence of effective chemotherapy.[1,2] At select centers, surgical templates involved bilateral dissections of retroperitoneal (RP) nodal tissues surrounding the aorta and vena cava, extending caudally to include the interiliac and cranially to the suprahilar regions.[3] However, significant morbidity was reported.[4] After several publications elucidating the regional spread of disease based on laterality of the primary lesion, a better understanding of the nodal distribution in low-stage and high-stage disease allowed for more thoughtful assessments of the surgical boundaries of dissection.[5–7] Through this, downscaling of the template could be performed without jeopardizing the accuracy of staging or therapeutic efficacy in early-stage disease. Additionally, with the advent of more effective chemotherapy, interest in reducing surgical morbidity became more relevant.[8] One of the major issues surrounding RP lymph node dissection (RPLND) at the time was loss of seminal emission and bladder neck closure resulting in anejaculation and secondary infertility.[4,9] It was recognized that, through ipsilateral or contralateral preservation of postganglionic sympathetic lumbar nerves coursing through the RP, ejaculatory function could be preserved.

Initial strategies involved the exclusion of nodal dissections contralaterally.[5,7,10,11] Eventually, prospective identification of ipsilateral (or bilateral) postganglionic nerves was introduced.[12–14] This article describes the anatomic and physiologic basis for, indications and technical aspects of, and functional and oncologic outcomes reported after nerve-sparing RPLND in early and advanced stage testicular cancer. Discussions regarding the indications for surgery in lieu of chemotherapy or observations in early-stage nonseminoma are beyond the scope of this article.

ANATOMY AND PHYSIOLOGY OF EJACULATION

An improved understanding of the anatomy and physiology of ejaculation has allowed men to maintain normal antegrade ejaculation following nerve-sparing RPLND. The ability to obtain an erection is controlled through the parasympathetic pathway. This arises in S2 to S4 of the sacral spinal cord and sends preganglionic fibers in the pelvic nerves to the pelvic plexus. The pelvic plexus branches to form the cavernous nerves that innervate the penis. Stimulation of the pelvic plexus and cavernous nerves induces erections.

The course of these nerve fibers is not at risk during an RPLND.

The process of ejaculation involves 3 main sequential events: (1) tightening of the bladder neck, (2) seminal emission, and (3) expulsion of semen by rhythmic contraction of the ischiocavernosus and bulbocavernosus muscles. This process involves both the sympathetic and somatic nervous pathways. The sympathetic pathway originates in the preganglionic fibers from thoracic (T) 10 to lumbar (L) 2 vertebrae, which synapses in the sympathetic chain of ganglia, then exits as postganglionic fibers from L1 to L4 and coalesces near the bifurcation of the aorta into the superior hypogastric plexus. The right and left sympathetic chains course on either side of the vertebral column (**Fig. 1**). The right sympathetic chain lies posterior to the inferior vena cava (IVC; see **Fig. 1**A), whereas the left chain lies posterior lateral to the abdominal aorta (see **Fig. 1**B). Prospective identification and preservation of the postganglionic fibers exiting the sympathetic chain is the objective of the nerve-sparing RPLND. The L2 and L3 postganglionic fibers are usually fused and take a more anterior course along the aorta, whereas L1 usually originates near the renal hilum and, therefore, takes a more caudal and oblique course (see **Fig. 1**C; **Fig. 2**). Intraoperative electrostimulation of the postganglionic sympathetic fibers results in intraoperative ejaculation.[15,16] On electrostimulation of these nerve fibers, emission begins with bladder neck closure, contraction of the seminal vesicles, and emission of semen from the prostatic ejaculatory ducts into the prostatic urethra, which can be directly visualized with suprapubic ultrasound and urethroscopy. These efforts have consistently shown the L3 postganglionic fiber to be of most importance in preserving seminal emission. The pudendal nerve then sends impulses to the ischiocavernosus and bulbocavernosus muscles to produce rhythmic contractions for ejaculation of the seminal emission. The anatomy and physiology of the ejaculatory process was characterized during the 1980s. However, the importance of the sympathetic chain of ganglia and superior hypogastric plexus were recognized as early as the 1950s during sympathectomies for various medical conditions.[17]

PATIENT SELECTION FOR NERVE-SPARING TECHNIQUES

Although there remains some debate regarding indications for and template of RPLND, there is little controversy regarding the importance of strict adherence to the tenets of this surgery. Although some surgeons may view the remarkable

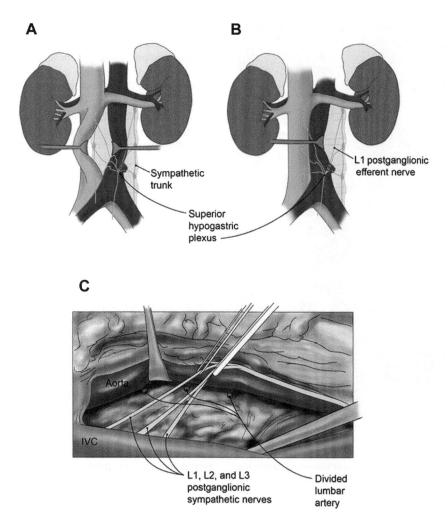

Fig. 1. The lumbar sympathetic nervous system and its relation to the great vessels. (*A*) Interaortocaval exposure of right-sided lumbar nerves. (*B*) Paraaortic exposure of left-sided lumbar nerves. (*C*) Course of postganglionic sympathetic nerve fibers L1 to L3 toward hypogastric plexus near the inferior mesenteric artery. (© 2015 Indiana University School of Medicine. All Rights Reserved.)

chemosensitivity of germ cell tumors as a safety net for challenging resections, this characteristic should not be a prime consideration once the decision has been made to proceed to RPLND. The strongest argument for primary RPLND in clinical stage I patients is that chemotherapy can be avoided in 90% of patients with pathologic stage I disease and 50% to 70% of patients with pathologic stage II disease.[18,19] Postchemotherapy RPLND is performed because residual teratoma is not chemosensitive and residual viable malignancy is rarely cured with salvage chemotherapy alone. Thus, the rationale for resection is that chemotherapy can be avoided or is unlikely to deliver a durable cure. Finally, the surgeon must consider the substantial financial burden that assisted reproductive technologies can place on

young couples that desire fertility after a non–nerve-sparing RPLND. This is particularly germane in the cases of primary RPLND, a surgery that is rarely absolutely indicated.

Principal to any surgical modification or restriction to the boundaries of dissection is ensuring that no compromise is made in oncologic outcomes. A feature unique among solid malignancies, testicular cancer remains curable in most patients with marker-negative, low-volume RP nodal involvement.[2,18,20] Therefore, inappropriate deviations from strict surgical principles subject patients to the potential of an unnecessary risk of relapse. A recent report demonstrated that intact lumbar vessels, as well as presence of ipsilateral gonadal vessels at reoperative RPLND, are associated with infield recurrences.[21] Similarly, a

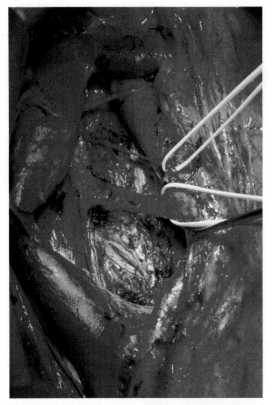

Fig. 2. Right-sided sympathetic nerves enveloped with vessel loops coursing through the interaortocaval space toward the hypogastric plexus intraoperatively. (© 2015 Indiana University School of Medicine. All Rights Reserved.)

previous series reported retroaortic and/or retrocaval recurrence in approximately half of patients undergoing reoperative RPLND.[22]

Although the optimal template that offers the greatest balance between oncologic control and minimization of morbidity in the setting of low-volume nodal metastasis remains controversial, the importance of sparing postganglionic sympathetic nerves for preservation of ejaculatory function is not. Depending on the philosophy of the operating surgeon, reduction of the surgical template in early-stage disease allows for nerve sparing through the exclusion of dissection around the contralateral postganglionic nerve fibers in early-stage patients. Given the ability of current imaging modalities to accurately stage disease preoperatively, the need for expansion of unilateral modified templates in clinical stage I and IIa patients are now uncommon. However, conversion of unilateral templates to bilateral dissections should be performed in the presence of any radiographic or palpable disease outside the primary landing zone. In appropriately selected patients, RP recurrences should be rare after either

unilateral modified template or bilateral nerve-sparing RPLND if properly performed.

Preservation of ejaculatory function with unilateral modified templates in early series were approximately 75%. In more contemporary reports, these rates exceed 95%.[23] Therefore, the decision to perform ipsilateral, prospective nerve sparing in the setting of a unilateral template is at the discretion of the operating surgeon and patient.

In centers where bilateral modified templates are performed routinely in all patients, nerve-sparing RPLND should be considered the standard of care for those individuals wishing to preserve ejaculatory function and/or fertility. In these cases, the incorporation of unilateral or bilateral nerve preservation is based on technical feasibility. Exclusions of ipsilateral or contralateral prospective nerve sparing would include any circumstance in which complete eradication of nodal disease would be compromised. Therefore, surgeon experience and intraoperative judgment are of the utmost importance to avoid RP recurrences.

In the postchemotherapy setting, similar arguments can be made with regard to the appropriate incorporation of unilateral, modified templates and/or nerve-sparing approaches in patients indicated for surgery. Patient selection is of the greatest importance, and safe utilization of these templates in the postchemotherapy setting is imperative. Patients may be considered for modified, unilateral templates in the postchemotherapy setting if they meet the following criteria:

1. Well-defined lesions less than or equal to 5 cm confined to the primary landing zone of the primary tumor on both prechemotherapy and postchemotherapy imaging
2. Normal postchemotherapy serum tumor markers
3. International Germ Cell Cancer Collaborative Group classification of low or intermediate risk of disease.

The standard of care remains a full bilateral, infrahilar template dissection to remove all residual macroscopic disease after chemotherapy. Therefore, when a modified, unilateral-template postchemotherapy RPLND is considered, strict adherence to these criteria is required to avoid relapses.[24]

TECHNIQUE

Preoperative imaging should occur within 4 to 6 weeks of surgery. When reviewing images, the surgeon should note of the size and location of masses, vascular anatomy, and renal or ureteral anatomy. Serum tumor markers should be checked within 2 weeks of surgery. Blood products should be reserved at the discretion of the surgeon. The anesthesia provider should be made aware of prior receipt of bleomycin if applicable. With few exceptions, the template of dissection to be used should be decided preoperatively. The boundaries of the templates can be found in **Fig. 3**.

The patient is placed in the supine position and a ventral midline incision is made. A thorough inspection of the abdomen and viscera is performed to assess for metastatic and incidental disease. A self-retaining retractor is placed. The RP is entered through the root of the small bowel mesentery for right-sided and bilateral dissections. The extent of this incision depends of the size and location of disease. Access to the RP can be gained through the left white line of Toldt in modified left-template dissections (**Fig. 4**). The bowels (including the third and fourth segments of the duodenum) and the mesentery are dissected off of the RP and placed behind retractors.

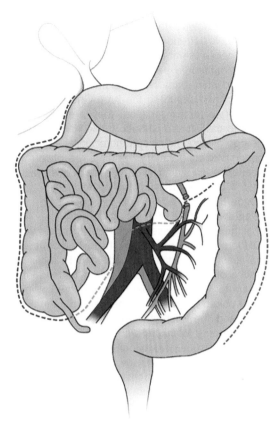

Fig. 4. Surgical approach to the retroperitoneum. Bilateral and right-template approaches (*green* and *purple dotted lines*). Left-template approaches (*red dotted line*). (© 2015 Indiana University School of Medicine. All Rights Reserved.)

The split and roll is then performed over the great vessels. Splitting over the aorta first is thought to avoid accidental injury to accessory right lower pole renal arteries not identified on preoperative imaging. Splitting over the IVC first is thought to avoid injury to the right-sided postganglionic sympathetic fibers. Whichever sequence is chosen, it is important to prospectively identify and preserve the postganglionic sympathetic fibers crossing anterior to the aorta below the level of the inferior mesenteric artery (IMA). The IMA is preserved in unilateral dissections versus ligation and division in some bilateral dissections.

The anatomy of the postganglionic sympathetic nerve fibers is variable due to fusion of adjacent roots and caliber variability. The L1 through L4 roots exit the ipsilateral sympathetic trunk, course obliquely toward the anterior surface of the distal aorta, and fuse with contralateral fibers in the superior hypogastric plexus. Right-sided postganglionic sympathetic fibers are identified coursing through the interaortocaval packet as it is rolled medially off the IVC. They are carefully dissected

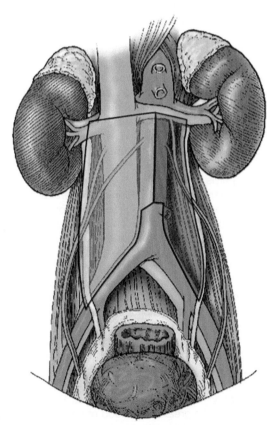

Fig. 3. Modified unilateral templates for right (*yellow shading*) and left (*blue shading*) dissections. (© 2015 Indiana University School of Medicine. All Rights Reserved.)

out of the packet and tagged with vessel loops and then traced down to their origins in the right sympathetic trunk. Left-sided nerve sparing is more difficult because the fibers run through the center of the left paraaortic packet. They are most easily identified where they cross the anterior surface of the aorta just caudal to the IMA. Once identified and tagged at this location, they are dissected down to the left sympathetic trunk. Patients who undergo bilateral nerve sparing or unilateral nerve sparing with contralateral complete resection may experience an anejaculatory period postoperatively.[12] This likely results from neuropraxia.

Once the lymphatic tissue has been split over the anterior surface of the great vessels, it is rolled off of the sides of these structures. All lumbar vessels located between the renal hilum and common iliac vessels are ligated and divided to facilitate removal of all lymphatic tissue within the template. The anatomy of the lumbar arteries is predictable, with 3 paired vessels found between the renal arteries and the bifurcation of the aorta. Lumbar vein anatomy is highly variable. Thus, careful attention must be paid to identify these structures in order to avoid hemorrhage. Before harvest, the superior aspect of the packets must be rolled inferiorly off of the renal hilum. Additionally, the paraaortic and paracaval packets must be dissected medially off of the lower pole of the ipsilateral kidney and ureter. These structures can then be placed behind a retractor to prevent injury during harvesting of the packet. The ipsilateral gonadal vein should be resected from its termination in the left renal vein or IVC down to the internal inguinal ring where the suture from the orchiectomy should be retrieved if possible.

The lymphatic packets are harvested off of the posterior body wall (psoas muscles and anterior spinous ligament). Perforating vessels are controlled with clips and/or electrocautery. Care should be taken to identify and ligate large lymphatics in order to prevent postoperative lymphatic or chylous ascites. These are often encountered coursing over and under the renal vessels and through the crus of the diaphragm. They can also be found at the most inferior tip of the paracaval and paraaortic packets where these join the ipsilateral common iliac lymph nodes. The cisterna chyli is located posteromedial to the aorta and is usually just cranial to the right renal artery. Thus, special attention should be paid to ligation of lymphatics this area in order to prevent chylous ascites. Care should be taken to preserve the genitofemoral nerve and sympathetic trunk whenever possible.

After all of the packets within the chosen template are removed, the resection beds are inspected for hemostasis and lymph leaks. The mesenteric incision is closed with an absorbable suture to prevent postoperative adhesion of the peritoneal viscera to the great vessels and RP. This may also prevent volvulus in cases of extensive intestinal mobilization. Surgical drains are only required in high-volume resections in which massive postoperative intraabdominal third spacing can be expected.

OUTCOMES
Antegrade Ejaculation

Oncologic and functional outcomes of nerve sparing are central to the appropriateness of this technique. Tenants remain that any compromise in cancer control warrants a close evaluation of whether the template or technique contributed. For primary RPLND, oncologic outcomes have proven to be excellent. **Table 1** summarizes the relapse rates and cancer outcomes after primary nerve-sparing RPLND. Importantly, they demonstrate that nerve-sparing approaches do not compromise oncologic outcomes, while maintaining high rates of ejaculatory preservation or recovery. In a recent study from Indiana, Beck and colleagues[23] demonstrated that with unilateral-template operations without ipsilateral nerve sparing, 97% preserved ejaculatory function. In those patients undergoing concomitant, ipsilateral nerve sparing, rates of preservation equal 99.2%. This is a significant improvement compared with the previously reported outcomes from the same institution demonstrating 75% preservation. This discrepancy likely reflects better patient selection and improvement along a surgical learning curve regarding the neuroanatomy of the postganglionic nerve fibers as they course from their origins to the pelvis.

In centers routinely performing bilateral dissections in the primary setting, ipsilateral or bilateral nerve sparing results in antegrade ejaculation rates of 90% to 100%. However, due to the presumed effects of neuropraxia and trauma of the nerves at the time of dissection, most of these patients reported temporary anejaculation that recovered over time.[12] Among those undergoing modified unilateral templates, a period of anejaculation is rarely encountered.[25]

In the postchemotherapy setting, far fewer patients are deemed candidates for template approaches or formal nerve sparing. Patients with left-sided primary testicular tumors and postchemotherapy RP residual masses less than 5 cm experienced a greater likelihood of preserving antegrade ejaculation with nerve sparing at time of postchemotherapy RPLND.[26] Several institutions have investigated to ability to safely incorporate modified unilateral templates in this setting.

Table 1
Selected primary nerve-sparing retroperitoneal lymphadenectomy series

Study	Number of Subjects	Study Period	Infield RP Recurrence (%)	Preservation of Ejaculation (%)	Median Follow-up (mo)	CSS (%)
Jewett et al,[12] 1988	13	NR	0 (0)	84.6	13.6	100
Donohue et al,[13] 1990	75	1984–1988	1 (1)	100	24–48	100
Weissbach et al,[40] 1990	168	1982–1987	4 (2)	74	30	NR
Richie,[41] 1990	85	1982–1989	NR	94	38	NR
de Bruin et al,[42] 1993	34	NA	0 (0)	91	17	100
Hobisch et al,[43] 1993	56	1988–1992	0 (0)	84	29	NR
Heidenreich et al,[44] 2003	239	1995–2000	1 (<1)	93.3	44	100%
Donohue et al,[35] 1998	402	NR	3 (0.4)	100	NR	99.6
Beck et al,[23] 2010	132[a] 34[b]	2000–2005	NR	99[a] 97[b]	68	NR

Abbreviations: CSS, cancer-specific survival; NA, not available; NR, not reported; RP, retroperitoneum.
[a] Unilateral modified template with ipsilateral nerve sparing.
[b] Unilateral modified template without ipsilateral nerve sparing.
Data from Refs.[12,13,23,35,40–44]

Table 2 outlines a summary of published outcomes of postchemotherapy RPLND modified templates regarding oncologic and functional endpoints. With proper selection of patients for unilateral templates, RP relapses are less than 1%, preservation of ejaculation is present in greater than 85%, and disease-specific survival rates exceed 98%.[24,27–29] Nevertheless, tempered enthusiasm for improving functional outcomes needs to be maintained if they come at the expense of compromised oncologic outcomes.

Fertility

Although the preservation of ejaculatory function remains a rate-limiting step in maintaining fertility, its maintenance does not guarantee successful paternity. Subfertility rates among men presenting

Table 2
Select nerve-sparing postchemotherapy retroperitoneal lymphadenectomy series

Study	Number of Subjects	Study Period	Infield RP Recurrence (%)	Preservation of Ejaculation (%)	Median Follow-up (mo)	CSS (%)
Wahle et al,[45] 1994	38	1988–1991	0 (0)	89.5	12	NR
Coogan et al,[46] 1996	81	1988–1995	0 (0)	76.5	35.5	NR
Rabbani et al,[27] 1998	8	1985–1995	0 (0)	50	55	100
Jacobsen et al,[47] 1999	85	1980–1994	4 (5)	89	96	NR
Nonomura et al,[48] 2002	26	1995–2000	1 (4)	86	26	NR
Steiner et al,[49] 2008	19	2004–2007	0 (0)	84	17.2	100
Heidenreich et al,[29] 2009	98[a] 54[b]	1999–2007	1 (1.9)	85[a] 25[b]	39	93[a] 79[b]
Pettus et al,[26] 2009	136	1995–2005	NR	79%	39	98
Steiner et al,[28] 2013	71[a] 21[b]	1993–2010	0 (0)	100[a] 95[b]	74	100

Abbreviations: CSS, cancer-specific survival; NR, not reported; RP, retroperitoneum.
[a] Ipsilateral or bilateral nerve sparing.
[b] Unilateral modified template.
Data from Refs.[26–29,45–49]

across all stages of testicular cancer range from 30% to 60%.[30–34] Therefore, baseline abnormalities on semen analysis before any intervention need to be considered when evaluating posttreatment fertility. Accordingly, limited data exist regarding paternity rates after intervention. In the primary setting of nerve-sparing RPLND, Indiana University has reported normal postoperative semen parameters in greater than 70% of men and successful paternity rates ranging from of 73% to 84%.[18,23,30,31,35,36] Fertility in the postchemotherapy setting proves even more challenging to determine because the negative effects of chemotherapy on spermatogenesis can persist for years following completion of treatment.[37] See elsewhere in this issue for a full discussion of fertility issues.

SUMMARY

Through the utilization of modified unilateral templates and nerve-sparing techniques, preservation of antegrade ejaculation can be expected in nearly all patients undergoing primary RPLND without compromise of oncologic outcomes. In doing so, nerve-sparing RPLND offers the most accurate way to identify micrometastatic disease that is present in 26% to 30% of early-stage nonseminoma patients, while proving therapeutic in 80% to 90% and avoiding any long-term morbidity. These conclusions are further supported by sexual quality of life, risk-benefit, and cost-benefit studies.[38,39] Similar success rates for ejaculatory preservation are possible after postchemotherapy RPLND when either or both of these techniques can be incorporated. Therefore, this approach offers the potential to reduce the morbidity of necessary surgery in a patient population in which limited therapeutic options exist for residual disease after chemotherapy.

REFERENCES

1. Cooper JF, Leadbetter WF, Chute R. The thoracoabdominal approach for retroperitoneal gland dissection: its application to testis tumors. 1950. J Urol 2002;167(2 Pt 2):920–6 [discussion: 927].
2. Patton JF, Hewitt CB, Mallis N. Diagnosis and treatment of tumors of the testis. JAMA 1959;171(16):2194–8.
3. Donohue JP. Retroperitoneal lymphadenectomy: the anterior approach including bilateral suprarenal-hilar dissection. Urol Clin North Am 1977;4(3):509–21.
4. Donohue JP, Rowland RG. Complications of retroperitoneal lymph node dissection. J Urol 1981;125(3):338–40.
5. Donohue JP, Zachary JM, Maynard BR. Distribution of nodal metastases in nonseminomatous testis cancer. J Urol 1982;128(2):315–20.
6. Ray B, Hajdu SI, Whitmore WF. Proceedings: distribution of retroperitoneal lymph node metastases in testicular germinal tumors. Cancer 1974;33(2):340–8.
7. Weissbach L, Boedefeld EA. Localization of solitary and multiple metastases in stage II nonseminomatous testis tumor as basis for a modified staging lymph node dissection in stage I. J Urol 1987;138(1):77–82.
8. Einhorn LH, Donohue JP. Improved chemotherapy in disseminated testicular cancer. J Urol 1977;117(1):65–9.
9. Narayan P, Lange PH, Fraley EE. Ejaculation and fertility after extended retroperitoneal lymph node dissection for testicular cancer. J Urol 1982;127(4):685–8.
10. Pizzocaro G, Zanoni F, Salvioni R, et al. Surveillance or lymph node dissection in clinical stage I nonseminomatous germinal testis cancer? Br J Urol 1985;57(6):759–62.
11. Rowland RG, Donohue JP. Testicular cancer: innovations in diagnosis and treatment. Semin Urol 1988;6(3):223–32.
12. Jewett MA, Kong YS, Goldberg SD, et al. Retroperitoneal lymphadenectomy for testis tumor with nerve sparing for ejaculation. J Urol 1988;139(6):1220–4.
13. Donohue JP, Foster RS, Rowland RG, et al. Nerve-sparing retroperitoneal lymphadenectomy with preservation of ejaculation. J Urol 1990;144(2 Pt 1):287–91 [discussion: 291–2].
14. Colleselli K, Poisel S, Schachtner W, et al. Nerve-preserving bilateral retroperitoneal lymphadenectomy: anatomical study and operative approach. J Urol 1990;144(2 Pt 1):293–7 [discussion: 297–8].
15. Dieckmann KP, Huland H, Gross AJ. A test for the identification of relevant sympathetic nerve fibers during nerve sparing retroperitoneal lymphadenectomy. J Urol 1992;148(5):1450–2.
16. Recker F, Tscholl R. Monitoring of emission as direct intraoperative control for nerve sparing retroperitoneal lymphadenectomy. J Urol 1993;150(5 Pt 1):1360–4.
17. Whitelaw GP, Smithwick RH. Some secondary effects of sympathectomy. N Engl J Med 1951;245(4):121–30.
18. Donohue JP, Thornhill JA, Foster RS, et al. Primary retroperitoneal lymph node dissection in clinical stage a non-seminomatous germ cell testis cancer review of the Indiana University experience 1965–1989. Br J Urol 1993;71(3):326–35.
19. Donohue JP, Thornhill JA, Foster RS, et al. The role of retroperitoneal lymphadenectomy in clinical stage

B testis cancer: the Indiana University experience (1965 to 1989). J Urol 1995;153(1):85–9.

20. Stephenson AJ, Bosl GJ, Motzer RJ, et al. Retroperitoneal lymph node dissection for nonseminomatous germ cell testicular cancer: impact of patient selection factors on outcome. J Clin Oncol 2005;23(12): 2781–8.

21. Pedrosa JA, Masterson TA, Rice KR, et al. Reoperative retroperitoneal lymph node dissection for metastatic germ cell tumors: analysis of local recurrence and predictors of survival. J Urol 2014; 191(6):1777–82.

22. Willis SF, Winkler M, Savage P, et al. Repeat retroperitoneal lymph-node dissection after chemotherapy for metastatic testicular germ cell tumour. Br J Urol 2007;100(4):809–12.

23. Beck SDW, Bey AL, Bihrle R, et al. Ejaculatory status and fertility rates after primary retroperitoneal lymph node dissection. J Urol 2010;184(5):2078–80.

24. Beck SDW, Foster RS, Bihrle R, et al. Is full bilateral retroperitoneal lymph node dissection always necessary for postchemotherapy residual tumor? Cancer 2007;110(6):1235–40.

25. Donohue JP, Thornhill JA, Foster RS, et al. Retroperitoneal lymphadenectomy for clinical stage A testis cancer (1965 to 1989): modifications of technique and impact on ejaculation. J Urol 1993;149(2): 237–43.

26. Pettus JA, Carver BS, Masterson T, et al. Preservation of ejaculation in patients undergoing nerve-sparing postchemotherapy retroperitoneal lymph node dissection for metastatic testicular cancer. Urology 2009;73(2):328–31 [discussion: 331–2].

27. Rabbani F, Goldenberg SL, Gleave ME, et al. Retroperitoneal lymphadenectomy for post-chemotherapy residual masses: is a modified dissection and resection of residual masses sufficient? Br J Urol 1998;81(2):295–300.

28. Steiner H, Leonhartsberger N, Stoehr B, et al. Postchemotherapy laparoscopic retroperitoneal lymph node dissection for low-volume, stage II, nonseminomatous germ cell tumor: first 100 patients. Eur Urol 2013;63(6):1013–7.

29. Heidenreich A, Pfister D, Witthuhn R, et al. Postchemotherapy retroperitoneal lymph node dissection in advanced testicular cancer: radical or modified template resection. Eur Urol 2009;55(1):217–26.

30. Foster RS, McNulty A, Rubin LR, et al. Fertility considerations in nerve-sparing retroperitoneal lymph-node dissection. World J Urol 1994;12(3): 136–8.

31. Foster RS, McNulty A, Rubin LR, et al. The fertility of patients with clinical stage I testis cancer managed by nerve sparing retroperitoneal lymph node dissection. J Urol 1994;152(4):1139–42 [discussion: 1142–3].

32. Lange PH, Chang WY, Fraley EE. Fertility issues in the therapy of nonseminomatous testicular tumors. Urol Clin North Am 1987;14(4):731–47.

33. Lange PH, Narayan P, Fraley EE. Fertility issues following therapy for testicular cancer. Semin Urol 1984;2(4):264–74.

34. Hansen PV, Glavind K, Panduro J, et al. Paternity in patients with testicular germ cell cancer: pretreatment and post-treatment findings. Eur J Cancer 1991;27(11):1385–9.

35. Donohue JP, Foster RS. Retroperitoneal lymphadenectomy in staging and treatment. Urol Clin North Am 1998;25(3):461–8.

36. Foster RS, Bennett R, Bihrle R, et al. A preliminary report: postoperative fertility assessment in nerve-sparing RPLND patients. Eur Urol 1993;23(1):165–7 [discussion: 168].

37. Lampe H, Horwich A, Norman A, et al. Fertility after chemotherapy for testicular germ cell cancers. J Clin Oncol 1997;15(1):239–45.

38. Aass N, Grünfeld B, Kaalhus O, et al. Pre- and posttreatment sexual life in testicular cancer patients: a descriptive investigation. Br J Cancer 1993;67(5):1113.

39. Baniel J, Roth BJ, Foster DRS, et al. Cost- and risk-benefit considerations in the management of clinical stage I nonseminomatous testicular tumors. Ann Surg Oncol 1996;3(1):86–93.

40. Weissbach L, Boedefeld EA, Horstmann-Dubral B. Surgical treatment of stage-I non-seminomatous germ cell testis tumor. Final results of a prospective multicenter trial 1982-1987. Testicular Tumor Study Group. Eur Urol 1990;17(2):97–106.

41. Richie JP. Clinical stage 1 testicular cancer: the role of modified retroperitoneal lymphadenectomy. J Urol 1990;144(5):1160–3.

42. de Bruin MJ, Oosterhof GO, Debruyne FM. Nerve-sparing retroperitoneal lymphadenectomy for low stage testicular cancer. Br J Urol 1993;71(3):336–9.

43. Hobisch A, Colleselli K, Ennemoser O, et al. Modified retroperitoneal lymph node excision in testicular tumors. Anatomy, surgical technique and results. Urologe A 1993;32(3):194–200 [in German].

44. Heidenreich A, Albers P, Hartmann M, et al. Complications of primary nerve sparing retroperitoneal lymph node dissection for clinical stage I nonseminomatous germ cell tumors of the testis: experience of the German Testicular Cancer Study Group. J Urol 2003;169(5):1710–4.

45. Wahle GR, Foster RS, Bihrle R, et al. Nerve sparing retroperitoneal lymphadenectomy after primary chemotherapy for metastatic testicular carcinoma. J Urol 1994;152(2 Pt 1):428–30.

46. Coogan CL, Hejase MJ, Wahle GR, et al. Nerve sparing post-chemotherapy retroperitoneal lymph node dissection for advanced testicular cancer. J Urol 1996;156(5):1656–8.

47. Jacobsen KD, Ous S, Waehre H, et al. Ejaculation in testicular cancer patients after post-chemotherapy retroperitoneal lymph node dissection. Br J Cancer 1999;80(1–2):249–55.

48. Nonomura N, Nishimura K, Takaha N, et al. Nerve-sparing retroperitoneal lymph node dissection for advanced testicular cancer after chemotherapy. Int J Urol 2002;9(10):539–44.

49. Steiner H, Zangerl F, Stöhr B, et al. Results of bilateral nerve sparing laparoscopic retroperitoneal lymph node dissection for testicular cancer. J Urol 2008;180(4):1348–52 [discussion: 1352–3].

Minimally Invasive Retroperitoneal Lymphadenectomy: Current Status

Thomas Kunit, FEBU, Günter Janetschek, MD*

KEYWORDS

- Laparoscopy • Testicular cancer • Retroperitoneal • Lymph node • Dissection • RPLND

KEY POINTS

- In patients with nonseminomatous germ cell tumor (NSGCT), clinical stage I retroperitoneal lymphadenectomy (RLA) is considered the only method that can immediately and reliably identify lymph nodes suspected of metastatic involvement.
- In well-defined residual masses smaller than 5 cm, strictly unilateral before chemotherapy, a modified unilateral template does not interfere with oncologic outcome.
- Recommendation for minimally invasive RLA and postchemotherapy RLA (PC) can only be given to tertiary centers with experience in laparoscopy and managing testicular cancer. No recommendation can be given for laparoscopic bilateral PC-RLA because of the lack of available data.

INTRODUCTION

Testicular cancer typically occurs in men between 15 and 35 years of age. The incidence is low, with 3 to 10 new cases per 100,000 men per year in the Western world. In total, testicular cancer represents 5% of urologic tumors[1] and only 2% of all human malignancies.[2] On the other hand, the incidence of germ cell tumors (GCTs) has been rising over the last 30 years in industrialized countries.[3] GCTs are divided in 2 major groups, seminomatous germ cell tumors (SGCTs) and nonseminomatous germ cell tumors (NSGCTs), consisting of teratoma, embryonal carcinoma, yolk sac tumor, and choriocarcinoma.[4]

Testicular cancer is eminently treatable with radiotherapy and chemotherapy, with excellent cure rates even in advanced cases provided that correct staging, early adequate treatment, and strict follow-up is carried out. If indicated, RCA in clinical stage I (CS I) or postchemotherapy (PC) is done as an open procedure at most centers. Nowadays, with the increased routine use of laparoscopy, the minimally invasive approach is gaining more interest. The first laparoscopic RLA was described for clinical stage I cancer in 1995 by Janetschek and colleagues,[5] who reported a case of laparoscopic PC-RLA in a patient with a left-sided stage IIb tumor. The operation was successful without major complications.

INDICATIONS FOR RETROPERITONEAL LYMPHADENECTOMY
Clinical Stage I Nonseminomatous Germ Cell Tumor

CS I NSGCT is defined as tumor involvement that is limited to the testis, normal serum tumor markers after inguinal orchiectomy, and no retroperitoneal lymph node metastasis.[6] However, up to 30% of these patients have occult metastases and will relapse if only surveillance is chosen after orchiectomy.[7] In large studies with high patient numbers, 80% of relapses occur during the first year of follow-up.[8,9]

Conflict of Interest: The authors have nothing to declare.
Department of Urology, Paracelsus Medical University Salzburg, Müllnerhauptstr 48, Salzburg 5020, Austria
* Corresponding author.
E-mail address: g.janetschek@salk.at

urologic.theclinics.com

Several studies have shown that vascular invasion of the tumor is a reproducible risk factor for relapse in CS I.[10,11] For this reason, the European Association of Urology (EAU) and the European Germ Cell Cancer Consensus Group (EGCCCG) recommend risk-adapted treatment in their guidelines. For patients with vascular invasion, PEB (cisplatin/etoposide/bleomycin) chemotherapy is the treatment of choice, and for those without vascular invasion surveillance should be chosen.[4,12]

RLA in CS I patients is preserved for those who are not suitable for chemotherapy or surveillance in the risk-adapted treatment according to EAU guidelines.[4] Also, the EGCCCG suggest RLA only for patients who do not agree to or qualify for the aforementioned options.[13] These recommendations are in contrast to those in the United States. The National Cancer Institute suggests postorchiectomy surveillance as the standard treatment option for CS I with no vascular invasion. On the other hand, RLA is considered the only method that can immediately and reliably identify lymph nodes suspected of metastatic involvement without the potential for false-positive results. If no retroperitoneal metastases are found, only 10% of these patients will relapse, and therefore no further treatment is needed.

In the guidelines of the National Comprehensive Cancer Network (NCCN), RLA-CS I has to be done within 4 weeks after imaging, with normal tumor markers not older than 7 days. This strict regime is chosen to ensure correct clinical staging.[2] RLA in NSGCT CS I has proved to be the most sensitive and specific method for testicular cancer staging in helping to choose the best treatment option for the patient. In 30% of patients testicular metastases are found, which leads to an upgrading to stage II disease.[14]

Clinical Stage IIa Nonseminomatous Germ Cell Tumor Without Elevated Tumor Marker: S0

In all advanced stages of NSGCT, initial cisplatin-based chemotherapy is the standard of care; this is one of the few treatment recommendations to reach general consensus in all guidelines.[2,4,15] Only in patients with very small lymph nodes (<2 cm) and negative tumor markers does the EAU suggest surveillance for 6 weeks, at which point a computed tomography (CT) scan should be repeated to clarify whether the lesion is stable, shrinking, or growing.[4] A shrinking lesion is due to a nonmalignant origin, so no further treatment is needed. A stable or progressive lymph node without marker evaluation indicates teratoma or tumor. In this case, nonseminomatous RLA should be performed.[15] On the other hand, in patients

with simultaneous increase of tumor markers surgery is obsolete. These patients require PEB chemotherapy according to the International Germ Cell Cancer Cooperative Group (IGCCCG) treatment algorithm.[16]

INDICATIONS FOR POSTCHEMOTHERAPY RETROPERITONEAL LYMPHADENECTOMY
Postchemotherapy Retroperitoneal Lymphadenectomy in Advanced Seminomas

A residual tumor after cisplatin-based chemotherapy in advanced stages of seminoma should not be primarily resected, irrespective of the size. A residual tumor smaller than 3 cm almost never contains viable cancer. Therefore, PC-RLA is not indicated in these cases.[17] After cisplatin-based chemotherapy in advanced seminoma, viable cancer was observed histologically only in 12% to 30% of patients after PC-RLA, even though the residual tumor was larger than 3 cm.[18–20] Hence PC-RLA is an overtreatment in about 80% of patients, harming them with needless morbidity.

To solve this problem, ^{18}F-labeled fluorodeoxyglucose PET (FDG-PET) scanning was included in the EAU guidelines in 2005, based on the SEMPET trial.[21,22] FDG-PET was affiliated into the EAU guidelines for patients with residual tumors larger than 3 cm to clarify viability. However, the scan must not be performed before 6 weeks after the last course of chemotherapy to reduce false-positive rates.[21,22] After this period, false positives are rare on FDG-PET. In patients with a positive FDG-PET scan, PC-RLA is indicated.

FDG-PET is an option in patients with residual tumors smaller than 3 cm according to EAU guidelines.[4] No further treatment besides observation is necessary in patients with a negative FDG-PET scan.[23]

Postchemotherapy Retroperitoneal Lymphadenectomy in Advanced Nonseminomatous Germ Cell Tumor

Overall, only 10% of residual masses contain viable cancer following PEB induction chemotherapy in NSGCT; 50% contain mature teratoma, and 40% contain necrotic-fibrotic tissue.[18,24,25] Even today no imaging investigation, including PET, or prognosis model can predict histologic differentiation of NSGCT residual tumor. Therefore in the case of any visible residual mass and marker normalization, surgical resection is indicated in accordance with EAU guidelines.[4,18]

However, there is still an increased risk of viable cancer or teratoma in patients with residual tumor smaller than 1 cm.[26] Mature teratoma was found in up to 22% and viable cancer in 9.4%.[27] In cases with teratoma in the primary orchiectomy specimen, these numbers increase to 41% and 16%.[28] Therefore, PC-RLA for residual tumors smaller than 1 cm may be considered for patients with teratoma in their primary histology.[29] However, PC-RLA in this setting is controversial.

This controversy begins with the critical size of lymph nodes in the retroperitoneum. Today there is no clear-cut consensus on nodal size. Therefore, it is mandatory that an expert surgeon reviews the prechemotherapy and postchemotherapy imaging to determine the extent and size of residual disease in relation to the initial tumor extension.[23] In contrast to the aforementioned increased risk in small residual tumors, the EGCCCG and Ehrlich and colleagues[30] from Indiana University recommended surveillance of patients with residual tumors smaller than 1 cm.[13] Ehrlich and colleagues[30] published data from 141 patients, and found relapse in only 12 patients (9%) after a long median follow-up of 15.5 years. Eight patients currently have no evidence of disease. However, 4 patients died of testicular cancer. The estimated 15-year recurrence-free survival (RFS) and cancer-specific survival (CSS) rates were 90% and 97%, respectively. The initial IGCCCG risk classification was found to be the only predictor of relapse and CSS.

TECHNIQUE
Template

The anatomic extent of RLA has been under consideration for many years. The traditional approach was to perform a full bilateral template dissection. In the 1980s this approach was the choice for patients with high-volume disease. However, the bilateral template leads to damage of the sympathetic trunks, hypogastric plexus, and postganglionic efferent nerves. To reduce morbidity, a modified unilateral template dissection was developed.[31]

A small residual tumor is the best indication for laparoscopic RLA because the dissection can be restricted to a unilateral template. Such a template can be chosen because the primary landing site of lymph node metastasis of a testicular cancer is unilateral. The primary tumor site of the testicle does not make a difference. Therefore, Weissbach and colleagues[32] defined the extent of surgery in a unilateral template for both sides. Studies have also shown that the primary landing site is always ventral to the lumbar vessels.[33] Regarding the extent of retroperitoneal metastasis, the tumor spreads to the contralateral side or behind the aorta and vena cava.

To clarify the best indication for a unilateral template, several investigators published data comparing unilateral templates with bilateral surgery. The Cologne Study Group[29] assessed 152 patients who underwent PC-RLA. A modified template was chosen for residual tumors smaller than 5 cm in 98 patients. A full bilateral template resection was done in 54 patients with larger lesions. Eight recurrences (5.2%) were observed after a mean follow-up of 39 months. All but one recurrence were outside of a bilateral template. Hence the investigators did not find a correlation with the extent of surgery.[29] In 2014, Vallier and colleagues[34] validated these selection criteria in a prospective study.

Bilateral nerve-sparing PC-RLA can also be done safely by means of laparoscopy, as reported by Steiner and colleagues.[35] The surgery was successfully finished in all 19 of their patients and no conversion was necessary, and there was no recurrence after a mean follow-up of 17.2 months. Another study compared the unilateral template with a bilateral template in PC-RLA. All operations were done laparoscopically, and 19 patients with a unilateral template were compared with 20 patients with a bilateral resection. The investigators did not find any difference in oncologic outcome and, surprisingly, morbidity.[36]

However, selection for a unilateral template is crucial. Not only the size of the residual tumor is important; it is also important to focus on tumor size and unilaterality before chemotherapy.[29,34] A safe but too restrictive approach was chosen by some investigators,[27,37] who decided to include only CS IIb (tumors <5 cm before chemotherapy) in unilateral template dissection.

In the United States the unilateral left template often includes the interaortocaval space, in contrast to the template described by Weissbach and colleagues[32]; this leads to damage of both sympathetic nerves (**Fig. 1**). Donohue and colleagues[38] first described nerve sparing using such a large left template. However, more recently they changed their template in terms of sparing the interaortocaval space. Hence, nerve sparing was provided by the template without compromising oncologic outcome.[39]

The data presented indicate that it is not always necessary to choose a full bilateral template. In well-defined residual masses smaller than 5 cm and strictly unilateral before chemotherapy, a modified unilateral template does not interfere with oncologic outcome. Moreover, full bilateral PC-RLA can be done laparoscopically, although it should be mentioned that in this procedure the position of the patient has to be changed with consequent loss of the advantages of laparoscopy.

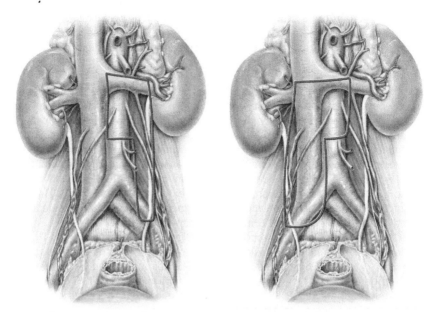

Fig. 1. Left-sided and right-sided modified template. (*From* Lattouf JB, Jeschke S, Janetschek G. Laparoscopic retroperitoneal lymph node dissection: technique. BJU Int 2007;100(6):1415–29; with permission.)

APPROACH
Laparoscopic Transperitoneal

Most published data concerns a transperitoneal approach with the patient in lateral decubitus position.[27,36,40–45] This approach provides exposure comparable with open surgery. A wide dissection and complete displacement of the bowel is crucial to obtain good exposure of the retroperitoneum. There is no difference between RLA and PC-RLA in terms of exposure. On the other hand, laparoscopic PC-RLA is one of the most technically challenging procedures because of the fibrosis and desmoplastic reaction caused by the chemotherapy, especially in seminoma where severe

fibrosis can be observed. However, less desmoplastic reaction is found in residual tumors caused by teratoma.

Laparoscopic Extraperitoneal

The first data on the laparoscopic extraperitoneal approach were published by LeBlanc and coleagues[46] in 2001, in which the approach was used in CS I patients. Nowadays it is also used for PC-RLA by several groups.[37,47–49] In contrast to the transperitoneal approach, the patient is in supine position. The surgical team is located on the ipsilateral side. Just as in retroscopic nephrectomy, a sufficient extraperitoneal

Table 1
Oncologic results for retroperitoneal lymphadenectomy

Authors,[Ref.] Year	No. of Patients	Age (y)	Upstaging to CS II	Relapse
Janetschek et al,[51] 1994	15	27 (16–43)	2/15	0
LeBlanc et al,[46] 2001	20	28 (19–41)	6/20	0
Steiner et al,[45] 2004	120	NR	24/120	0
Albqami & Janetschek,[56] 2005	103	29.9 (16–51)	26/103	0
Corvin et al,[57] 2005	18	35.5 (22–47)	7/18	0
Nielsen et al,[43] 2007	120	NR	45/120	2
Cresswell et al,[54] 2008	87	33.3 (17–69)	22/87	2
Castillo et al,[58] 2011	164	28 (24–33)	32/164	9
Basiri et al,[59] 2013	55	32.8 (19.41)	14/55	0

Abbreviations: CS, clinical stage; NR, not reported.
Data from Refs.[43,45,46,51,54,56–59]

Table 2
Oncologic results for postchemotherapy retroperitoneal lymphadenectomy

Authors,[Ref.] Year	No. of Patients	Age (y)	Histology	Relapse
Rassweiler et al,[44] 1996	8	NR	Necrosis 8/8	0
Bales et al,[60] 1997	1	42	NR	NR
Janetschek et al,[27] 1999	24	29.4 (15–48)	Necrosis 17/24 Teratoma 6/24 Active tumor 1/24	0
Palese et al[50] 2002	7	36.6 (35–55)	Necrosis 2/7 Teratoma 3/7 Active tumor 2/7	NR
Hara et al,[48] 2004	3	22 (20–27)	Necrosis 3/3	NR
Steiner et al,[45] 2004	68	NR	Necrosis 41/68 Teratoma 26/68 Active tumor 1/68	1
Tobias-Machado et al,[61] 2004	2	27 (NR)	NR	NR
Albqami & Janetschek,[56] 2005	59	29.2 (15–56)	Necrosis 36/59 Teratoma 21/59 Active tumor 2/59	1
Corvin et al,[57] 2005	7	30 (24–47)	Necrosis 3/7 Teratoma 3/7 Active tumor 1/7	0
Lima et al,[62] 2005	1	23	Active tumor 1/1	0
Castillo et al,[63] 2006	1	18	NR	NR
Maldonado-Valadez et al,[42] 2007	16	31.4 (20–49)	Necrosis 7/16 Teratoma 6/16 Active tumor 3/16	2
Permpongkosol et al,[53] 2007	16	34 (16–55)	Necrosis 6/16 Teratoma 5/16 Active tumor 5/16	0
Skolarus et al,[64] 2008	4	31 (NR)	Teratoma 3/4 Active tumor 1/4	0
Spermon & Witjes,[65] 2008	1	27	Active tumor 1/1	1
Tanaka et al,[49] 2008	5	NR	NR	2
Calestroupat et al,[41] 2009	26	31 (26–34)	Necrosis 14/26 Teratoma 9/26 Active tumor 3/26	0
Busch et al,[40] 2012	44	32.0 (26.5–37.5)	Necrosis 26/44 Teratoma 11/44 Active tumor 7/44	4
Arai et al,[37] 2012	20	27 (18–49)	Necrosis 16/20 Teratoma 2/29 Active tumor 2/20	0
Aufderklamm et al,[36] 2013	19	30.8 (NR)	Necrosis 8/19 Teratoma 8/19 Active tumor 3/19	5
Aufderklamm et al,[36] 2013 (bilateral)	20	31.5 (NR)	Necrosis 12/20 Teratoma 7/20 Active tumor 1/20	2
Basiri et al,[66] 2010	4	31.5 (28–35)	Teratoma 4/4	0
Kimura et al,[47] 2013	6	31 (19–48)	Necrosis 4/6 Teratoma 2/6	0
Steiner et al,[55] 2013	100	29.6 (11.4–52)	Necrosis 60/100 Teratoma 38/100 Active tumor 2/100	1

Abbreviation: NR, not reported.
Data from Refs.[27,36,37,40,42,44,45,47–50,53,55–57,60–66]

space is developed by blunt dissection and insufflation, or a distending balloon is used. However, a major concern is that in contrast to a transperitoneal approach, chylous ascites in extraperitoneal RLA will result in large lymphoceles.

Follow-up

There is no consensus on the exact protocol for follow-up. All follow-up recommendations suggest tumor markers and CT scans as the methods of choice.[4,15] The recurrence rate after RLA in CS I NSGCT patients is low. Therefore the EAU, in contrast to surveillance policy in CS I, recommend only 1 CT scan per year to avoid unnecessary radiation, increasing the risk of a radiation-induced second cancer.[4] Of course, CT could be replaced by MRI to reduce radiation depending on national and institutional facilities.

Certainly CSS in advanced GCT correlates with the extent of disease and the primary response to therapy. Also, the primary objective of follow-up is to detect relapse in these patients as soon as possible. Therefore, CT scans are recommended twice a year in the first 2 years. Tumor markers should be determined every 3 months.[4]

OUTCOMES
Complications

To summarize complications arising from minimally invasive RLA-CSI or PC-RLA is difficult because the first reported data were published 20 years ago, so complications are not classified according to the Clavien system in every publication. Certainly complication rates are decreasing with experience. Overall complication rates were described in early series in up to 46.7% of RLA-CS I and 57.1% of PC-RLA procedures.[50,51] These numbers are decreasing in later series, to 15.6% on average.[52]

In RLA CS I, vascular injury and hemorrhage were the most commonly reported complications. Clavien grade IV complications were described rarely. In PC-RLA, however, injury to the renal artery requiring vascular bypass or nephrectomy, duodenal perforation, intestinal segment resection because of intestinal lesion, and transection of the iliac artery have been described.[41,50,53] Conversion to open surgery should not been seen as a complication per se; furthermore, it could be due to wrong patient selection. The highest conversion rate was described by Rassweiler and colleagues[44] in 7 of 9 patients. In recent series only 1.1% for RLA and not a single conversion for PL-RLA were described.[54,55]

A frequent postoperative finding is chylous ascites. In most of these cases, conservative treatment with a low-fat or medium-chain triglyceride diet is effective.[27] As mentioned earlier, the transperitoneal approach should prevent lymphocele formation. However, 2 symptomatic lymphoceles requiring drainage after PC-RLA have been described.[45] By contrast, for the retroperitoneal approach lymphorrhea rates of 30%–40% have been reported.[37,47,48]

The sympathetic nerves are crucial for antegrade ejaculation. On full bilateral dissection, these nerves are destroyed. Therefore, nerve-sparing techniques are mandatory to preserve antegrade ejaculation.[39] Steiner and colleagues[35] have published data showing that nerve sparing is also feasible in laparoscopy. Using the modified template for unilateral RLA, nerve sparing is provided by the template as mentioned earlier (**Tables 1 and 2**).[39]

FUTURE CONSIDERATIONS ON ROBOTIC RETROPERITONEAL LYMPHADENECTOMY

Davol and colleagues,[67] the first investigators to describe a robot-assisted RLA in 2006, performed the surgery in an 18-year-old boy using a full bilateral template. The first series of 3 consecutive patients were published by Williams and colleagues,[68] who performed a modified template approach in NSGCT CS I patients. The initial series of PC-RLA done by robot-assisted laparoscopy was published by Cheney and colleagues,[69] in which bilateral RLA was done without repositioning in 18 patients (8 PC-RLA and 10 RLA). After a follow-up of 22 months, no retroperitoneal recurrences were found.

SUMMARY

RLA and PC-RLA by means of laparoscopy are challenging but feasible procedures. The published data indicate that oncologic results are comparable with those of the open approach. On the other hand, there is not a single prospective randomized trial comparing laparoscopy with open surgery. The highest level of evidence published to date is 3. In well-selected cases, unilateral template resection can be done in minimally invasive fashion to reduce morbidity, but with a risk of severe complications. Therefore, recommendation can only be given to tertiary centers with experience in laparoscopy and managing testicular cancer. No recommendation can be given for laparoscopic bilateral PC-RLA because of the lack of available data.

REFERENCES

1. Engholm G, Ferlay J, Christensen N, et al. Nord-can—a Nordic tool for cancer information, planning, quality control and research. Acta Oncol 2010;49(5): 725–36.
2. Motzer RJ, Agarwal N, Beard C, et al. NCCN clinical practice guidelines in oncology: testicular cancer. J Natl Compr Cancer Netw 2009;7(6):672–93.
3. Jemal A, Siegel R, Ward E, et al. Cancer statistics, 2009. CA Cancer J Clin 2009;59(4):225–49.
4. Albers P, Albrecht W, Algaba F, et al, European Association of Urology. EAU guidelines on testicular cancer: 2011 update. European Association of Urology. Actas Urol Esp 2012;36(3):127–45 [in Spanish].
5. Janetschek G, Reissigl A, Peschel R, et al. Diagnostic laparoscopic retroperitoneal lymph node dissection for non seminomatous testicular tumor. Ann Urol (Paris) 1995;29(2):81–90.
6. Yuvaraja TB. Current update of management of clinical stage I non seminomatous germ cell tumors of testis. Indian J Surg Oncol 2012;3(2):101–6.
7. Freedman LS, Parkinson MC, Jones WG, et al. Histopathology in the prediction of relapse of patients with stage I testicular teratoma treated by orchidectomy alone. Lancet 1987;2(8554):294–8.
8. Colls BM, Harvey VJ, Skelton L, et al. Late results of surveillance of clinical stage I nonseminoma germ cell testicular tumours: 17 years' experience in a national study in New Zealand. BJU Int 1999;83(1):76–82.
9. Read G, Stenning SP, Cullen MH, et al. Medical Research Council prospective study of surveillance for stage I testicular teratoma. Medical Research Council testicular tumors working party. J Clin Oncol 1992;10(11):1762–8.
10. Ondrus D, Matoska J, Belan V, et al. Prognostic factors in clinical stage I nonseminomatous germ cell testicular tumors: rationale for different risk-adapted treatment. Eur Urol 1998;33(6):562–6.
11. Maroto P, Garcia del Muro X, Aparicio J, et al. Multi-centre risk-adapted management for stage I non-seminomatous germ cell tumours. Ann Oncol 2005; 16(12):1915–20.
12. Krege S, Beyer J, Souchon R, et al. European consensus conference on diagnosis and treatment of germ cell cancer: a report of the second meeting of the European Germ Cell Cancer Consensus Group (EGCCCG): part I. Eur Urol 2008;53(3): 478–96.
13. Krege S, Beyer J, Souchon R, et al. European consensus conference on diagnosis and treatment of germ cell cancer: a report of the second meeting of the European Germ Cell Cancer Consensus Group (EGCCCG): part II. Eur Urol 2008;53(3): 497–513.
14. Heidenreich A, Albers P, Hartmann M, et al, German Testicular Cancer Study Group. Complications of primary nerve sparing retroperitoneal lymph node dissection for clinical stage I nonseminomatous germ cell tumors of the testis: Experience of the German Testicular Cancer Study Group. J Urol 2003;169(5):1710–4.
15. Oldenburg J, Fossa SD, Nuver J, et al. Testicular seminoma and non-seminoma: ESMO clinical practice guidelines for diagnosis, treatment and follow-up. Ann Oncol 2013;24(Suppl 6):vi125–32.
16. Winter C, Pfister D, Busch J, et al. Residual tumor size and IGCCCG risk classification predict additional vascular procedures in patients with germ cell tumors and residual tumor resection: a multicenter analysis of the German Testicular Cancer Study Group. Eur Urol 2012;61(2):403–9.
17. Heidenreich A, Thuer D, Polyakov S. Postchemotherapy retroperitoneal lymph node dissection in advanced germ cell tumours of the testis. Eur Urol 2008;53(2):260–72.
18. Oldenburg J, Alfsen GC, Lien HH, et al. Postchemotherapy retroperitoneal surgery remains necessary in patients with nonseminomatous testicular cancer and minimal residual tumor masses. J Clin Oncol 2003;21(17):3310–7.
19. Puc HS, Heelan R, Mazumdar M, et al. Management of residual mass in advanced seminoma: results and recommendations from the Memorial Sloan-Kettering Cancer Center. J Clin Oncol 1996;14(2):454–60.
20. Ravi R, Ong J, Oliver RT, et al. The management of residual masses after chemotherapy in metastatic seminoma. BJU Int 1999;83(6):649–53.
21. De Santis M, Becherer A, Bokemeyer C, et al. 2-[18]Fluoro-deoxy-d-glucose positron emission tomography is a reliable predictor for viable tumor in postchemotherapy seminoma: an update of the prospective multicentric SEMPET trial. J Clin Oncol 2004;22(6):1034–9.
22. Bachner M, Loriot Y, Gross-Goupil M, et al. 2-(1)(8) Fluoro-deoxy-d-glucose positron emission tomography (FDG-PET) for postchemotherapy seminoma residual lesions: a retrospective validation of the SEMPET trial. Ann Oncol 2012;23(1):59–64.
23. Daneshmand S, Albers P, Fossa SD, et al. Contemporary management of postchemotherapy testis cancer. Eur Urol 2012;62(5):867–76.
24. Albers P, Weissbach L, Krege S, et al, German Testicular Cancer Study Group. Prediction of necrosis after chemotherapy of advanced germ cell tumors: results of a prospective multicenter trial of the German Testicular Cancer Study Group. J Urol 2004;171(5):1835–8.
25. Albers P, Melchior D, Muller SC. Surgery in metastatic testicular cancer. Eur Urol 2003;44(2):233–44.
26. Tarin T, Carver B, Sheinfeld J. The role of lymphadenectomy for testicular cancer: indications, controversies, and complications. Urol Clin North Am 2011;38(4):439–49, vi.

27. Janetschek G, Hobisch A, Hittmair A, et al. Laparoscopic retroperitoneal lymphadenectomy after chemotherapy for stage IIb nonseminomatous testicular carcinoma. J Urol 1999;161(2):477–81.

28. Toner GC, Panicek DM, Heelan RT, et al. Adjunctive surgery after chemotherapy for nonseminomatous germ cell tumors: recommendations for patient selection. J Clin Oncol 1990;8(10):1683–94.

29. Heidenreich A, Pfister D, Witthuhn R, et al. Postchemotherapy retroperitoneal lymph node dissection in advanced testicular cancer: radical or modified template resection. Eur Urol 2009;55(1):217–24.

30. Ehrlich Y, Brames MJ, Beck SD, et al. Long-term follow-up of cisplatin combination chemotherapy in patients with disseminated nonseminomatous germ cell tumors: is a postchemotherapy retroperitoneal lymph node dissection needed after complete remission? J Clin Oncol 2010;28(4):531–6.

31. Wood DP Jr, Herr HW, Heller G, et al. Distribution of retroperitoneal metastases after chemotherapy in patients with nonseminomatous germ cell tumors. J Urol 1992;148(6):1812–5 [discussion: 1815–16].

32. Weissbach L, Boedefeld EA. Localization of solitary and multiple metastases in stage II nonseminomatous testis tumor as basis for a modified staging lymph node dissection in stage I. J Urol 1987; 138(1):77–82.

33. Holtl L, Peschel R, Knapp R, et al. Primary lymphatic metastatic spread in testicular cancer occurs ventral to the lumbar vessels. Urology 2002;59(1):114–8.

34. Vallier C, Savoie PH, Delpero JR, et al. External validation of the Heidenreich criteria for patient selection for unilateral or bilateral retroperitoneal lymph node dissection for post-chemotherapy residual masses of testicular cancer. World J Urol 2014; 32(6):1573–8.

35. Steiner H, Zangerl F, Stohr B, et al. Results of bilateral nerve sparing laparoscopic retroperitoneal lymph node dissection for testicular cancer. J Urol 2008;180(4):1348–52 [discussion: 1352–3].

36. Aufderklamm S, Todenhofer T, Hennenlotter J, et al. Bilateral laparoscopic postchemotherapy retroperitoneal lymph-node dissection in nonseminomatous germ cell tumors—a comparison to template dissection. J Endourol 2013;27(7):856–61.

37. Arai Y, Kaiho Y, Yamada S, et al. Extraperitoneal laparoscopic retroperitoneal lymph node dissection after chemotherapy for nonseminomatous testicular germ-cell tumor: surgical and oncological outcomes. Int Urol Nephrol 2012;44(5):1389–95.

38. Donohue JP, Foster RS, Rowland RG, et al. Nerve-sparing retroperitoneal lymphadenectomy with preservation of ejaculation. J Urol 1990;144(2 Pt 1):287–91 [discussion 291–80].

39. Donohue JP, Thornhill JA, Foster RS, et al. Retroperitoneal lymphadenectomy for clinical stage a testis cancer (1965 to 1989): modifications of technique and impact on ejaculation. J Urol 1993;149(2): 237–43.

40. Busch J, Magheli A, Erber B, et al. Laparoscopic and open postchemotherapy retroperitoneal lymph node dissection in patients with advanced testicular cancer—a single center analysis. BMC Urol 2012; 12:15.

41. Calestroupat JP, Sanchez-Salas R, Cathelineau X, et al. Postchemotherapy laparoscopic retroperitoneal lymph node dissection in nonseminomatous germ-cell tumor. J Endourol 2009;23(4):645–50.

42. Maldonado-Valadez R, Schilling D, Anastasiadis AG, et al. Post-chemotherapy laparoscopic retroperitoneal lymph-node dissection in testis cancer patients. J Endourol 2007;21(12): 1501–4.

43. Nielsen ME, Lima G, Schaeffer EM, et al. Oncologic efficacy of laparoscopic RPLND in treatment of clinical stage I nonseminomatous germ cell testicular cancer. Urology 2007;70(6):1168–72.

44. Rassweiler JJ, Henkel TO, Stock C, et al. Retroperitoneal laparoscopic lymph node dissection for staging non-seminomatous germ cell tumors before and after chemotherapy. Lymphology 1996;29(1):36–44.

45. Steiner H, Peschel R, Janetschek G, et al. Long-term results of laparoscopic retroperitoneal lymph node dissection: a single-center 10-year experience. Urology 2004;63(3):550–5.

46. LeBlanc E, Caty A, Dargent D, et al. Extraperitoneal laparoscopic para-aortic lymph node dissection for early stage nonseminomatous germ cell tumors of the testis with introduction of a nerve sparing technique: description and results. J Urol 2001;165(1): 89–92.

47. Kimura Y, Nakamura T, Kawauchi A, et al. Postchemotherapy nerve-sparing laparoscopic retroperitoneal lymph node dissection in stage IIb testicular cancer. Int J Urol 2013;20(8):837–41.

48. Hara I, Kawabata G, Yamada Y, et al. Extraperitoneal laparoscopic retroperitoneal lymph node dissection in supine position after chemotherapy for advanced testicular carcinoma. Int J Urol 2004;11(10):934–9.

49. Tanaka K, Hara I, Takenaka A, et al. Incidence of local and port site recurrence of urologic cancer after laparoscopic surgery. Urology 2008;71(4): 728–34.

50. Palese MA, Su LM, Kavoussi LR. Laparoscopic retroperitoneal lymph node dissection after chemotherapy. Urology 2002;60(1):130–4.

51. Janetschek G, Reissigl A, Peschel R, et al. Laparoscopic retroperitoneal lymph node dissection for clinical stage I nonseminomatous testicular tumor. Urology 1994;44(3):382–91.

52. Rassweiler JJ, Scheitlin W, Heidenreich A, et al. Laparoscopic retroperitoneal lymph node dissection: does it still have a role in the management of clinical stage I nonseminomatous testis cancer?

A European perspective. Eur Urol 2008;54(5): 1004–15.

53. Permpongkosol S, Lima GC, Warlick CA, et al. Post-chemotherapy laparoscopic retroperitoneal lymph node dissection: evaluation of complications. Urology 2007;69(2):361–5.

54. Cresswell J, Scheitlin W, Gozen A, et al. Laparoscopic retroperitoneal lymph node dissection combined with adjuvant chemotherapy for pathological stage II disease in nonseminomatous germ cell tumours: a 15-year experience. BJU Int 2008; 102(7):844–8.

55. Steiner H, Leonhartsberger N, Stoehr B, et al. Post-chemotherapy laparoscopic retroperitoneal lymph node dissection for low-volume, stage II, nonseminomatous germ cell tumor: first 100 patients. Eur Urol 2013;63(6):1013–7.

56. Albqami N, Janetschek G. Laparoscopic retroperitoneal lymph-node dissection in the management of clinical stage I and II testicular cancer. J Endourol 2005;19(6):683–92 [discussion: 692].

57. Corvin S, Sturm W, Schlatter E, et al. Laparoscopic retroperitoneal lymph-node dissection with the waterjet is technically feasible and safe in testis-cancer patient. J Endourol 2005;19(7):823–6.

58. Castillo OA, Sanchez-Salas R, Secin FP, et al. Primary laparoscopic retroperitoneal lymph node dissection for clinical stage I nonseminomatous germ-cell testis tumor. Actas Urol Esp 2011;35(1): 22–8 [in Spanish].

59. Basiri A, Ghaed MA, Simforoosh N, et al. Is modified retroperitoneal lymph node dissection alive for clinical stage I non-seminomatous germ cell testicular tumor? Urol J 2013;10(2):873–7.

60. Bales GT, Gerber GS, Rukstalis DB. Laparoscopic post-chemotherapy retroperitoneal dissection of residual mass. Br J Urol 1997;80(2):349–50.

61. Tobias-Machado M, Zambon JP, Ferreira AD, et al. Retroperitoneal lymphadenectomy by videolaparoscopic transperitoneal approach in patients with non-seminomatous testicular tumor. Int Braz J Urol 2004;30(5):389–96 [discussion: 396–7].

62. Lima GC, Kohanim S, Rais-Bahrami S, et al. Laparoscopic retroperitoneal lymph node dissection after prior open retroperitoneal lymphadenectomy and chemotherapy. Urology 2005;66(6):1319.

63. Castillo OA, Litvak JP, Kerkebe M, et al. Case report: laparoscopic management of massive chylous ascites after salvage laparoscopic retroperitoneal lymph-node dissection. J Endourol 2006; 20(6):394–6.

64. Skolarus TA, Bhayani SB, Chiang HC, et al. Laparoscopic retroperitoneal lymph node dissection for low-stage testicular cancer. J Endourol 2008;22(7): 1485–9.

65. Spermon JR, Witjes JA. Case report: the danger of postchemotherapy laparoscopic retroperitoneal lymph node dissection for nonseminomatous testicular carcinoma. J Endourol 2008;22(5):1013–6.

66. Basiri A, Asl-Zare M, Sichani MM, et al. Laparoscopic bilateral retroperitoneal lymph node dissection in stage II testis cancer. Urol J 2010;7(3): 157–60.

67. Davol P, Sumfest J, Rukstalis D. Robotic-assisted laparoscopic retroperitoneal lymph node dissection. Urology 2006;67(1):199.

68. Williams SB, Lau CS, Josephson DY. Initial series of robot-assisted laparoscopic retroperitoneal lymph node dissection for clinical stage I nonseminomatous germ cell testicular cancer. Eur Urol 2011; 60(6):1299–302.

69. Cheney SM, Andrews PE, Leibovich BC, et al. Robot-assisted retroperitoneal lymph node dissection: technique and initial case series of 18 patients. BJU Int 2015;115(1):114–20.

The Role of Postchemotherapy Surgery in Germ Cell Tumors

Lisly Chéry, MD*, Atreya Dash, MD

KEYWORDS

- Germ cell tumors • Chemotherapy • Lymph node dissection • Testicular cancer

KEY POINTS

- Retroperitoneal lymph node dissection (RPLND) after chemotherapy has a proved role in the staging and treatment of metastatic testicular cancer.
- Complete removal of all postchemotherapy residual masses in nonseminomatous germ cell tumor (NSGCT) should be performed.
- Complete removal of positron emission tomography (PET)-avid masses greater than 3 cm in pure seminoma should be performed.
- Outcomes depend on patient selection and extent of surgery.

The first retroperitoneal lymph node dissection (RPLND) was performed in Paris in 1905.[1] Its use did not become popularized until the 1940s, when the results of young men treated at Walter Reed Army Medical Center were published. Since then, the use of RPLND in the treatment of testis cancer has evolved. RPLND was once associated with substantial complications, but the technique has since been refined, with improvement in patient outcomes. Additionally, older chemotherapy treatments for metastatic testicular cancer had significant toxicity. The introduction of cisplatin-based chemotherapy in the treatment of metastatic testicular cancer resulted in improved patient survival. Recent data have demonstrated that a stage migration has occurred, with more patients presenting with clinical stage I disease.[2,3] Additionally, active surveillance has become the standard treatment of clinical stage I disease, resulting in fewer therapies aimed at regional treatment, such as primary RPLND, performed for NSGCT or adjuvant radiotherapy for seminoma.[4]

A substantial number of men with metastatic testicular cancer, however, have residual disease after the administration of chemotherapy. The majority of this residual disease is located in the retroperitoneum. Another subset of men are those with clinical stage I disease on surveillance who relapse and are treated with induction chemotherapy and possibly require subsequent resection. As such, a majority of RPLNDs performed today are in the postchemotherapy setting. This article focuses on the rationale, approach, outcome, morbidity, and follow-up of postchemotherapy RPLND (PC-RPLND).

CLASSIFYING POSTCHEMOTHERAPY RETROPERITONEAL LYMPH NODE DISSECTION

The Indiana University provided definitions of categories of PC-RPLND that are clinically useful and allow meaningful comparisons of outcome.[5] Standard RPLND is performed in patients presenting

Department of Urology, University of Washington School of Medicine, 1959 Northeast Pacific, Box 356510, Seattle, WA 98195, USA
* Corresponding author.
E-mail address: lislyj@uw.edu

Urol Clin N Am 42 (2015) 331–342
http://dx.doi.org/10.1016/j.ucl.2015.04.007

urologic.theclinics.com

with disseminated disease that after chemotherapy have normal serum tumor markers (STMs) and only retroperitoneal residual disease on imaging. Other situations are more complex. Salvage RPLND refers to cases of patients having received second-line chemotherapy, either with other cisplatin-based chemotherapy regimen or high-dose chemotherapy with bone marrow support, and having normal STMs. Desperation RPLND refers to cases of, despite second-line chemotherapy, RPLND performed in a setting of persistently elevated STMs. Redo RPLND is resection performed after previous surgery for an in-field recurrence. Lastly, unresectable RPLND is the setting where disease found at time of surgery itself is determined as unresectable.

RATIONALE FOR SURGERY AFTER CHEMOTHERAPY

The rationale for PC-RPLND is based on 4 principles. PC-RPLND (1) is diagnostic of the histology of the residual mass, (2) has therapeutic benefit, (3) is the preferred management of teratoma, and (4) has decreasing morbidity.

PC-RPLND establishes if the residual mass contains (1) necrosis/fibrosis, (2) teratoma, (3) viable germ cell carcinoma, or (4) non–germ cell carcinoma. The frequency of the histology varies, as depicted in **Table 1**, but in general necrosis/fibrosis is found in 40% to 50%, teratoma in 35% to 40%, viable germ cell carcinoma in 10% to 15% and non–germ cell carcinoma in less than 1%. Currently, there are no clinical tools that can reliably predict the histology of a postchemotherapy mass in the preoperative setting. Because further treatment and follow-up regimens depend on the histology of residual masses, PC-RPLND is necessary.

Recent studies have examined if the choice of induction chemotherapy has an effect on residual tumor at time of PC-RPLND. Cary and colleagues[6] from Indiana examined the difference in final pathology for patients receiving 4 cycles of etoposide and cisplatin (EP) (47 patients) versus 3 cycles of bleomycin, etoposide, and cisplatin (BEP) (179 patients). They found a higher rate of active tumor in the EP group (22.9%) than in the BEP group (7.8%). Kundu and colleagues[7] from Memorial Sloan Kettering (MSK) reported on 505 patients who received EP × 4 and compared them with 74 patients who received BEP × 3. The BEP group was found to have teratoma more often (53% vs 32%) than the EP group. There was no difference in the frequency of active tumor between the groups (BEP 5%, EP 6%).

The results of these 2 retrospective analyses may be attributable to differences other than the choice of chemotherapy regimen.[8] In the study by Cary and colleagues, the majority of patients who received chemotherapy at Indiana University received 3 cycles of BEP (48 patients) rather than 4 cycles of EP (1 patient). The differences in active tumor at PC-RPLND may be a reflection of a higher dose intensity of chemotherapy given at Indiana University than at community chemotherapy centers who then referred patients to Indiana for surgery. In the study by Kundu and colleagues, the differences in teratoma at PC-RPLND may be due to differences in the size of residual masses in the 2 groups. The majority of the EP group received chemotherapy at MSK and had smaller residual masses at time of surgery. The majority of the BEP group received chemotherapy outside of MSK and had larger residual masses at time of surgery. Therefore, factors, such as possible differences in chemotherapy intensity at community versus tertiary centers and referral patterns to tertiary centers for surgery may at least partially explain these apparently conflicting results.

A complete resection of all residual masses during PC-RPLND can be therapeutic. Patients in the International Germ Cell Consensus Classification Group (IGCCCG) good prognosis group with complete resection of residual masses and less than 10% viable tumor cells in the resected specimen can be observed without further chemotherapy, but postoperative chemotherapy should be directed to those with less favorable characteristics.[9] Fox and colleagues[10] from Indiana University reported on 580 men who underwent PC-RPLND; 417 (72%) were after primary chemotherapy and 163 (28%) were after salvage chemotherapy; 43 (10%) of the primary chemotherapy patients and 90 (55%) of the salvage chemotherapy patients had viable germ cell carcinoma. This study demonstrated a survival advantage for those patients with viable germ cell tumor who had a complete resection, even if they did not receive further chemotherapy.

The role of RPLND in the management of teratoma is well established. Teratoma, by definition, is resistant to chemotherapy and radiotherapy. First described by Logothetis and colleagues,[11] growing teratoma syndrome can result in local morbidity and may compromise adjacent structures. Although teratoma itself is benign, a somatic teratoma component of a germ cell tumor may undergo malignant transformation, referred to as teratoma with malignant transformation. This transformation, usually to sarcoma or adenocarcinoma, like teratoma is resistant to chemotherapy.[12–14]

RPLND has developed from a procedure with limited long-term survival in the early 1900s[1] to the current state of limited mortality.[15] This

Table 1
Histologic findings for standard post-chemotherapy retroperitoneal lymph node dissection studies

Study, Year	N	Clinical Stage	Chemotherapy	Tumor Markers	Residual Mass(es) (cm)	Necrosis, N (%)	Teratoma, N (%)	Carcinoma, N (%)	Median Follow-Up, months	Survival (%)
Donohue et al,[63] 1982	51	II–IV	Induction	Normal	NS	16 (31)	16 (31)	19 (37)	NS	Fibrosis—15/16 NED Teratoma—15/16 NED Tumor—10/19 NED
Bracken et al,[64] 1983	45	III	Induction	Normal	22 Not palpable 23 Palpable	14 (64) 8 (35)	3 (14) 7 (30)	5 (23) 7 (30)	60 33	13/22 (59) NED 18/23 (78) NED
Freiha et al,[65] 1984	40	IIc—10 III—30	Induction	Normal	NS	21 (52)	18 (45)	1 (3)	36	37 NED 3 Relapse
Pizzocaro et al,[66] 1985	36	II–III	Induction	Normal	NS	16 (44)	10 (28)	10 (28)	36	11/18 (61) NED
Fossa et al,[67] 1989	101	II–IV	Induction	Normal	NS	52 (51)	37 (37)	12 (12)	55	Fibrosis/teratoma—83/89 (93) NED Tumor—7/12 (58) NED
Gelderman et al,[68] 1988	35	III–IV	Induction	Normal	NS	17 (49)	14 (40)	4 (11)	65	25/35 (66) NED
Williams et al,[69] 1989	29	II	Induction • 4 Second line • 3 Radiotherapy	6 Elevated 23 Normal	NS	13 (52)	9 (36)	3 (12)	33	29/29 NED
Harding et al,[70] 1989	42	IIb–IV	Induction	Normal	>1.5	19 (45)	14 (33)	9 (21)	36	36/42 (86) NED
Mulders,[71] 1990	55	IIc–IV	Induction	Normal	>1	31 (56)	12 (22)	12 (22)	36	Fibrosis (93) Teratoma (92) Tumor (27)
Aass et al,[72] 1991	173	II–IV	Induction	Normal	None – 30 <2 – 6 2-5 – 107 >5 – 57	85 (49)	50 (25)	38 (29)	75	160/173 (92) NED (82) CSS
Kulkarni et al,[73] 1991	67	IIb–IV	Induction	Elevated: 37% NS Normal: 63%	NS	18 (27)	29 (43)	20 (30)	50	55/67 (82) NED
Aprikian et al,[74] 1994	40	IIb–III	Induction • 5 Second line	Normal	Stage II <5-2 (5%) >5-17 (42%) Stage III—NS	18 (45)	17 (43)	5 (13)	36	32/40 (80) NED 8/40 (20) Relapse

(continued on next page)

Table 1
(continued)

Study, Year	N	Clinical Stage	Chemotherapy	Tumor Markers	Residual Mass(es) (cm)	Necrosis, N (%)	Teratoma, N (%)	Carcinoma, N (%)	Median Follow-Up, months	Survival (%)
Steyerberg et al,[75] 1995	556	II–IV	Induction	Normal	NS	250 (45)	236 (42)	70 (13)	NS	NS
Brenner et al,[76] 1996	24	II–IV	Induction • 21 Salvage • 5 BM Transplant	2 Elevated 22 Normal	2–20	13 (54)	8 (33)	3 (13)	NS	(79) 5-Y overall survival
Stenning et al,[77] 1998	153	II–III	Induction	Normal	≥2	45 (29)	85 (56)	23 (15)	84	Fibrosis (90) 2-y NED Teratoma (88) 2-y NED Tumor (43) 2-y NED
Donohue et al,[78] 1998	414	II–IV	Induction	Normal	NS	25	52	23	108	(11.8) Relapse (95) CSS
Napier et al,[79] 2000	48	II–IV	Induction	Normal	NS	15 (31)	24 (50)	9 (19)	66	37/48 (77) NED
Hendry et al,[38] 2002	330	II–IV	Induction	46% Normal 54% Elevated	≥1	84 (25)	218 (66)	28 (8)	77	(83) 5-y NED (89) 5-y overall survival
Oldenburg et al,[30] 2003	87	II	Induction	19 Elevated 68 Normal	≤2	58 (67)	23 (26)	6 (7)	80	(94) 5-y NED (96) 5-y overall survival
Albers et al,[80] 2004	193	II–III	Induction	Normal	NS	35	34	31	NS	NS
Muramaki et al,[81] 2004	24	II–III	Induction • 12 Second line	Normal	<3-62.5% >3-37.5%	15 (63)	6 (25)	3 (12)	NS	Complete resection (100) 3-y CSS Incomplete resection (50) 3-y CSS
Carver et al,[31] 2006	532	II–III	Induction 85% Salvage 15%	89% Normal 11% Elevated	≤1–30% 1–5–50% >5–20%	263 (49)	210 (40)	59 (11)	NS	NS
Spiess et al,[82] 2007	198	II–III	Induction	Normal	3.5	86 (43%)	79 (40)	33 (17)	53	(87) 5-y CSS
Heidenreich et al,[50] 2009	152	II–III	Induction	80% Normal 20% Elevated	6	84 (55)	45 (30)	23 (15)	39	144/152 (95) NED
Luz et al,[83] 2010	73	II–III	Induction	Normal	4	27 (37)	30 (41)	16 (22)	47	66/73 (90) NED
Busch et al,[84] 2012	67	II–III	Induction	10 Elevated 57 Normal	2.2 Lap 6.7 Open	38 (57)	17 (25)	15 (22)	30 Lap 54 Open	57/67 (85) NED
Steiner et al,[55] 2013	100	II	Induction	Normal	1.4	60 (60)	38 (38)	2 (2)	74	99/100 (99) NED

Abbreviations: BM, bone marrow; NED, no evidence of disease; NS, not specified.
Data from Refs.[30,31,38,50,55,63–84]

advancement is due to improvement in operative techniques, such as limitation of suprahilar dissection, use of modified templates, and identification of hypogastric nerves. Optimization of perioperative care has also resulted in decreased morbidity.[16,17]

INDICATIONS FOR POSTCHEMOTHERAPY RETROPERITONEAL LYMPH NODE DISSECTION

The indication for PC-RPLND depends primarily on the primary tumor histology, and the presence and size of residual masses. These characteristics guide clinicians and patients in decision making.

The major branch point in determining the need for a PC-RPLND is the histology of the primary tumor. Pure seminoma is treated differently from NSGCT. Seminoma is rarely associated with teratoma; therefore, the risk of growing teratoma syndrome or teratoma with malignant transformation is low. Additionally, PC-RPLND is more technically challenging for pure seminoma due to the adherence to the great vessels of postchemotherapy residual seminoma masses.[18] This increases the morbidity of the procedure. There is evidence that not all postchemotherapy residual seminoma masses harbor viable germ cell carcinoma. Herr and colleagues[19] initially published that 30% of residual masses greater than 3 cm in the retroperitoneum harbored viable tumor, whereas no masses smaller than 3 cm had viable tumor. Ravi and colleagues[20] had similar findings, with 28% of residual masses greater than 3 cm in the retroperitoneum having viable tumor and no viable tumor found in masses less than 3 cm. Flechon and colleagues[21] found viable tumor in 13% of residual masses greater than 3 cm in the retroperitoneum, with no viable tumor in masses less than 3 cm.

Recently, the use of 2-[18]fluoro-deoxy-D-glucose PET (FDG PET) was shown to discriminate whether a residual mass after chemotherapy for pure seminoma harbors viable tumor. FDG is a glucose analog, and thus tumor cells, which have high glucose metabolism, absorb FDG at a higher rate than normal tissue. FDG PET can be combined with conventional CT to provide both functional and spatial information.

In the largest prospective trial to date, De Santis and colleagues[22] examined 51 patients with pure seminoma and residual masses in the retroperitoneum after chemotherapy. They reported that FDG PET has a sensitivity of 80% and specificity of 100%, with a positive predictive value of 100% and a negative predictive value of 96%. This was compared with conventional CT size criteria, with a sensitivity of 70%, specificity of 74%, positive

predictive value of 37%, and negative predictive value of 97%. These findings were supported by Johns Putra and colleagues[23] as well as a recent meta-analysis.[24] As such, the use of FDG PET or PET/CT is indicated in patients with pure seminoma with negative STMs and retroperitoneal residual masses greater than 3 cm after chemotherapy and has been incorporated into National Comprehensive Cancer Network guidelines.[25] FDG PET should be performed at least 6 weeks after completion of chemotherapy to allow for resolution of inflammation, which can cause a false-positive result.

In contrast to pure seminoma, FDG PET imaging is not useful for NSGCT. This is due to the presence of teratoma. Teratoma can be FDG PET avid, giving the same appearance as viable tumor.[26] The vast majority of teratoma is not FDG PET avid, however, and thus a negative FDG PET does not exclude the presence of teratoma in postchemotherapy NSGCT masses.[27] The largest study to date examining FDG PET in NSGCT comes from the German Multicenter PET Study Group.[28] This study examined 121 patients with stage IIC or III NSGCT after chemotherapy and prior to RPLND. Regarding tumor viability, the study revealed a sensitivity of 70%, specificity of 48%, positive predictive value of 59%, and negative predictive value of 83%. FDG PET was able to predict tumor viability in 56% of patients, but this was no better than standard CT (55%) or STMs (56%).

PATIENT SELECTION

Approximately 70% of patients who present with NSGCT with metastatic spread to the retroperitoneum have a complete response to chemotherapy. For the remaining 30% with persistent radiographic masses and negative STMs, there is agreement that surgical resection is the treatment of choice, because these masses can harbor viable germ cell tumor or teratoma. The definition of a persistent radiographic mass, however, is not standard. Additionally, there is debate as to the management of patients who exhibit a complete response to chemotherapy.

Mass Less Than 1 cm

There is no uniform standard size criteria for normal retroperitoneal lymph nodes. As CT imaging techniques have improved, the ability to detect lymph nodes smaller than 1 cm in maximal diameter has increased. Fossa and colleagues[29] examined 37 patients who had NSGCT with a complete response to chemotherapy (lymph nodes <10 mm); 11 patients (30%) had teratoma and 1 patient (3%) had viable tumor. Oldenburg and colleagues[30] examined 54 patients with lymph nodes less than 10 mm after chemotherapy; 5 (9%) had viable tumor and 11 (20%) had teratoma. A study by Carver and colleagues[31] included 154 patients with lymph nodes less than 10 mm after chemotherapy for NSGCT; 35 patients (22%) had teratoma and 1 patient had viable tumor. The exact behavior of viable tumor or teratoma less than 1 cm is unknown; however, the potential for unpredictable or aggressive behavior has convinced several centers to recommend PC-RPLND even for those patients with a complete response to chemotherapy.[32]

There are data to support the observation of postchemotherapy residual masses less than 1 cm in size. Ehrlich and colleagues[33] published a report on 141 patients who underwent surveillance after a complete radiographic and tumor marker response to chemotherapy for NSGCT. During a median follow-up of 15.5 years, 12 patients (9%) recurred, with a median time to recurrence of 11 months; 6 of the 12 had recurrence in the retroperitoneum. Of those 12 recurrences, 8 had a durable response to subsequent treatment with chemotherapy and PC-RPLND after a median of 11 years of follow-up. The remaining 4 patients died within 12 months of chemotherapy; 2 of these patients had recurrence in the retroperitoneum. This study found the only predictor of cancer-specific survival (CSS) or relapse was initial IGCCCG risk classification. Kollmannsberger and colleagues[34] reported on 161 patients who underwent surveillance after a complete radiographic and tumor marker response to chemotherapy for NSGCT; 10 patients (6%) relapsed, with 9 of these relapses in the retroperitoneum. All retroperitoneal relapses were treated with PC-RPLND, with 100% CSS at 52 months of follow-up.

There is universal acceptance that NSGCT post-chemotherapy residual masses greater than 1 cm should be resected due to the potential for viable tumor or teratoma. There is debate about the extent of dissection that is necessary and the surgical approach to PC-RPLND. The standard technique for a full bilateral template is well established and described.[35]

Refractory Germ Cell Tumor

Of the 30% of patients with a persistent mass after first-line chemotherapy, approximately 10% to 15% have persistently elevated STMs.[36] Patients with elevated but stable or declining STMs should undergo PC-RPLND.[37] Unfortunately, if STMs are clearly rising, the options are for salvage chemotherapy versus complete surgical resection. After salvage chemotherapy, however, resection of residual disease is indicated. Compared with standard PC-RPLND, the surgical procedure may require more extensive and surgery with adjunctive procedures. The histology in resected masses after salvage chemotherapy is more likely to harbor viable GCT,[10,38,39] and these patients are more likely to suffer worse outcomes.[40] Additional salvage chemotherapy does not offer greater benefit after complete resection in this setting.[41] Receipt of taxane-based chemotherapy regimens compared with other regimens was associated with a similar rate of teratoma in the resected residual mass but with a lower rate of viable GCT.[40] Another circumstance requiring complex PC-RPLND is the growing teratoma syndrome with continued growth often of a residual retroperitoneal mass despite normal STMs. Although unusual, resection is imperative due to its insensitivity to chemotherapy and radiation. The growth of the mass to a large size may involve adjacent structures and make resection a demanding procedure possibly requiring adjunctive procedures.[42] Late relapse is a recurrence of tumor 2 years after curative treatment, and some investigators advocate this definition to be further distinguished by chemotherapy treatment.[43] Histology of late relapse may be of viable GCT, teratoma, or teratoma with malignant transformation.[43,44] Late relapse is infrequent and ranges from 1.4% to 3%.[45,46] The treatment and management of late relapse are addressed in an article elsewhere in this issue, but those patients with elevated markers should undergo additional chemotherapy before resection, whereas those with teratoma or teratoma with malignant transformation should undergo complete resection.[42,43]

EXTENT OF DISSECTION

The consideration of the extent of operation in PC-RPLND remains controversial; however, in the contemporary era, there is uniform agreement to limiting operations to an infrahilar dissection in the absence of known suprahilar disease. The debate centers on whether a more extended dissection, such as a full bilateral template, has improved oncologic efficacy at the expense of potential loss of antegrade ejaculation. Conversely, does limiting the extent of dissection with a modified template to better preserve ejaculation compromise oncologic outcome? In the setting of stage I disease, a modified template applied to primary RPLND has some supporting rationale. There is known risk, however, of disease outside a modified template, and with some broadening of the modified template, the recurrence risk may be reduced to 3%.[47] With the diminished disease burden at presentation and with a wider use of induction chemotherapy, some investigators have considered limiting the extent of dissection in the postchemotherapy setting as a way of preserving sympathetic nerve tissue. The modified template may have some surgical benefits over a nerve-sparing approach by avoiding some nerve rich areas altogether, and the operation may be shorter and technically less demanding. In the setting of lower-volume disease, however, it is also more feasible to perform PC-RPLND after a bilateral template using a nerve-sparing technique. Currently there are few studies to address these issues. The published literature is mainly of single-institution case series with varying inclusion criteria and methods that preclude direct comparisons, but important points are gleaned from these studies.

The MSK group evaluated a cohort of 269 patients with known viable germ cell tumor or teratoma after chemotherapy.[32] This study compared 5 different surgical templates for incidence of extratemplate disease. Depending on the modified template, between 7% and 32% of patients would have viable GCT or teratoma beyond the boundaries of the template. Patients who presented with clinical stage III disease had a greater incidence of extratemplate disease in the retroperitoneum. And in patients where there was no radiographic disease outside the template, the incidence of disease outside the template increased with increasing size of mass resected within the template up to 29% for residual masses 2 to 5 cm in size. In a separate study from the same institution of 341 PC-RPLND patients who underwent dissection according to the full MSK template, 40% underwent a dissection with nerve sparing.[48] The patients who underwent nerve sparing had fewer right-sided primary tumors, smaller masses, and better IGCCGC risk disease. Of the 141 men who underwent nerve sparing, 79% had preservation of ejaculation, including 4/9 (44%) with masses greater than 5 cm. In a multivariable analysis, right-sided primary and mass size 5 cm were negatively associated with recovery of ejaculation.

Indiana University reported the outcomes from 100 patients who underwent PC-RPLND after a modified template dissection.[49] Inclusion criteria were patients who had retroperitoneal masses within the primary landing zone of the affected testis before and after chemotherapy. The pathology of the resected masses was 2% viable germ cell tumor but a high rate of teratoma of 62%, and 94% of patients had prechemotherapy and postchemotherapy masses less than 5 cm. The

median follow-up for the 100 patients was 31.9 months and for those 62 patients with teratoma it was 25.5 months. There were 4 recurrences, all with teratoma, within 12 months, and outside the boundaries of a full bilateral template. The findings of disease outside the modified template in the study from MSK may have reflected a cohort with worse disease than those included in the study from Indiana University; therefore, the favorable results from Indiana were consistent with their study population. Antegrade ejaculation rates were not discussed.

Heidenreich and colleagues[50] analyzed 152 patients who underwent modified versus full template PC-RPLND. The choice of dissection was based on mass location in the landing zone and size less than 5 cm. Patients who underwent full dissection had worse disease by IGCCCG classification (29.6% poor risk) than patients who underwent modified dissection (15.3% poor risk). Average follow-up was 39 months, and there were 8 recurrences, 7 of which were outside the full template. Antegrade ejaculation was preserved in 85% of patients who underwent modified versus only 25% of patients who underwent full dissection.

There is broad agreement in the context of gross disease that the extent of dissection and aggressiveness of dissection should not be compromised to better preserve nerves. When feasible and technically reasonable, however, there are approaches to preserving sympathetic nerve tissue either by performing PC-RPLND within a modified template or with a nerve-sparing approach. These approaches are less likely to occur and succeed with worse cancer by IGCCCG risk criteria and or with a larger postchemotherapy mass. Therefore, such patients should be prepared preoperatively for loss of ejaculation and have banked sperm if future fertility is considered.

MINIMALLY INVASIVE POSTCHEMOTHERAPY–RETROPERITONEAL LYMPH NODE DISSECTION

Minimally invasive (laparoscopic or robotic) RPLND in the postchemotherapy setting has been reported from several institutions. Rassweiler and colleagues[51] reported on laparoscopic PC-RPLND for 9 patients with residual masses after chemotherapy for NSGCT. Only 2 of 9 patients successfully underwent laparoscopic PC-RPLND, the rest were converted to open procedures. Palese and colleagues[52] reported on 7 patients undergoing laparoscopic PC-RPLND; 5 of 7 patients had the procedure completed laparoscopically and 3 of the 7 patients had major complications, including renal artery mural hematoma requiring bypass graft, external iliac transection requiring grafting, delayed renal artery thrombus requiring nephrectomy, and duodenal perforation requiring hepaticojejunostomy. Calestroupat and colleagues[53] reported on 26 patients undergoing laparoscopic PC-RPLND. Three procedures (12%) were converted to open. There were 7 minor vascular complications and 1 patient required a bowel resection, which was completed laparoscopically. At a median on 27 months, there were no recurrences. Cheney and colleagues[54] recently published on 8 patients undergoing robotic PC-RPLND. Two patients (25%) were converted to open procedures. There were no major complications and no recurrences in the retroperitoneum on a mean follow-up of 22 months of the overall 18 patient cohort. Steiner and colleagues[55] reported on the largest laparoscopic PC-RPLND study to date; 100 patients underwent laparoscopic PC-RPLND, 71 unilateral template and 29 bilateral template. There was 1 conversion to open for bleeding. There were 2 major complications (large lymphocele and chylous ascites). During a median follow-up of 74 months, 1 patient had a recurrence, but this was outside the operative field of a patient who had a unilateral template. The use of minimally invasive PC-RPLND has evolved over time, with a decrease in intraoperative complications. Its use should be reserved, however, for centers with extensive laparoscopic or robotic experience and selected patients with low-volume disease. A comprehensive discussion of these approaches, in both the primary and postchemotherapy settings, is the subject of another article in this issue.

ADJUVANT PROCEDURES

Patients undergoing PC-RPLND often require additional procedures. Nephrectomy and resection of the inferior vena cava (IVC) are the most common. Stephenson and colleagues[56] reported 32 of 647 (5%) of PC-RPLNDs required a nephrectomy. A majority of these were in the postsalvage chemotherapy, reoperative RPLND, or desperation RPLND setting. Disease was found in 66% of kidney specimens. Winter and colleagues[57] published a report where 40 of 402 patients required a major vascular procedure (IVC or aortic resection). They found that residual tumor greater than 5 cm and IGCCCG intermediate or poor prognosis classification was associated with the need for a vascular procedure. Djaladat and colleagues[58] report 28 of 85 patients (33%) undergoing PC-RPLND needed an adjuvant procedure, including vascular resection, nephrectomy, bowel

resection, and liver resection. In cases of the IVC completed obstructed prior to surgery, it can be resected without replacement due to the development of collateral circulation.[59] The role of additional procedures outside the retroperitoneum is discussed in another article elsewhere in this issue.

MORBIDITY

At the onset, RPLND was a procedure with high morbidity and low survival.[1] Safety improved with refinement of operative technique, and RPLND is no longer associated with high mortality. PC-RPLND remains a challenging operation, however, due to the inherent complexity of the procedure and the desmoplastic reaction created by chemotherapy. Overall morbidity for PC-RPLND ranges from 12% to 32%.[1,16,17,60] Complications from PC-RPLND can be divided into pulmonary, lymphatic, vascular, gastrointestinal, infectious, and reproductive. Reproductive and fertilities issues are addressed in articles elsewhere in this issue.

Pulmonary complications from PC-RPLND can occur in up to 8% of cases.[16] These include atelectasis, pneumonia, adult respiratory distress syndrome and pulmonary embolism. Early ambulation, incentive spirometry, adequate analgesia, and aggressive pulmonary hygiene can decrease pulmonary morbidity. Patients who receive bleomycin are at increased risk for pulmonary complications. Judicious use of intravenous fluids and limitation of supplemental oxygen are crucial in this patient population.[61]

Injury to the lymphatic system can result in chylous ascites, exhibited by abdominal distention and fluid wave on physical examination. This occurs in up to 3% of cases.[16] Risk of chylous ascites is increased by suprahilar dissection, resection of liver lesions, or resection of the IVC. Initiation of medium-chain triglyceride diet and diuretic therapy are the mainstays of nonoperative intervention. Patients may require paracentesis, parenteral nutrition, or octreotide to help resolve the lymphatic leak. Lymphatic leak can also result in a lymphocele, which becomes clinically significant if it causes bowel obstruction or urinary obstruction or becomes infected. Symptomatic lymphoceles require percutaneous drainage and antibiotics if infection is suspected.

Injury to the aorta or IVC can occur during PC-RPLND. This can be addressed via primary repair, vascular patch, or interposition graft. If the IVC was completely occluded preoperatively, it can often be resected with minimal consequence due to venous collateralization that occurred prior to surgery.[59] Injury to renal vasculature requires careful repair to avoid renal infarction. Hemorrhage and anemia requiring transfusion are rare in high-volume centers. Injury to the anterior spinal artery is a rare occurrence that can result in spinal ischemia. There is a higher risk of this injury with advancing patient age. This can be avoided by judicious resection of lumbar arterial branches around the area of T8. Risk of deep venous thrombosis can be reduced by early ambulation, use of sequential compression devices, and subcutaneous heparin.

Prolonged ileus and small bowel obstruction are the most common gastrointestinal complications. These can usually be managed conservatively. Pancreatitis, ischemic bowel, and gastrointestinal hemorrhage are rare complications.

Infectious complications include urinary tract infection, infected lymphocele, and pneumonia. Wound infection is the most common infectious complication and rarely causes long-term sequelae.

OUTCOMES

Outcomes after standard PC-RPLND depend on multiple factors, including initial IGCCCG prognostic category, prior treatment, completeness of resection, pathology of RPLND specimens, and subsequent treatment. The utility of receiving additional chemotherapy in patients with residual viable tumor found on PC-RPLND was demonstrated by Fox and colleagues.[10] This is generally in the form of 2 additional cycles of chemotherapy. Fizazi and colleagues[9] published a study challenging the need for additional chemotherapy. This study examined 238 patients with viable germ cell tumor after PC-RPLND. Patients were stratified based on IGCCCG risk group, complete resection, and greater than 10% viable tumor. Postoperative chemotherapy only improved survival in the intermediate prognostic group. These finding have not been reproduced, and most organizations advocate for additional chemotherapy if viable tumor is found.

FOLLOW-UP

Continued follow-up of patients after treatment is to detect recurrence early to intervene and to identify toxicities of treatment, including secondary malignancy and cardiovascular disease.[62] Several different organizations have published recommendations for follow-up based on expert opinion rather than evidence-based findings. In general, the guidelines recommend follow-up with periodic physical examinations, STMs, chest radiographs, and CT scans, with decreasing frequency of these evaluations over a greater interval of follow-up. Some experts suggest that patients who have undergone PC-RPLND may require less frequent abdominal imaging than patients who have not.[37]

REFERENCES

1. Hinman F. The operative treatment of tumors of the testicles. JAMA 1914;58:2008.
2. Kollmannsberger C, Moore C, Chi KN, et al. Non-risk-adapted surveillance for patients with stage I nonseminomatous testicular germ-cell tumors: diminishing treatment-related morbidity while maintaining efficacy. Ann Oncol 2010;21(6):1296–301.
3. Sturgeon JF, Moore MJ, Kakiashvili DM, et al. Non-risk-adapted surveillance in clinical stage I nonseminomatous germ cell tumors: the Princess Margaret Hospital's experience. Eur Urol 2011;59(4):556–62.
4. Kollmannsberger C, Tyldesley S, Moore C, et al. Evolution in management of testicular seminoma: population-based outcomes with selective utilization of active therapies. Ann Oncol 2011;22(4):808–14.
5. Foster RS, Donohue JP. Can retroperitoneal lymphadenectomy be omitted in some patients after chemotherapy? Urol Clin North Am 1998;25(3):479–84.
6. Cary KC, Pedrosa JA, Kaimakliotis HZ, et al. The impact of bleomycin on retroperitoneal histology at post-chemotherapy retroperitoneal lymph node dissection of good risk germ cell tumors. J Urol 2015;193(2):507–12.
7. Kundu SD, Feldman DR, Carver BS, et al. Rates of teratoma and viable cancer at post-chemotherapy retroperitoneal lymph node dissection after induction chemotherapy for good risk nonseminomatous germ cell tumors. J Urol 2015;193(2):513–8.
8. de Wit R. Optimal management of germ cell cancer: more a matter of expertise than of chemotherapy regimen. J Urol 2015;193(2):391–3.
9. Fizazi K, Tjulandin S, Salvioni R, et al. Viable malignant cells after primary chemotherapy for disseminated nonseminomatous germ cell tumors: prognostic factors and role of postsurgery chemotherapy–results from an international study group. J Clin Oncol 2001;19(10):2647–57.
10. Fox EP, Weathers TD, Williams SD, et al. Outcome analysis for patients with persistent nonteratomatous germ cell tumor in postchemotherapy retroperitoneal lymph node dissections. J Clin Oncol 1993;11(7):1294–9.
11. Logothetis CJ, Samuels ML, Trindade A, et al. The growing teratoma syndrome. Cancer 1982;50(8):1629–35.
12. Ahmed T, Bosl GJ, Hajdu SI. Teratoma with malignant transformation in germ cell tumors in men. Cancer 1985;56(4):860–3.

13. Donadio AC, Motzer RJ, Bajorin DF, et al. Chemotherapy for teratoma with malignant transformation. J Clin Oncol 2003;21(23):4285–91.

14. Motzer RJ, Amsterdam A, Prieto V, et al. Teratoma with malignant transformation: diverse malignant histologies arising in men with germ cell tumors. J Urol 1998;159(1):133–8.

15. Williams SB, McDermott DW, Winston D, et al. Morbidity of open retroperitoneal lymph node dissection for testicular cancer: contemporary perioperative data. BJU Int 2010;105(7):918–21.

16. Baniel J, Foster RS, Rowland RG, et al. Complications of post-chemotherapy retroperitoneal lymph node dissection. J Urol 1995;153(3 Pt 2):976–80.

17. Mosharafa AA, Foster RS, Koch MO, et al. Complications of post-chemotherapy retroperitoneal lymph node dissection for testis cancer. J Urol 2004; 171(5):1839–41.

18. Mosharafa AA, Foster RS, Leibovich BC, et al. Is post-chemotherapy resection of seminomatous elements associated with higher acute morbidity? J Urol 2003;169(6):2126–8.

19. Herr HW, Sheinfeld J, Puc HS, et al. Surgery for a post-chemotherapy residual mass in seminoma. J Urol 1997;157(3):860–2.

20. Ravi R, Ong J, Oliver RT, et al. The management of residual masses after chemotherapy in metastatic seminoma. BJU Int 1999;83(6):649–53.

21. Flechon A, Bompas E, Biron P, et al. Management of post-chemotherapy residual masses in advanced seminoma. J Urol 2002;168(5):1975–9.

22. De Santis M, Becherer A, Bokemeyer C, et al. 2-18fluoro-deoxy-D-glucose positron emission tomography is a reliable predictor for viable tumor in postchemotherapy seminoma: an update of the prospective multicentric SEMPET trial. J Clin Oncol 2004;22(6):1034–9.

23. Johns Putra L, Lawrentschuk N, Ballok Z, et al. 18F-fluorodeoxyglucose positron emission tomography in evaluation of germ cell tumor after chemotherapy. Urology 2004;64(6):1202–7.

24. Treglia G, Sadeghi R, Annunziata S, et al. Diagnostic performance of fluorine-18-fluorodeoxyglucose positron emission tomography in the postchemotherapy management of patients with seminoma: systematic review and meta-analysis. Biomed Res Int 2014;2014:852681.

25. Motzer RJ, Agarwal N, Beard C, et al. Testicular cancer. J Natl Compr Canc Netw 2012;10(4):502–35.

26. Suh YJ, Kim MJ, Lee MJ. Increased 18F-FDG uptake by a retroperitoneal mature cystic teratoma in an infant. Clin Nucl Med 2014;39(4):352–4.

27. Pfannenberg AC, Oechsle K, Bokemeyer C, et al. The role of [(18)F] FDG-PET, CT/MRI and tumor marker kinetics in the evaluation of post chemotherapy residual masses in metastatic germ cell tumors–prospects for management. World J Urol 2004;22(2):132–9.

28. Oechsle K, Hartmann M, Brenner W, et al. [18F]Fluorodeoxyglucose positron emission tomography in nonseminomatous germ cell tumors after chemotherapy: the German multicenter positron emission tomography study group. J Clin Oncol 2008; 26(36):5930–5.

29. Fossa SD, Ous S, Lien HH, et al. Post-chemotherapy lymph node histology in radiologically normal patients with metastatic nonseminomatous testicular cancer. J Urol 1989;141(3):557–9.

30. Oldenburg J, Alfsen GC, Lien HH, et al. Postchemotherapy retroperitoneal surgery remains necessary in patients with nonseminomatous testicular cancer and minimal residual tumor masses. J Clin Oncol 2003;21(17):3310–7.

31. Carver BS, Bianco FJ Jr, Shayegan B, et al. Predicting teratoma in the retroperitoneum in men undergoing post-chemotherapy retroperitoneal lymph node dissection. J Urol 2006;176(1):100–3 [discussion: 103–4].

32. Carver BS, Shayegan B, Eggener S, et al. Incidence of metastatic nonseminomatous germ cell tumor outside the boundaries of a modified postchemotherapy retroperitoneal lymph node dissection. J Clin Oncol 2007;25(28):4365–9.

33. Ehrlich Y, Brames MJ, Beck SD, et al. Long-term follow-up of Cisplatin combination chemotherapy in patients with disseminated nonseminomatous germ cell tumors: is a postchemotherapy retroperitoneal lymph node dissection needed after complete remission? J Clin Oncol 2010;28(4):531–6.

34. Kollmannsberger C, Daneshmand S, So A, et al. Management of disseminated nonseminomatous germ cell tumors with risk-based chemotherapy followed by response-guided postchemotherapy surgery. J Clin Oncol 2010;28(4):537–42.

35. Wein AJ, Kavoussi LR, Campbell MF. Campbell-Walsh urology. In: Wein AJ, Kavoussi LR, Novick AC, et al, editors. Surgery of Testicular Tumors. 10th edition. Philadelphia: Elsevier Saunders; 2012.

36. Beck SD, Foster RS, Bihrle R, et al. Outcome analysis for patients with elevated serum tumor markers at postchemotherapy retroperitoneal lymph node dissection. J Clin Oncol 2005;23(25):6149–56.

37. Daneshmand S, Albers P, Fossa SD, et al. Contemporary management of postchemotherapy testis cancer. Eur Urol 2012;62(5):867–76.

38. Hendry WF, Norman AR, Dearnaley DP, et al. Metastatic nonseminomatous germ cell tumors of the testis: results of elective and salvage surgery for patients with residual retroperitoneal masses. Cancer 2002;94(6):1668–76.

39. Rick O, Bokemeyer C, Weinknecht S, et al. Residual tumor resection after high-dose chemotherapy in patients with relapsed or refractory germ cell cancer. J Clin Oncol 2004;22(18):3713–9.

40. Eggener SE, Carver BS, Loeb S, et al. Pathologic findings and clinical outcome of patients undergoing

retroperitoneal lymph node dissection after multiple chemotherapy regimens for metastatic testicular germ cell tumors. Cancer 2007;109(3):528–35.

41. Donohue JP, Fox EP, Williams SD, et al. Persistent cancer in postchemotherapy retroperitoneal lymph-node dissection: outcome analysis. World J Urol 1994;12(4):190–5.

42. Daneshmand S. Role of surgical resection for refractory germ cell tumors. Urol Oncol 2015. [Epub ahead of print].

43. Sharp DS, Carver BS, Eggener SE, et al. Clinical outcome and predictors of survival in late relapse of germ cell tumor. J Clin Oncol 2008;26(34):5524–9.

44. Michael H, Lucia J, Foster RS, et al. The pathology of late recurrence of testicular germ cell tumors. Am J Surg Pathol 2000;24(2):257–73.

45. Oldenburg J, Martin JM, Fossa SD. Late relapses of germ cell malignancies: incidence, management, and prognosis. J Clin Oncol 2006;24(35):5503–11.

46. Ronnen EA, Kondagunta GV, Bacik J, et al. Incidence of late-relapse germ cell tumor and outcome to salvage chemotherapy. J Clin Oncol 2005;23(28):6999–7004.

47. Eggener SE, Carver BS, Sharp DS, et al. Incidence of disease outside modified retroperitoneal lymph node dissection templates in clinical stage I or IIA nonseminomatous germ cell testicular cancer. J Urol 2007;177(3):937–42 [discussion: 942–3].

48. Pettus JA, Carver BS, Masterson T, et al. Preservation of ejaculation in patients undergoing nerve-sparing postchemotherapy retroperitoneal lymph node dissection for metastatic testicular cancer. Urology 2009;73(2):328–31 [discussion: 331–2].

49. Beck SD, Foster RS, Bihrle R, et al. Is full bilateral retroperitoneal lymph node dissection always necessary for postchemotherapy residual tumor? Cancer 2007;110(6):1235–40.

50. Heidenreich A, Pfister D, Witthuhn R, et al. Postchemotherapy retroperitoneal lymph node dissection in advanced testicular cancer: radical or modified template resection. Eur Urol 2009;55(1):217–24.

51. Rassweiler JJ, Seemann O, Henkel TO, et al. Laparoscopic retroperitoneal lymph node dissection for nonseminomatous germ cell tumors: indications and limitations. J Urol 1996;156(3):1108–13.

52. Palese MA, Su LM, Kavoussi LR. Laparoscopic retroperitoneal lymph node dissection after chemotherapy. Urology 2002;60(1):130–4.

53. Calestroupat JP, Sanchez-Salas R, Cathelineau X, et al. Postchemotherapy laparoscopic retroperitoneal lymph node dissection in nonseminomatous germ-cell tumor. J Endourol 2009;23(4):645–50.

54. Cheney SM, Andrews PE, Leibovich BC, et al. Robot-assisted retroperitoneal lymph node dissection: technique and initial case series of 18 patients. BJU Int 2015;115(1):114–20.

55. Steiner H, Leonhartsberger N, Stoehr B, et al. Postchemotherapy laparoscopic retroperitoneal lymph node dissection for low-volume, stage II, nonseminomatous germ cell tumor: first 100 patients. Eur Urol 2013;63(6):1013–7.

56. Stephenson AJ, Tal R, Sheinfeld J. Adjunctive nephrectomy at post-chemotherapy retroperitoneal lymph node dissection for nonseminomatous germ cell testicular cancer. J Urol 2006;176(5):1996–9 [discussion: 1999].

57. Winter C, Pfister D, Busch J, et al. Residual tumor size and IGCCCG risk classification predict additional vascular procedures in patients with germ cell tumors and residual tumor resection: a multicenter analysis of the German Testicular Cancer Study Group. Eur Urol 2012;61(2):403–9.

58. Djaladat H, Nichols C, Daneshmand S. Adjuvant surgery in testicular cancer patients undergoing postchemotherapy retroperitoneal lymph node dissection. Ann Surg Oncol 2012;19(7):2388–93.

59. Duty B, Daneshmand S. Resection of the inferior vena cava without reconstruction for urologic malignancies. Urology 2009;74(6):1257–62.

60. Subramanian VS, Nguyen CT, Stephenson AJ, et al. Complications of open primary and postchemotherapy retroperitoneal lymph node dissection for testicular cancer. Urol Oncol 2010;28(5):504–9.

61. Goldiner PL, Schweizer O. The hazards of anesthesia and surgery in bleomycin-treated patients. Semin Oncol 1979;6(1):121–4.

62. Haugnes HS, Bosl GJ, Boer H, et al. Long-term and late effects of germ cell testicular cancer treatment and implications for follow-up. J Clin Oncol 2012;30(30):3752–63.

63. Donohue JP, Roth LM, Zachary JM, et al. Cytoreductive surgery for metastatic testis cancer: tissue analysis of retroperitoneal masses after chemotherapy. J Urol 1982;127(6):1111–4.

64. Bracken RB, Johnson DE, Frazier OH, et al. The role of surgery following chemotherapy in stage III germ cell neoplasms. J Urol 1983;129(1):39–43.

65. Freiha FS, Shortliffe LD, Rouse RV, et al. The extent of surgery after chemotherapy for advanced germ cell tumors. J Urol 1984;132(5):915–7.

66. Pizzocaro G, Salvioni R, Pasi M, et al. Early resection of residual tumor during cisplatin, vinblastine, bleomycin combination chemotherapy in stage III and bulky stage II nonseminomatous testicular cancer. Cancer 1985;56(2):249–55.

67. Fossa SD, Aass N, Ous S, et al. Histology of tumor residuals following chemotherapy in patients with advanced nonseminomatous testicular cancer. J Urol 1989;142(5):1239–42.

68. Gelderman WA, Schraffordt Koops H, Sleijfer DT, et al. Results of adjuvant surgery in patients with stage III and IV nonseminomatous testicular tumors

after cisplatin-vinblastine-bleomycin chemotherapy. J Surg Oncol 1988;38(4):227–32.

69. Williams SN, Jenkins BJ, Baithun SI, et al. Radical retroperitoneal node dissection after chemotherapy for testicular tumours. Br J Urol 1989;63(6):641–3.

70. Harding MJ, Brown IL, MacPherson SG, et al. Excision of residual masses after platinum based chemotherapy for non-seminomatous germ cell tumours. Eur J Cancer Clin Oncol 1989;25(12):1689–94.

71. Mulders PF, Oosterhof GO, Boetes C, et al. The importance of prognostic factors in the individual treatment of patients with disseminated germ cell tumours. Br J Urol 1990;66(4):425–9.

72. Aass N, Klepp O, Cavallin-Stahl E, et al. Prognostic factors in unselected patients with nonseminomatous metastatic testicular cancer: a multicenter experience. J Clin Oncol 1991;9(5):818–26.

73. Kulkarni RP, Reynolds KW, Newlands ES, et al. Cytoreductive surgery in disseminated nonseminomatous germ cell tumours of testis. Br J Surg 1991;78(2):226–9.

74. Aprikian AG, Herr HW, Bajorin DF, et al. Resection of postchemotherapy residual masses and limited retroperitoneal lymphadenectomy in patients with metastatic testicular nonseminomatous germ cell tumors. Cancer 1994;74(4):1329–34.

75. Steyerberg EW, Keizer HJ, Fossa SD, et al. Prediction of residual retroperitoneal mass histology after chemotherapy for metastatic nonseminomatous germ cell tumor: multivariate analysis of individual patient data from six study groups. J Clin Oncol 1995;13(5):1177–87.

76. Brenner PC, Herr HW, Morse MJ, et al. Simultaneous retroperitoneal, thoracic, and cervical resection of postchemotherapy residual masses in patients with metastatic nonseminomatous germ cell tumors of the testis. J Clin Oncol 1996;14(6):1765–9.

77. Stenning SP, Parkinson MC, Fisher C, et al. Postchemotherapy residual masses in germ cell tumor patients: content, clinical features, and prognosis. Medical Research Council Testicular Tumour Working Party. Cancer 1998;83(7):1409–19.

78. Donohue JP, Leviovitch I, Foster RS, et al. Integration of surgery and systemic therapy: results and principles of integration. Semin Urol Oncol 1998; 16(2):65–71.

79. Napier MP, Naraghi A, Christmas TJ, et al. Longterm follow-up of residual masses after chemotherapy in patients with non-seminomatous germ cell tumours. Br J Cancer 2000;83(10):1274–80.

80. Albers P, Weissbach L, Krege S, et al. Prediction of necrosis after chemotherapy of advanced germ cell tumors: results of a prospective multicenter trial of the German Testicular Cancer Study Group. J Urol 2004;171(5):1835–8.

81. Muramaki M, Hara I, Miyake H, et al. Clinical outcome of retroperitoneal lymph node dissection after induction chemotherapy for metastatic nonseminomatous germ cell tumors. Int J Urol 2004; 11(9):763–7.

82. Spiess PE, Brown GA, Liu P, et al. Recurrence pattern and proposed surveillance protocol following post-chemotherapy retroperitoneal lymph node dissection. J Urol 2007;177(1):131–8.

83. Luz MA, Kotb AF, Aldousari S, et al. Retroperitoneal lymph node dissection for residual masses after chemotherapy in nonseminomatous germ cell testicular tumor. World J Surg Oncol 2010;8:97.

84. Busch J, Magheli A, Erber B, et al. Laparoscopic and open postchemotherapy retroperitoneal lymph node dissection in patients with advanced testicular cancer–a single center analysis. BMC Urol 2012;12:15.

Desperation Postchemotherapy Retroperitoneal Lymph Node Dissection for Metastatic Germ Cell Tumors

CrossMark

Brett S. Carver, MD

KEYWORDS

- Postchemotherapy • Retroperitoneal lymph node dissection • Germ cell tumors
- Serum tumor markers

KEY POINTS

- Patients with persistently elevated serum tumor markers should be monitored for marker kinetics and evaluated for nonviable cancer causes of marker elevation.
- Desperation postchemotherapy retroperitoneal lymph node dissection is performed in select patients following second-line chemotherapy.
- Adjuvant postoperative chemotherapy is not indicated in patients following second-line chemotherapy.

INTRODUCTION

Patients with advanced germ cell tumors (GCTs) of the testis (cIIB–cIII) and those with persistently elevated serum tumor markers (STM) following radical orchiectomy (cIS) are initially treated with platinum-based chemotherapy according to the International Germ Cell Cancer Collaborative Group risk classification.[1] Approximately 70% to 80% are rendered free of disease following first-line chemotherapy and adjunctive resection of all residual sites of disease.[2] Despite the profound sensitivity of GCTs to platinum-based chemotherapy regimens, approximately 20% to 30% of patients will not achieve undetectable STMs following first-line risk-appropriate chemotherapy or will relapse early following a serologic complete response.[2] With rare exception, these patients are managed with conventional second-line chemotherapy regimens or high-dose chemotherapy with autologous stem cell replacement. With this approach, approximately 50% to 60% of patients will achieve a complete clinical response and long-term freedom from relapse following surgical resection of all sites of residual disease. However, a subset of patients will continue to have persistently elevated STMs and proceed directly to surgical resection, known as a desperation postchemotherapy retroperitoneal lymph node dissection (PC-RPLND), or third-line systemic therapies. In the current article, the indications for and therapeutic outcomes following PC-RPLND and resection of extra-retroperitoneal sites of disease in patients with persistently elevated STMs following chemotherapy are reviewed.

ELEVATED SERUM TUMOR MARKERS FOLLOWING FIRST-LINE CHEMOTHERAPY FOR GERM CELL TUMOR

Although most patients with elevated STMs following first-line chemotherapy for metastatic

Department of Surgery, Division of Urology, Memorial Sloan-Kettering Cancer Center, 1275 York Avenue, New York, NY 10065, USA
E-mail address: carverb@mskcc.org

Urol Clin N Am 42 (2015) 343–346
http://dx.doi.org/10.1016/j.ucl.2015.04.008
0094-0143/15/$ – see front matter © 2015 Elsevier Inc. All rights reserved.

GCT will be managed with second-line chemotherapy, a highly select group of patients will benefit from immediate PC-RPLND. This highly select group represents patients in whom the elevated STMs are associated with nonviable tumor causes of marker elevations (**Table 1**). Generally, this includes patients who have low-level serum elevations of human chorionic gonadotrophin (b-HCG) or α-fetoprotein (AFP) that are stable and not increasing over time. For patients with a stable but persistently elevated b-HCG following chemotherapy, hypogonadism and test cross-reactivity with luteinizing hormone should be suspected and further evaluated with a testosterone suppression test.[3] In addition, hepatic dysfunction related to hepatitis and alcohol abuse has been shown to be associated with increase serum levels of AFP.[4]

Furthermore, it has been shown that in patients with residual disease consistent with cystic teratoma, these cystic lesions may contain high quantities of AFP or b-HCG that slowly leak back into the serum, leading to low-level elevations of these STMs.[5] In a study from Memorial Sloan-Kettering, select patients with residual retroperitoneal masses that were cystic in nature underwent PC-RPLND. Intraoperatively, the fluid from the cysts was aspirated and analyzed for AFP and b-HCG concentrations. In all cases, the cystic fluid was positive for b-HCG (9/9 cases) or AFP (9/11 cases). Retroperitoneal histology revealed teratomatous elements in all patients and no evidence of viable GCT. Of these patients, 3 patients also had elevated STMs. In 2 patients with elevated serum AFP, both patients had elevated levels of AFP in the cystic fluid and their serum AFP levels returned to normal following surgery. One patient with elevated serum b-HCG had increasing b-HCG levels and progressive disease following RPLND despite having increased b-HCG levels in the cystic mass. This data suggest that carefully selected patients with stable low levels of serum AFP and residual cystic teratomatous disease in

the retroperitoneum may benefit from immediate PC-RPLND and avoid second-line chemotherapy.

ELEVATED SERUM TUMOR MARKERS FOLLOWING SECOND-LINE CHEMOTHERAPY FOR GERM CELL TUMOR

In patients undergoing PC-RPLND following second-line chemotherapy in the setting of normal STMs, the rates of viable GCT are approximately 50%.[6,7] However, with improved risk stratification and refinements of second-line chemotherapy regimens, including taxane-based regimens and high-dose chemotherapy, the rate of persistent viable GCT has been declining.[7] Previous studies have demonstrated that although 2 cycles of adjuvant chemotherapy for patients with residual viable GCT following PC-RPLND (normal STMs) after first-line chemotherapy reduces relapse rates, there is no therapeutic benefit for adjuvant chemotherapy after second-line chemotherapy.[8]

For patients with persistently elevated STMs following second-line chemotherapy, the therapeutic options include third-line systemic therapies or, for select patients, PC-RPLND with surgical resection of all residual sites of disease, also known as a desperation RPLND.[2] The selection criteria used to determine acceptable candidates for desperation RPLND highly depends on the individual patient, but ideally these are patients with (1) slowly rising STMs, (2) limited number of residual sites of disease, and (3) disease that is amendable to surgical resection whereby the surgical intent is to cure.

Histologic Findings at the Time of Desperation Retroperitoneal Lymph Node Dissection

The incidence of viable GCT at RPLND in patients undergoing desperation surgery is reported to range between 40% and 80% across several studies (**Table 2**).[9–11] However, most of these studies include patients undergoing PC-RPLND

Table 1
Cause of elevated serum tumor markers in patients not associated with viable germ cell tumors

Clinical Scenario	Clinical Evaluation
Hypogonadism associated with elevated b-HCG	1. Measurement of serum testosterone 2. Testosterone suppression test
Hepatic dysfunction associated with elevated AFP	1. Measurement of liver function tests 2. Hepatic ultrasound/computed tomographic (CT) imaging 3. Hepatitis panel
Cystic teratoma associated with increased AFP ± b-HCG	1. CT abdomen/pelvis reveals findings consistent with teratoma 2. STMs remain mildly elevated but stable

Table 2
Retroperitoneal histologic findings in patients undergoing postchemotherapy retroperitoneal lymph node dissection with persistently elevated serum tumor markers

Retroperitoneal Histology	Eastham et al,[9] 1994	Beck et al,[10] 2005	Ravi et al,[11] 1998
Viable GCT	13/16 (81%)	61/114 (54%)	14/30 (46%)
Teratoma	2/16 (13%)	39/114 (34%)	8/30 (27%)
Fibrosis	1/16 (6%)	14/114 (12%)	8/30 (27%)

with elevated STMs following first- or second-line chemotherapy. When evaluating only patients undergoing true desperation PC-RPLND after second-line chemotherapy, the incidence of viable GCT is approximately 80%, and 20% of cases are found to harbor teratoma or fibrosis.[10] The findings of teratoma or fibrosis in the retroperitoneum, and not viable GCT, suggest that viable GCT elements responsible for the persistently rising STMs may reside in extra-retroperitoneal sites, be the result of systemic disease, or be associated with pathologic sample error of large retroperitoneal masses. Pathologic sample error has been observed in select patients wherein STMs have normalized following PC-RPLND despite the histologic finding of fibrosis.

Clinical Outcome Following Desperation Retroperitoneal Lymph Node Dissection

The 5-year survival rates for patients undergoing PC-RPLND following first-line chemotherapy with elevated STMs or patients treated with second-line chemotherapy whose STMs have normalized are quite similar and range from 70% to 80%.[2,7] However, there is a dramatic decline in 5-year survival rates for patients undergoing true desperation PC-RPLND after second-line chemotherapy wherein only approximately 30% of patients are 5-year survivors (**Table 3**).[9–11] These results

highlight the aggressive chemorefractory nature of these cancers for patients undergoing desperation surgery. Risk factors associated with a poor survival include increasing b-HCG and AFP levels, reoperative surgery, and the histologic finding of viable GCT in the resected specimen.[10] For patients with progressive disease following desperation surgery, third-line and experimental systemic therapies are used based on patient performance status and tolerability.

SUMMARY

Although most patients with GCTs are sensitive to chemotherapy, a subset of approximately 20% harbors chemorefractory disease to first-line chemotherapy regimens. With improvements in risk stratification and chemotherapy regimens, more than half of these patients are now rendered free of disease following adjunctive surgical resection. Patients with persistently elevated STMs following chemotherapy should be evaluated for tumor marker kinetics and the potential to harbor nonviable cancer causes of their STM elevation. Following second-line chemotherapy, men with persistently elevated STMs represent a unique population of patients with a relatively poor prognosis. Surgical resection or desperation RPLND is performed in select patients deemed to be potentially curable and overall survival rates are approximately 30%. This cohort of patients is highly selected based on STM kinetics and surgical respectability.

Table 3
Clinical outcome following postchemotherapy retroperitoneal lymph node dissection in the setting of elevated serum tumor markers

	Median Follow-up (mo)	Clinical Outcome
Eastham et al,[9] 1994	74	6/16 (37%) alive free of disease
Beck et al,[10] 2005	72	61/114 (54%) alive free of disease
Ravi et al,[11] 1998	57	17/30 (57%) alive free of disease

REFERENCES

1. International Germ Cell Consensus Classification: a prognostic factor-based staging system for metastatic germ cell cancers. International Germ Cell Cancer Collaborative Group. J Clin Oncol 1997;15:594–603.
2. Voss MH, Feldman DR, Bosl GJ, et al. A review of second-line chemotherapy and prognostic models for disseminated germ cell tumors. Hematol Oncol Clin North Am 2011;25:557–76.
3. Catalona WJ, Vaitukaitis JL, Fair WR. Falsely positive specific human chorionic gonadotropin assays in patients with testicular tumors: conversion to

negative with testosterone administration. J Urol 1979;122:126–8.

4. Doherty AP, Bower M, Christmas TJ. The role of tumour markers in the diagnosis and treatment of testicular germ cell cancers. Br J Urol 1997;79: 247–52.

5. Beck SD, Patel MI, Sheinfeld J. Tumor marker levels in post-chemotherapy cystic masses: clinical implications for patients with germ cell tumors. J Urol 2004;171:168–71.

6. Calabro F, Albers P, Bokemeyer C, et al. The contemporary role of chemotherapy for advanced testis cancer: a systematic review of the literature. Eur Urol 2012;61:1212–21.

7. Eggener SE, Carver BS, Loeb S, et al. Pathologic findings and clinical outcome of patients undergoing retroperitoneal lymph node dissection after multiple chemotherapy regimens for metastatic germ cell tumors. Cancer 2007;109:528–35.

8. Fox EP, Weathers TD, Williams SD, et al. Outcome analysis for patients with persistent nonteratomatous germ cell tumor in postchemotherapy retroperitoneal lymph node dissections. J Clin Oncol 1993; 11:1294–9.

9. Eastham JA, Wilson TG, Russell C, et al. Surgical resection in patients with nonseminomatous germ cell tumor who fail to normalize serum tumor markers after chemotherapy. Urology 1994;43:74–80.

10. Beck SD, Foster RS, Bihrle R, et al. Post chemotherapy desperation retroperitoneal lymph node dissection for patients with elevated tumor markers. Urol Oncol 2005;23:423–30.

11. Ravi R, Ong J, Oliver RT, et al. Surgery as salvage therapy in chemotherapy resistant nonseminomatous germ cell tumours. Br J Urol 1998;81:884–8.

Chemotherapy for Good-Risk Nonseminomatous Germ Cell Tumors
Current Concepts and Controversies

Gino In, MD, MPH, Tanya Dorff, MD*

KEYWORDS

- Germ cell tumor • Cisplatin • Bleomycin • Etoposide

KEY POINTS

- Combination chemotherapy results in a high rate of cure for good-risk GCT.
- Surgery is part of the cure process for a significant proportion of patients.
- Three cycles of BEP remains the gold standard, with four cycles of EP an alternative option depending on individual concerns about patient comorbidity and toxicity.
- As data emerge regarding late chemotherapy toxicity, studies of interventions to improve survivorship will be needed.

The rate of diagnosis of germ cell tumors (GCT) has remained fairly constant, and in 2015 it is estimated that 8,430 men will be diagnosed with, and 380 deaths will be attributed to, GCTs.[1] By the International Germ Cell Cancer Consensus Classification, roughly 60% of all metastatic GCTs are classified as good risk.[2] The criteria defining good risk are presented in **Table 1**. This group of patients has an excellent prognosis, with greater than 90% expectation of cure. Treatment standards have not changed much in recent years. This article focuses on key concepts in the development of the currently accepted first-line regimens and addresses some evolving areas of interest, if not controversy.

CONCEPT 1: CISPLATIN COMBINATION CHEMOTHERAPY CAN CURE EVEN ADVANCED GERM CELL PATIENTS

Cisplatin, also known as *cis*-diamminedichloroplatinum, is a platinum alkylating agent that gained considerable attention in testicular cancer because of its significant activity in refractory disease. In 1974, Einhorn and Donohue[3] at Indiana University investigated cisplatin in combination with vinblastine and bleomycin (PVB) with dosing summarized in **Table 2**. A total of 50 patients with disseminated GCT were treated with four cycles of PVB followed by 21 months of maintenance vinblastine, resulting in 74% complete remissions and 26% partial remissions. Five patients with partial remissions were also able achieve disease-free status following surgical resection of residual disease, resulting in an overall 85% disease-free status.

Etoposide, a semisynthetic epipodophyllotoxin derivative, was found to induce complete remissions in patients with cisplatin-refractory GCT,[4–6] leading to study of this active agent in the first-line setting, in combination with cisplatin. From 1981 to 1984 the Southeastern Cancer Study Group and Mid-Atlantic Oncology Program conducted a phase III study to compare PVB with

Division of Medical Oncology, USC Keck School of Medicine, USC Norris Comprehensive Cancer Center, 1441 Eastlake Avenue, Los Angeles, CA 90033, USA
* Corresponding author.
E-mail address: dorff@usc.edu

Table 1
Criteria defining good-, intermediate-, and poor-risk germ cell tumors

	AFP	HCG	LDH	
Good risk	<1000 ng/ml	<5000 mU/ml	<1.5 × ULN	Gonadal or retroperitoneal primary
Intermediate risk	1000–10,000 ng/ml	5000–50,000 mU/ml	1.5–10.0 × ULN	Gonadal or retroperitoneal primary
Poor risk	≥10,000 ng/ml	≥50,000 mU/ml	≥10 × ULN	Mediastinal primary site; nonpulmonary visceral metastases

Abbreviations: AFP, alpha-fetoprotein; HCG, human chorionic gonadotropin; LDH, lactate dehydrogenase; ULN, upper limit of normal.
Data from International Germ Cell Consensus Classification. A prognostic factor-based staging system for metastatic germ cell cancers. International Germ Cell Cancer Collaborative Group. J Clin Oncol 1997;15(2):594–603.

cisplatin, bleomycin, and etoposide (BEP). A total of 261 patients with disseminated GCTs were randomized to four cycles of cisplatin, 20 mg/m² intravenous (IV) daily Days 1 to 5; bleomycin, 30 U IV on Days 2, 9, and 16; and either IV vinblastine, 0.15 mg/kg on Days 1 and 2 or IV etoposide, 100 mg/m² on Days 1 to 5.[7] Among those receiving BEP, 83% achieved complete remission, compared with 74% of those receiving PVB. Survival was higher among patients on the etoposide arm (P = .048). Both regimens showed similar myelosuppression and pulmonary toxicity, but BEP-treated patients experienced significantly less neuromuscular and gastrointestinal toxicity. As such, four cycles of BEP replaced PVB as the new standard.

It should be noted that resection of residual disease is important toward the cure of GCTs, and often requires coordinated multidisciplinary efforts to achieve optimal outcomes. Incomplete

Table 2
Doses for established chemotherapy regimens for germ cell patients, with a summary of efficacy data

Regimen (Citation)	Agents and Doses	N	Response Rates
PVB × 3 Einhorn & Donohue,[3] 1977	Cisplatin, 20 mg/m² Days 1–5 Vinblastine, 0.4 mg/kg Days 1 and 2 Bleomycin, 30 U Days 2, 9, 16 Every 3 wk × 3 cycles	N = 50	CR 85% Durable CR 64%
BEP × 4 Williams et al,[7] 1987	Bleomycin, 30 U Days 2, 9, 16 Etoposide, 100 mg/m² Days 1–5 Cisplatin, 20 mg/m² Days 1–5 Every 3 wk × 4 cycles	N = 123	CR 83% Durable CR 78%
BEP × 3 Einhorn et al,[11] 1989	Bleomycin, 30 U Days 2, 9, 16 Etoposide, 100 mg/m² Days 1–5 Cisplatin, 20 mg/m² Days 1–5 Every 3 wk × 3 cycles	N = 88	CR 98% Durable CR 92%
EP × 4 Bosl et al,[17] 1988	Etoposide, 100 mg/m² Days 1–5 Cisplatin, 20 mg/m² Days 1–5 Every 3 wk × 4 cycles	N = 82	CR 93% Durable CR 82%
BEC × 4 Horwich et al,[37] 2010	Bleomycin, 30 U Day 2 Etoposide, 120 mg/m² Days 1–3 Carboplatin, area under the curve 5 Every 3 wk × 4 cycles	N = 260	CR 87% Durable CR 77%
EC × 4 Bajorin et al,[38] 1997	Etoposide, 100 mg/m² Days 1–5 Carboplatin, 500 mg/m² Days 1 Every 4 wk × 4 cycles	N = 131	CR 88% Durable CR 76%

Abbreviations: BEP, cisplatin, bleomycin, and etoposide; CR, complete remission.

resection is associated with increased risk of relapse.[8] Late relapses are often more resistant to chemotherapy[9] and thus the need for surgical resection becomes even more important. Malignant transformation of residual teratoma also may be resistant to standard chemotherapy. Studies have shown that community low-volume centers have higher rates of recurrence following retroperitoneal lymph node dissection.[10] In contrast, tertiary referral centers achieve the lowest recurrence rates, and thus should be used as a resource for these patients when possible.

CONCEPT 2: THREE CYCLES OF COMBINED CISPLATIN, BLEOMYCIN, AND ETOPOSIDE IS ASSOCIATED WITH HIGH CURE RATES FOR GOOD-RISK NONSEMINOMATOUS GERM CELL TUMORS

In 1989, Einhorn and colleagues[11] sought to decrease BEP toxicity by reducing the number of total cycles. A phase III study of 184 patients with Indiana criteria good-risk disseminated GCTs were randomized to four cycles of BEP or three cycles of BEP. The disease-free rate was similar between arms; 98% for three cycles of BEP compared with 97% for four cycles of BEP. An additional, noninferiority study was conducted by de Wit and colleagues[12] to compare three cycles of BEP versus 4 cycles in International Germ Cell Cancer Consensus Classification good-risk patients. The study also compared a 5-day versus 3-day schedule for BEP, using a 2 × 2 factorial design. Three cycles of BEP and four cycles of BEP showed equivalence (projected 2-year progression-free survival, 90.4% and 89.4%, respectively) and the 5-day and 3-day regimens were also equivalent, with projected 2-year progression-free survival, 88.8% and 89.7%. A subsequent study by the Australian and New Zealand Germ Cell Trial Group compared standard BEP with a reduced-dose BEP.[13] A total of 166 Memorial Sloan Kettering Cancer Center criteria good-risk patients were randomized to receive either three cycles of standard BEP or four cycles of a modified BEP 3-day regimen (cisplatin, 100 mg/m^2 IV daily Day 1; bleomycin, 30 U IV on Day 1; and etoposide, 120 mg/m^2 on Days 1–3). Standard BEP showed significantly better overall survival compared with the modified BEP (3 vs 13 deaths, respectively; hazard ratio, 0.22; 95% confidence interval [CI], 0.06–0.77; $P = .008$) highlighting the importance of the full 500 mg/m^2 of etoposide and 90 U bleomycin per cycle. These results increased confidence

that three cycles of BEP is adequate therapy for good-risk patients.

CONTROVERSY 1: IS BLEOMYCIN NECESSARY?

Bleomycin, a glycopeptide antibiotic originally isolated from *Streptomyces verticillus*[14] in 1966, has been shown to have significant antitumor activity in solid and hematologic neoplasms. Its antineoplastic activity results from oxygen-free radical formation and in the induction of double-stranded DNA breakage.[15] A study by the Australasian Germ Cell Trial Group comparing PVB with vinblastine and cisplatin alone (PV) found that cancer-related deaths were significantly greater for patients on PV (15% compared with 5%) compared with PVB ($P = .02$).[16] Although 34% of patients receiving bleomycin experienced pulmonary toxicity, the authors pointed out that this risk was greatly outweighed by the improved survival noted for patients who received bleomycin.

The bleomycin-free cisplatin and etoposide (EP) regimen was first tested against an older five-drug regimen: bleomycin, vinblastine, cisplatin, cyclophosphamide, and dactinomycin (VAB-6). Among patients on VAB-6, 96% achieved complete remission at 2 years compared with 93% on EP, with a 12% relapse rate for both arms. Because of its equivalent efficacy and lower toxicity, the authors recommended four cycles of EP as an alternate treatment regimen for good-risk GCT.[17] Subsequently, three cycles of BEP was compared with four cycles of EP in a study conducted by the Genito-Urinary Group of the French Federation of Cancer Centers (GETUG). A total of 270 patients with nonseminomatous germ cell tumors (NSGCT) were randomized to receive three cycles of BEP or four cycles of EP.[18] With median follow-up of 53 months the 4-year event-free survival for the 256 patients categorized as good risk was 93% for BEP compared with 86% for EP, with hazard ratio of 0.46 ($P = .052$). Overall survival was 96% for men treated with BEP and 92% for those treated with EP (hazard ratio, 0.42; $P = .096$). Although this did not reach statistical significance, it contributes to the evidence that bleomycin is an important component of curative therapy for patients with GCT.

Given its excellent cure rates, it is our practice to offer three cycles of BEP as first-line therapy for good-risk NSGCT whenever possible. Although four cycles of EP is accepted by National Comprehensive Cancer Network guidelines[19] and others as an equivalent alternative first-line regimen, we usually reserve four cycles of EP for those patients who are otherwise unfit for bleomycin (ie, those patients with underlying lung disease), or who develop toxicity related to bleomycin after starting BEP.

CONCEPT 3: BLEOMYCIN PULMONARY TOXICITY IS RELATIVELY RARE AND SOME FACTORS MAY FACILITATE SELECTION OF PATIENTS AT HIGHER RISK FOR ALTERNATE REGIMENS

Bleomycin pulmonary toxicity has been a driving concern in the search for an alternative to BEP. Pulmonary toxicity presents with a multitude of syndromes, including bronchiolitis obliterans with organizing pneumonia,[20] eosinophilic hypersensitivity,[21] and interstitial pneumonitis with progression to pulmonary fibrosis.[22] Mortality from bleomycin interstitial pneumonitis is estimated at 3%.[23]

Monitoring for bleomycin pulmonary toxicity has been difficult because of a lack of uniform characteristics and defining criteria. Initial studies identified decreased carbon monoxide diffusing capacity as an indicator for subclinical bleomycin toxicity in the absence of other clinical findings.[24] However, a prospective study comparing 27 patients receiving four cycles of BEP with 27 patients receiving four cycles of EP found that carbon monoxide diffusing capacity was significantly decreased with both regimens, whereas vital capacity and pulmonary capillary blood volume were decreased only in patients treated with BEP. This suggests that it may be more appropriate to use vital capacity and pulmonary capillary blood volume as measures for identifying early bleomycin pulmonary toxicity.[25] Additional methods are needed to optimize the early identification of pulmonary toxicity, which could include high-resolution chest computed tomography.

Early studies suggested that there is a dose-related effect between bleomycin and pulmonary toxicity; fatal bleomycin pulmonary toxicity occurred in less than 1% of patients at lower doses, but increased to 10% in the doses greater than 550 U.[26] However, toxicity has been reported with doses less than 100 U.[27] A retrospective analysis of 194 patients receiving bleomycin for GCT identified additional potential risk factors.[23] Based on five deaths (2.8%) it seemed that bleomycin toxicity was influenced by reduced glomerular filtration rate (GFR) ($P<.001$) and by older age ($P<.001$), with increased toxicity for each decade of life older than 30 years old. These risk factors were confirmed in a larger series of 835 patients with GCT treated at the Royal Mardsen; in addition to GFR and age, cumulative bleomycin dose greater than 300 U predicted risk of pulmonary toxicity.[28] Additional factors associated with pulmonary toxicity include high-dose chemotherapy, pulmonary surgery,[29] and smoking.[30]

Importantly, the suggestion that use of granulocyte colony–stimulating factor may increase the risk of bleomycin pulmonary toxicity has not been confirmed. A large MRC/EORTC trial of 263 patients receiving BEP or bleomycin, vincristine, cisplatin (BOP)/etoposide, ifosfamide, cisplatin (VIP) showed no increased bleomycin pulmonary toxicity in patients receiving granulocyte colony–stimulating factor.[31] A retrospective study also identified no difference in bleomycin pulmonary toxicity between patients with GCT who did and did not receive granulocyte colony–stimulating factor.[32]

CONTROVERSY 2: IS THE TOXICITY PROFILE OF FOUR CYCLES OF BLEOMYCIN-FREE CISPLATIN AND ETOPOSIDE BETTER THAN THREE CYCLES OF COMBINED CISPLATIN, BLEOMYCIN, AND ETOPOSIDE?

Toxicities associated with the increased cumulative dose of cisplatin and etoposide in four cycles of EP must be weighed against the risk of pulmonary toxicity from bleomycin in three cycles of BEP. To help put this in perspective, three cycles of BEP includes bleomycin, 270 U; cisplatin, 300 mg/m^2; and etoposide, 1500 mg/m^2. Four cycles of EP includes cisplatin, 400 mg/m^2 and etoposide, 2000 mg/m^2.

Studies have shown an increased risk of infertility associated with a cumulative cisplatin dose of 400 mg/m^2.[33] Peripheral neuropathy is a significant dose-limiting toxicity that occurs in as many as 80% of patients following cisplatin-based chemotherapy. Reversible cisplatin-induced neuropathy usually begins at cumulative doses greater than 300 mg/m^2,[34] but persistent neuropathy occurs at cumulative doses greater than 400 mg/m^2.[35] The incidence of cardiovascular events, including myocardial infarction, cerebrovascular accident, and arterial thrombosis, occurring during chemotherapy is estimated to be 0.3%.[36]

The aforementioned GETUG trial of three cycles of BEP compared with four cycles of EP provides direct comparative toxicity data.[18] Patients receiving BEP experienced more neurotoxicity ($P<.006$) and dermatitis, and Raynaud phenomenon ($P<.0001$). Patients receiving EP experienced more grade 3 to 4 neutropenia ($P = .0002$), but there was no statistical difference in neutropenic fever compared with BEP ($P = .44$). There was no significant difference in pulmonary toxicity

(9% for BEP vs 6% for EP; $P = .38$), and there were no toxic deaths for either arm. Based on the data currently available, neither regimen seems clearly superior in terms of toxicity at this time.

CONCEPT 4: CARBOPLATIN IS INFERIOR IN ACHIEVING CURE FOR NONSEMINOMATOUS GERM CELL TUMORS

The MRC/EORTC conducted a trial from 1989 to 1993, in which 598 patients with good-risk GCT were randomized to four cycles of either BEP or BEC (bleomycin, etoposide, and carboplatin).[37] Etoposide was dosed 120 mg/m^2 on Days 1 to 3, and bleomycin was dosed 30 U on Day 2. On the BEP arm, cisplatin was dosed either 20 mg/m^2 Days 1 to 5 or 50 mg/m^2 Days 1 to 2. On the BEC arm, carboplatin was administered at a dose of area under the curve 5 on Day 1 of each 21-day cycle. BEP showed statistically significant improvement in complete response rates: 94.4%, compared with 87.3% with BEC ($P = .009$). The 3-year survival rate for BEP was 97% compared with 90% for BEC.

A multi-institutional study conducted in the United States from 1986 to 1990 randomized 270 Memorial Sloan Kettering Cancer Center criteria good-risk NSGCT patients to receive either four cycles of EP or EC (etoposide, carboplatin).[38] Etoposide was dosed 100 mg/m^2 on Days 1 to 5. For the EP arm, cisplatin was dosed 20 mg/m^2 Days 1 to 5, whereas on the EC arm, carboplatin was dosed at 500 mg/m^2 on Day 1 alone. Complete response rates were 90% and 88% for EP and EC, respectively. Relapse rates were 3% for EP compared with 12% for EC. At median follow-up of 22.4 months, event-free and relapse-free survival were inferior for patients receiving EC ($P = .02$ and $P = .005$, respectively).

CONCEPT/CONTROVERSY 5: ADDRESSING SURVIVORSHIP NEEDS OF PATIENTS WITH GERM CELL TUMOR

Germ cell tumors affect young men at a vulnerable time period, during college or early in their career, and often before fatherhood. This results in unique psychosocial considerations, sources of stress, and survivorship concerns. Cardiovascular disease and malignancy represent major causes of mortality for survivors. Long-term complications of treatment of GCTs are also significant and must be considered. These are summarized in **Table 3** and explored in detail next. Although increasing data have become available about the long-term consequences of chemotherapy for GCT, much less is known about how to mitigate

these effects, and whether specific surveillance practices are effective.

Cardiovascular Effects

Major cardiac events, including myocardial infarction or angina pectoris with proved myocardial ischemia, are estimated to occur among 5% to 7% of patients receiving chemotherapy for GCT.[39–43] A long-term follow-up study of 990 testicular cancer survivors in Norway found that survivors treated with BEP had a 5.7 times (95% CI, 1.9–17.1) higher risk of coronary arterial disease compared with survivors treated with surgery alone, and a 3.1 times higher risk (95% CI, 1.2–7.7) of myocardial infarction compared with age-matched men from the general population.[43] A longitudinal study of serial echocardiography among 37 patients with GCT treated with cisplatin-containing chemotherapy demonstrated a gradual decline in diastolic function over 7 years.[44] Mechanisms for cisplatin-related cardiovascular disease include inflammation induced by cytokine release[45] and reactive oxygen species.[46] Animal models suggest that cisplatin impairs cardiac contractility and coronary flow,[47] with the potential for direct myocardial injury.[48] Thrombosis may be induced via platelet aggregation and thromboxane formation,[49] and release of plasminogen activator inhibitor, von Willebrand factor, and tissue-type plasminogen activator.[50,51] Chemotherapy has been shown to cause vasoconstriction and arterial narrowing,[52] as seen in patients who develop Raynaud phenomenon. These effects have been reported up to 20 years after treatment.[53,54] Although classically associated with bleomycin, cisplatin may also contribute to Raynaud phenomenon.[55]

Further contribution to cardiovascular risk occurs via chemotherapy effects on hypertension, obesity, dyslipidemia, and insulin resistance. Studies indicate that survivors of GCT receiving chemotherapy have at least double the risk of metabolic syndrome compared with those who received other treatment modalities.[56,57] A study of 1289 survivors of GCT with median follow-up of 11.2 years identified higher rates of hypertension and obesity in chemotherapy patients, with higher risk in the group receiving greater than 850 mg cisplatin.[58] Low testosterone levels may also contribute to the development of metabolic syndrome in patients with GCT treated with chemotherapy.[59] Although studies are lacking, at a minimum, survivors of GCT should receive standard age-appropriate evaluation of cardiovascular risk factors, with counseling about diet and exercise. When to begin such evaluation and

Table 3
Chemotherapy-related long-term toxicities in survivors of germ cell cancer

	Causative Agent	Cumulative Dose	Incidence	Interventions to Mitigate Risk
Cardiovascular				
Coronary artery disease (MI, angina, SCD)	Cisplatin	—	5%–7%[38-42]	Lifestyle modifications (diet, exercise); smoking cessation; control blood pressure, glucose, and lipids; weight management; consider aspirin (based on CHD risk)
Raynaud phenomenon	Bleomycin, cisplatin, vinblastine	—	15%–45%[51-54]	Role of calcium channel blockers has not been established
Thromboembolic events (arterial or venous)	Cisplatin	—	8%–19%	Prophylactic anticoagulation, mechanical thromboprophylaxis (compression stockings or devices)
Second Malignancy				
Solid tumors	Cisplatin	—	—	Age-appropriate screening, smoking cessation, consider MRI instead of CT to minimize radiation exposure (unproven)
Hematologic malignancies[a]	Etoposide[64]	<2 g/m^2	0.4%–0.6%	Consider MRI instead of CT to minimize radiation exposure (unproven)
	Cisplatin	≥2 g/m^2	1.3%–2%	
Neurologic				
Neuropathy	Cisplatin Bleomycin	300 mg/m^2	20%–30%[53]	Avoid neurotoxins, including alcohol; avoid hypomagnesemia; symptom management with duloxetine; consider complementary therapy (eg acupuncture, physical therapy)
Ototoxicity	Cisplatin	400 mg/m^2	20%–22%[70]	Avoid exposure to loud noise, consider audiogram if high risk or symptomatic
Cognitive impairment	Unknown	—	15%–29%[b]	Monitor for symptoms, early referral for neurologic testing, psychosocial support
Other				
Pulmonary toxicity	Bleomycin	>550 U	17%	Monitor pulmonary function tests, avoid high concentrations of inspired oxygen
Nephrotoxicity	Cisplatin	500 mg/m^2	10%–30%[76]	Slower infusion rate, saline diuresis; avoid nephrotoxins; monitor serum creatinine
Infertility	Cisplatin	>400 mg/m^2 or 850 mg	10%–40%[86-88]	Sperm banking, referral to reproductive specialist
Hypogonadism	Cisplatin	>400 mg/m^2	11%–53%[b,91,92]	Monitor for symptoms and consider routine monitoring for testosterone levels

Abbreviations: CHD, coronary heart disease; CT, computed tomography; MI, myocardial infarction; SCD, sudden cardiac death.
[a] Hematologic malignancies include acute leukemias and myelodysplastic syndromes.
[b] Reported incidence varies, depending on criteria used.

education, and how to effectively mitigate cardiac risk, remains undefined.

Secondary Malignancies

Second malignancy has been identified as a significant cause of mortality among survivors of testicular cancer. Aside from the 12-fold higher risk of contralateral testicular cancer,[60] a population-based study of 40,576 survivors of GCT found increased risk of solid tumors for patients with GCT treated with chemotherapy (relative risk, 1.8; 95% CI, 1.3–2.5).[61] This was confirmed by a separate study of 2707 survivors of GCT, with median follow-up of 17.6 years, reporting a 2.1 times increased risk of secondary cancer among those treated with cisplatin-containing chemotherapy.[42]

The risk of developing hematologic malignancies, particularly leukemia and myelodysplastic syndrome, is also increased by chemotherapy for GCT. Acute myeloid leukemia related to prior therapy with alkylating agents classically involves a preceding myelodysplastic syndrome with deletions in chromosomes 5 or 7, and a latency period of 5 to 10 years,[62] whereas leukemia related to topoisomerase II inhibitors has a shorter latency of 1 to 5 years, does not involve myelodysplastic syndrome, and is associated with balanced translocations of chromosome bands 11q23 (MLL gene) and 21q22 (RUNX1 gene).[63]

A case-control study of 18,567 survivors of GCT reported a dose-dependent association between cisplatin and secondary leukemia; the relative risk increased from 3.2 (95% CI, 1.5–8.4) for cumulative cisplatin dose of 650 mg to 5.9 (95% CI, 2.0–26) when cumulative cisplatin dose was greater than 1000 mg.[64] Treatment-related leukemia associated with etoposide also seems to be dose-dependent. For cumulative etoposide doses greater than 2 g/m^2, the reported incidence of secondary hematologic malignancy is 1.3%, which is two to three times higher than that of patients receiving cumulative etoposide less than 2 g/m^2.[65] No specific guidelines exist regarding surveillance for secondary solid or hematologic malignancies aside from clinical history and physical examination, which must include assessment of the contralateral testicle.

Neurologic Toxicities

Peripheral neuropathy typically manifests as "stocking-glove" pattern paresthesias and dysesthesias, or reduced proprioception and vibratory sensation, and can create significant long-term morbidity for survivors of GCT.[53] The mechanism of cisplatin neuropathy involves platinum-DNA binding, which preferentially binds to and causes apoptosis of dorsal root ganglion cells.[66] Cisplatin-induced neuropathy occurs in 20% to 30% of survivors of testicular cancer,[54] in a dose-dependent manner,[53,67] and usually beginning at cumulative doses greater than 300 mg/m^2.[68] Cisplatin neurotoxicity has been correlated with low serum magnesium levels.[69]

Similarly, cisplatin can damage the outer hair cells in the organ of Corti,[70] resulting in chronic tinnitus or high-frequency hearing loss. Ototoxicity occurs in a dose-dependent manner[53,67] with persistent ototoxicity affecting 20% of patients receiving standard dose cisplatin, but increasing to more than 50% with higher cisplatin doses greater than 400 mg/m^2.[71] Slow infusion rates may reduce the risk of cisplatin ototoxicity.[72] A third form of neurotoxicity may be cognitive impairment,[73] although the contribution of chemotherapy remains unclear.[74,75] At least one study suggested there may be a dose-dependent association between chemotherapy and cognitive decline at 12-month follow-up.[76] The lack of consensus regarding optimal instruments for evaluating cognitive function limits the ability to quantify risk, or to perform interventional studies to mitigate potential risk.

Renal Toxicity

Long-term renal toxicity occurs in approximately 20% to 30% of survivors of GCT following cisplatin therapy,[77] with multiple studies consistently demonstrating a 20% to 30% decrease in GFR.[77–79] The degree of renal dysfunction seems closely related to the cumulative cisplatin dose.[80,81] Multiple mechanisms have been described, including direct platinum damage to epithelial cells of the proximal tubule,[82] formation of reactive oxygen species,[46] renal vasoconstriction,[83] and proinflammatory effects.[45] Slower infusions,[84] saline hydration,[85] and diuresis[86] are beneficial in reducing the risk of nephrotoxicity.

Gonadal Effects

Fertility is an important issue for young men diagnosed with testicular cancer. Infertility occurs in 10% to 35% of patients with GCT,[87–89] and nearly half of patients with GCT have defective spermatogenesis before orchiectomy.[90] Cisplatin induces azospermia in a dose-dependent manner.[91] Conception rates are also lower among men receiving higher cumulative doses of cisplatin: 38% for men who received greater than 850 mg compared with 62% in men who received less than or equal to 850 mg.[87] Hypogonadism also occurs in survivors of GCT following chemotherapy.[92,93] In addition to infertility, hypogonadism negatively impacts sexual functioning.[88] All men with good-risk NSGCT should be offered sperm banking before chemotherapy treatment, and monitoring of testosterone levels should be considered part of standard surveillance.

Psychosocial Effects

Although survivors of GCT achieve equitable rates of employment[94] with the general population and report high quality of life,[95] they face significant psychological and social stressors. Compared with the general population, survivors of GCT experience higher rates of chronic cancer-related fatigue,[96] anxiety,[97] and sexual dysfunction.[88,98,99] Up to two-thirds of survivors report unmet needs including life stress and fear of cancer recurrence; this association is stronger with younger patients and those with chronic illnesses.[100] Adolescent and young adult programs are developing in cancer centers, with the goal of better understanding and addressing the needs of patients with GCT, and other young cancer survivors.

SUMMARY

Young men with good-risk GCTs have an excellent prognosis for cure with cisplatin-based chemotherapy and surgical resection. Risks of chemotherapy include short- and long-term toxicities, which may influence the decision to use three cycles of BEP or four cycles of EP. Further studies must investigate survivorship interventions for this unique population of long-term cancer survivors.

REFERENCES

1. Siegel RL, Miller KD, Jemal A, et al. Cancer statistics, 2015. CA Cancer J Clin 2015;65(1):5–29.
2. International Germ Cell Consensus Classification: a prognostic factor-based staging system for metastatic germ cell cancers. International Germ Cell Cancer Collaborative Group. J Clin Oncol 1997; 15(2):594–603.
3. Einhorn LH, Donohue J. Cis-diamminedichloroplatinum, vinblastine, and bleomycin combination chemotherapy in disseminated testicular cancer. Ann Intern Med 1977;87(3):293–8.
4. Williams SD, Einhorn LH, Greco FA, et al. VP-16-213 salvage therapy for refractory germinal neoplasms. Cancer 1980;46(10):2154–8.
5. Cavalli F, Klepp O, Renard J, et al. A phase II study of oral VP-16-213 in non-seminomatous testicular cancer. Eur J Cancer 1981;17(2):245–9.
6. Fitzharris BM, Kaye SB, Saverymuttu S, et al. VP16-213 as a single agent in advanced testicular tumors. Eur J Cancer 1980;16(9):1193–7.
7. Williams SD, Birch R, Einhorn LH, et al. Treatment of disseminated germ-cell tumors with cisplatin, bleomycin, and either vinblastine or etoposide. N Engl J Med 1987;316(23):1435–40.
8. Hendry WF, Norman AR, Dearnaley DP, et al. Metastatic nonseminomatous germ cell tumors of the testis: results of elective and salvage surgery for patients with residual retroperitoneal masses. Cancer 2002;94(6):1668–76.
9. Baniel J, Foster RS, Gonin R, et al. Late relapse of testicular cancer. J Clin Oncol 1995;13(5):1170–6.
10. Albers P, Siener R, Krege S, et al. Randomized phase III trial comparing retroperitoneal lymph node dissection with one course of bleomycin and etoposide plus cisplatin chemotherapy in the adjuvant treatment of clinical stage I nonseminomatous testicular germ cell tumors: AUO trial AH 01/94 by the German Testicular Cancer Study Group. J Clin Oncol 2008;26(18):2966–72.
11. Einhorn LH, Williams SD, Loehrer PJ, et al. Evaluation of optimal duration of chemotherapy in favorable-prognosis disseminated germ cell tumors: a Southeastern Cancer Study Group protocol. J Clin Oncol 1989;7(3):387–91.
12. de Wit R, Roberts JT, Wilkinson PM, et al. Equivalence of three or four cycles of bleomycin, etoposide, and cisplatin chemotherapy and of a 3- or 5-day schedule in good-prognosis germ cell cancer: a randomized study of the European Organization for Research and Treatment of Cancer Genitourinary Tract Cancer Cooperative Group and the Medical Research Council. J Clin Oncol 2001;19(6):1629–40.
13. Toner GC, Stockler MR, Boyer MJ, et al. Comparison of two standard chemotherapy regimens for good-prognosis germ-cell tumours: a randomised trial. Australian and New Zealand Germ Cell Trial Group. Lancet 2001;357(9258):739–45.
14. Umezawa H, Maeda K, Takeuchi T, et al. New antibiotics, bleomycin A and B. J Antibiot (Tokyo) 1966; 19(5):200–9.
15. Sausville EA, Peisach J, Horwitz SB. Effect of chelating agents and metal ions on the degradation of DNA by bleomycin. Biochemistry 1978; 17(14):2740–6.
16. Levi JA, Raghavan D, Harvey V, et al. The importance of bleomycin in combination chemotherapy for good-prognosis germ cell carcinoma. Australasian Germ Cell Trial Group. J Clin Oncol 1993;11(7):1300–5.
17. Bosl GJ, Geller NL, Bajorin D, et al. A randomized trial of etoposide + cisplatin versus vinblastine + bleomycin + cisplatin + cyclophosphamide + dactinomycin in patients with good-prognosis germ cell tumors. J Clin Oncol 1988;6(8):1231–8.

18. Culine S, Kerbrat P, Kramar A, et al. Refining the optimal chemotherapy regimen for good-risk metastatic nonseminomatous germ-cell tumors: a randomized trial of the Genito-Urinary Group of the French Federation of Cancer Centers (GETUG T93BP). Ann Oncol 2007;18(5):917–24.

19. Motzer RJ, Agarwal N, Beard C, et al. NCCN clinical practice guidelines in oncology: testicular cancer. J Natl Compr Canc Netw 2009;7(6):672–93.

20. Santrach PJ, Askin FB, Wells RJ, et al. Nodular form of bleomycin-related pulmonary injury in patients with osteogenic sarcoma. Cancer 1989; 64(4):806–11.

21. Holoye PY, Luna MA, MacKay B, et al. Bleomycin hypersensitivity pneumonitis. Ann Intern Med 1978;88(1):47–9.

22. Jules-Elysee K, White DA. Bleomycin-induced pulmonary toxicity. Clin Chest Med 1990;11(1):1–20.

23. Simpson AB, Paul J, Graham J, et al. Fatal bleomycin pulmonary toxicity in the west of Scotland 1991-95: a review of patients with germ cell tumours. Br J Cancer 1998;78(8):1061–6.

24. Comis RL, Kuppinger MS, Ginsberg SJ, et al. Role of single-breath carbon monoxide-diffusing capacity in monitoring the pulmonary effects of bleomycin in germ cell tumor patients. Cancer Res 1979; 39(12):5076–80.

25. Sleijfer S, van der Mark TW, Schraffordt Koops H, et al. Decrease in pulmonary function during bleomycin-containing combination chemotherapy for testicular cancer: not only a bleomycin effect. Br J Cancer 1995;71(1):120–3.

26. Blum RH, Carter SK, Agre K. A clinical review of bleomycin–a new antineoplastic agent. Cancer 1973;31(4):903–14.

27. Wilson KS, Worth A, Richards AG, et al. Low-dose bleomycin lung. Med Pediatr Oncol 1982;10(3): 283–8.

28. O'Sullivan JM, Huddart RA, Norman AR, et al. Predicting the risk of bleomycin lung toxicity in patients with germ-cell tumours. Ann Oncol 2003; 14(1):91–6.

29. Haugnes HS, Aass N, Fossa SD, et al. Pulmonary function in long-term survivors of testicular cancer. J Clin Oncol 2009;27(17):2779–86.

30. Lehne G, Johansen B, Fossa SD. Long-term follow-up of pulmonary function in patients cured from testicular cancer with combination chemotherapy including bleomycin. Br J Cancer 1993;68(3):555–8.

31. Fossa SD, Kaye SB, Mead GM, et al. Filgrastim during combination chemotherapy of patients with poor-prognosis metastatic germ cell malignancy. European Organization for Research and Treatment of Cancer, Genito-Urinary Group, and the Medical Research Council Testicular Cancer Working Party, Cambridge, United Kingdom. J Clin Oncol 1998;16(2):716–24.

32. Saxman SB, Nichols CR, Einhorn LH. Pulmonary toxicity in patients with advanced-stage germ cell tumors receiving bleomycin with and without granulocyte colony stimulating factor. Chest 1997; 111(3):657–60.

33. Pont J, Albrecht W. Fertility after chemotherapy for testicular germ cell cancer. Fertil Steril 1997;68(1): 1–5.

34. Thompson SW, Davis LE, Kornfeld M, et al. Cisplatin neuropathy. Clinical, electrophysiologic, morphologic, and toxicologic studies. Cancer 1984;54(7):1269–75.

35. von Schlippe M, Fowler CJ, Harland SJ. Cisplatin neurotoxicity in the treatment of metastatic germ cell tumour: time course and prognosis. Br J Cancer 2001;85(6):823–6.

36. Dieckmann KP, Gerl A, Witt J, et al. Myocardial infarction and other major vascular events during chemotherapy for testicular cancer. Ann Oncol 2010;21(8):1607–11.

37. Horwich A, Sleijfer DT, Fossa SD, et al. Randomized trial of bleomycin, etoposide, and cisplatin compared with bleomycin, etoposide, and carboplatin in good-prognosis metastatic nonseminomatous germ cell cancer: a Multiinstitutional Medical Research Council/European Organization for Research and Treatment of Cancer Trial. J Clin Oncol 1997;15(5):1844–52.

38. Bajorin DF, Sarosdy MF, Pfister DG, et al. Randomized trial of etoposide and cisplatin versus etoposide and carboplatin in patients with good-risk germ cell tumors: a multiinstitutional study. J Clin Oncol 1993;11(4):598–606.

39. Meinardi MT, Gietema JA, van der Graaf WT, et al. Cardiovascular morbidity in long-term survivors of metastatic testicular cancer. J Clin Oncol 2000; 18(8):1725–32.

40. Huddart RA, Norman A, Shahidi M, et al. Cardiovascular disease as a long-term complication of treatment for testicular cancer. J Clin Oncol 2003; 21(8):1513–23.

41. van den Belt-Dusebout AW, Nuver J, de Wit R, et al. Long-term risk of cardiovascular disease in 5-year survivors of testicular cancer. J Clin Oncol 2006; 24(3):467–75.

42. van den Belt-Dusebout AW, de Wit R, Gietema JA, et al. Treatment-specific risks of second malignancies and cardiovascular disease in 5-year survivors of testicular cancer. J Clin Oncol 2007;25(28):4370–8.

43. Haugnes HS, Wethal T, Aass N, et al. Cardiovascular risk factors and morbidity in long-term survivors of testicular cancer: a 20-year follow-up study. J Clin Oncol 2010;28(30):4649–57.

44. Altena R, Hummel YM, Nuver J, et al. Longitudinal changes in cardiac function after cisplatin-based chemotherapy for testicular cancer. Ann Oncol 2011;22(10):2286–93.

45. Ramesh G, Reeves WB. TNF-alpha mediates chemokine and cytokine expression and renal injury in cisplatin nephrotoxicity. J Clin Invest 2002; 110(6):835–42.

46. Davis CA, Nick HS, Agarwal A. Manganese superoxide dismutase attenuates cisplatin-induced renal injury: importance of superoxide. J Am Soc Nephrol 2001;12(12):2683–90.

47. Misic MM, Jakovljevic VL, Bugarcic ZD, et al. Platinum complexes-induced cardiotoxicity of isolated, perfused rat heart: comparison of Pt(II) and Pt(IV) analogues versus cisplatin. Cardiovasc Toxicol 2015;15(3):261–8.

48. El-Awady el SE, Moustafa YM, Abo-Elmatty DM, et al. Cisplatin-induced cardiotoxicity: mechanisms and cardioprotective strategies. Eur J Pharmacol 2011;650(1):335–41.

49. Togna GI, Togna AR, Franconi M, et al. Cisplatin triggers platelet activation. Thromb Res 2000; 99(5):503–9.

50. Nuver J, Smit AJ, Sleijfer DT, et al. Microalbuminuria, decreased fibrinolysis, and inflammation as early signs of atherosclerosis in long-term survivors of disseminated testicular cancer. Eur J Cancer 2004;40(5):701–6.

51. Nuver J, Smit AJ, van der Meer J, et al. Acute chemotherapy-induced cardiovascular changes in patients with testicular cancer. J Clin Oncol 2005; 23(36):9130–7.

52. Hansen SW, Olsen N. Raynaud's phenomenon in patients treated with cisplatin, vinblastine, and bleomycin for germ cell cancer: measurement of vasoconstrictor response to cold. J Clin Oncol 1989;7(7):940–2.

53. Brydoy M, Oldenburg J, Klepp O, et al. Observational study of prevalence of long-term Raynaud-like phenomena and neurological side effects in testicular cancer survivors. J Natl Cancer Inst 2009;101(24):1682–95.

54. Glendenning JL, Barbachano Y, Norman AR, et al. Long-term neurologic and peripheral vascular toxicity after chemotherapy treatment of testicular cancer. Cancer 2010;116(10):2322–31.

55. Vogelzang NJ, Bosl GJ, Johnson K, et al. Raynaud's phenomenon: a common toxicity after combination chemotherapy for testicular cancer. Ann Intern Med 1981;95(3):288–92.

56. Haugnes HS, Aass N, Fossa SD, et al. Components of the metabolic syndrome in long-term survivors of testicular cancer. Ann Oncol 2007;18(2):241–8.

57. Willemse PM, Burggraaf J, Hamdy NA, et al. Prevalence of the metabolic syndrome and cardiovascular disease risk in chemotherapy-treated testicular germ cell tumour survivors. Br J Cancer 2013;109(1):60–7.

58. Sagstuen H, Aass N, Fossa SD, et al. Blood pressure and body mass index in long-term survivors of testicular cancer. J Clin Oncol 2005;23(22): 4980–90.

59. Nuver J, Smit AJ, Wolffenbuttel BH, et al. The metabolic syndrome and disturbances in hormone levels in long-term survivors of disseminated testicular cancer. J Clin Oncol 2005;23(16):3718–25.

60. Fossa SD, Chen J, Schonfeld SJ, et al. Risk of contralateral testicular cancer: a population-based study of 29,515 U.S. men. J Natl Cancer Inst 2005;97(14):1056–66.

61. Travis LB, Fossa SD, Schonfeld SJ, et al. Second cancers among 40,576 testicular cancer patients: focus on long-term survivors. J Natl Cancer Inst 2005;97(18):1354–65.

62. Smith SM, Le Beau MM, Huo D, et al. Clinical-cytogenetic associations in 306 patients with therapy-related myelodysplasia and myeloid leukemia: the University of Chicago series. Blood 2003;102(1):43–52.

63. Pedersen-Bjergaard J, Daugaard G, Hansen SW, et al. Increased risk of myelodysplasia and leukaemia after etoposide, cisplatin, and bleomycin for germ-cell tumours. Lancet 1991;338(8763): 359–63.

64. Travis LB, Andersson M, Gospodarowicz M, et al. Treatment-associated leukemia following testicular cancer. J Natl Cancer Inst 2000; 92(14):1165–71.

65. Nichols CR, Breeden ES, Loehrer PJ, et al. Secondary leukemia associated with a conventional dose of etoposide: review of serial germ cell tumor protocols. J Natl Cancer Inst 1993;85(1):36–40.

66. Ta LE, Espeset L, Podratz J, et al. Neurotoxicity of oxaliplatin and cisplatin for dorsal root ganglion neurons correlates with platinum-DNA binding. Neurotoxicology 2006;27(6):992–1002.

67. Sprauten M, Darrah TH, Peterson DR, et al. Impact of long-term serum platinum concentrations on neuro- and ototoxicity in cisplatin-treated survivors of testicular cancer. J Clin Oncol 2012;30(3):300–7.

68. Tuxen MK, Hansen SW. Neurotoxicity secondary to antineoplastic drugs. Cancer Treat Rev 1994;20(2): 191–214.

69. Bokemeyer C, Berger CC, Kuczyk MA, et al. Evaluation of long-term toxicity after chemotherapy for testicular cancer. J Clin Oncol 1996;14(11):2923–32.

70. Rybak LP, Whitworth CA, Mukherjea D, et al. Mechanisms of cisplatin-induced ototoxicity and prevention. Hear Res 2007;226(1–2):157–67.

71. Bokemeyer C, Berger CC, Hartmann JT, et al. Analysis of risk factors for cisplatin-induced ototoxicity in patients with testicular cancer. Br J Cancer 1998;77(8):1355–62.

72. Reddel RR, Kefford RF, Grant JM, et al. Ototoxicity in patients receiving cisplatin: importance of dose and method of drug administration. Cancer Treat Rep 1982;66(1):19–23.

73. Skaali T, Fossa SD, Dahl AA. A prospective study of cognitive complaints in patients with testicular cancer. Clin Genitourin Cancer 2011;9(1):6–13.

74. Schagen SB, Boogerd W, Muller MJ, et al. Cognitive complaints and cognitive impairment following BEP chemotherapy in patients with testicular cancer. Acta Oncol 2008;47(1):63–70.

75. Skaali T, Fossa SD, Andersson S, et al. Self-reported cognitive problems in testicular cancer patients: relation to neuropsychological performance, fatigue, and psychological distress. J Psychosom Res 2011;70(5):403–10.

76. Wefel JS, Vidrine DJ, Marani SK, et al. A prospective study of cognitive function in men with non-seminomatous germ cell tumors. Psychooncology 2014;23(6):626–33.

77. Fossa SD, Aass N, Winderen M, et al. Long-term renal function after treatment for malignant germ-cell tumours. Ann Oncol 2002;13(2):222–8.

78. Meijer S, Sleijfer DT, Mulder NH, et al. Some effects of combination chemotherapy with cis-platinum on renal function in patients with nonseminomatous testicular carcinoma. Cancer 1983; 51(11):2035–40.

79. MacLeod PM, Tyrell CJ, Keeling DH. The effect of cisplatin on renal function in patients with testicular tumours. Clin Radiol 1988;39(2):190–2.

80. Aass N, Fossa SD, Aas M, et al. Renal function related to different treatment modalities for malignant germ cell tumours. Br J Cancer 1990;62(5): 842–6.

81. Cost NG, Adibi M, Lubahn JD, et al. Effect of testicular germ cell tumor therapy on renal function. Urology 2012;80(3):641–8.

82. Dobyan DC, Levi J, Jacobs C, et al. Mechanism of cis-platinum nephrotoxicity: II. Morphologic observations. J Pharmacol Exp Ther 1980;213(3):551–6.

83. Winston JA, Safirstein R. Reduced renal blood flow in early cisplatin-induced acute renal failure in the rat. Am J Physiol 1985;249(4 Pt 2):F490–496.

84. Reece PA, Stafford I, Russell J, et al. Creatinine clearance as a predictor of ultrafilterable platinum disposition in cancer patients treated with cisplatin: relationship between peak ultrafilterable platinum plasma levels and nephrotoxicity. J Clin Oncol 1987;5(2):304–9.

85. Dumas M, de Gislain C, d'Athis P, et al. Influence of hydration on ultrafilterable platinum kinetics and kidney function in patients treated with cis-diamminedichloroplatinum(II). Cancer Chemother Pharmacol 1990;26(4):278–82.

86. Hayes DM, Cvitkovic E, Golbey RB, et al. High dose cis-platinum diammine dichloride: amelioration of renal toxicity by mannitol diuresis. Cancer 1977;39(4):1372–81.

87. Brydoy M, Fossa SD, Klepp O, et al. Paternity following treatment for testicular cancer. J Natl Cancer Inst 2005;97(21):1580–8.

88. Huddart RA, Norman A, Moynihan C, et al. Fertility, gonadal and sexual function in survivors of testicular cancer. Br J Cancer 2005;93(2):200–7.

89. Kim C, McGlynn KA, McCorkle R, et al. Quality of life among testicular cancer survivors: a case-control study in the United States. Qual Life Res 2011;20(10):1629–37.

90. Petersen PM, Skakkebaek NE, Vistisen K, et al. Semen quality and reproductive hormones before orchiectomy in men with testicular cancer. J Clin Oncol 1999;17(3):941–7.

91. Petersen PM, Hansen SW, Giwercman A, et al. Dose-dependent impairment of testicular function in patients treated with cisplatin-based chemotherapy for germ cell cancer. Ann Oncol 1994; 5(4):355–8.

92. Sprauten M, Brydoy M, Haugnes HS, et al. Longitudinal serum testosterone, luteinizing hormone, and follicle-stimulating hormone levels in a population-based sample of long-term testicular cancer survivors. J Clin Oncol 2014;32(6):571–8.

93. Gerl A, Muhlbayer D, Hansmann G, et al. The impact of chemotherapy on Leydig cell function in long term survivors of germ cell tumors. Cancer 2001;91(7):1297–303.

94. de Boer AG, Taskila T, Ojajarvi A, et al. Cancer survivors and unemployment: a meta-analysis and meta-regression. JAMA 2009;301(7):753–62.

95. Rossen PB, Pedersen AF, Zachariae R, et al. Health-related quality of life in long-term survivors of testicular cancer. J Clin Oncol 2009;27(35): 5993–9.

96. Orre IJ, Fossa SD, Murison R, et al. Chronic cancer-related fatigue in long-term survivors of testicular cancer. J Psychosom Res 2008;64(4): 363–71.

97. Dahl AA, Haaland CF, Mykletun A, et al. Study of anxiety disorder and depression in long-term survivors of testicular cancer. J Clin Oncol 2005;23(10): 2389–95.

98. Nazareth I, Lewin J, King M. Sexual dysfunction after treatment for testicular cancer: a systematic review. J Psychosom Res 2001;51(6):735–43.

99. Dahl AA, Bremnes R, Dahl O, et al. Is the sexual function compromised in long-term testicular cancer survivors? Eur Urol 2007;52(5):1438–47.

100. Smith AB, King M, Butow P, et al. The prevalence and correlates of supportive care needs in testicular cancer survivors: a cross-sectional study. Psychooncology 2013;22(11):2557–64.

Late Relapse of Testicular Germ Cell Tumors

Matthew J. O'Shaughnessy, MD, PhD[a], Darren R. Feldman, MD[b], Brett S. Carver, MD[a], Joel Sheinfeld, MD[a],*

KEYWORDS

- Germ cell tumor • Late relapse • Retroperitoneal lymph node dissection

KEY POINTS

- Late relapse affects approximately 1% to 6% of patients with germ cell tumors and may develop after more than 30 years, necessitating long-term follow-up of patients with germ cell tumor.
- The most common site of late relapse is the retroperitoneum, possibly related to suboptimal treatment of the retroperitoneum at the time of initial diagnosis and management.
- The histology of late recurrence is distinct, with more aggressive biology, including somatic malignant transformation, than that found at retroperitoneal lymph node dissection for primary germ cell tumor.
- The overall prognosis of late relapse is poor, and treatment requires an experienced multidisciplinary team, and most often requires surgery.

INTRODUCTION

Germ cell tumors (GCTs) of the testis have favorable prognosis, with overall survival rates higher than 90% for all stages when properly managed by a multidisciplinary approach.[1] Because most GCT relapses occur within 24 months, it was historically considered that 2-year disease-free survival was equivalent to cure.[2] As the experience with GCT accrued, it was noted that late relapse (LR), defined as relapse after a 2-year disease-free interval in the absence of a second primary tumor, was a distinct clinical entity.[3] The incidence of LR in patients who have achieved complete response (CR) is reported to be 1% to 6%, although because most reports are from referral centers, it is difficult to precisely define the incidence.[3–9] In a pooled analysis of 7 studies comprising 5880 patients,[10] the estimated incidence of LR is 3.2% in nonseminomatous GCT (NSGCT) and 1.4% in seminoma, and based on referral patterns, the incidence of LR may be increasing.[11] Factors associated with LR of GCT include the presence of bulky adenopathy at the time of initial presentation[5–7] and teratoma at postchemotherapy retroperitoneal lymph node dissection (RPLND).[6,12,13]

LR is a distinct clinical entity based on clinical presentation, pattern of histology, and poor overall survival, and the successful management of LR is one of the important challenges of contemporary management of testicular GCT. In this review, the data regarding the clinical presentation and detection of LR, clinical outcomes, and predictors of survival in LR are presented, and the importance of a multidisciplinary treatment approach for successful management of LR is discussed.

Disclosures: the authors have nothing to disclose.
Funding: supported by The Richard E. Capri Foundation and The Sidney Kimmel Center for Prostate and Urologic Cancers.
[a] Urology Service, Department of Surgery, Memorial Sloan Kettering Cancer Center, 353 East 68th Street, New York, NY 10065, USA; [b] Genitourinary Oncology Service, Department of Medicine, Memorial Sloan Kettering Cancer Center, 353 East 68th Street, New York, NY 10065, USA
* Corresponding author.
E-mail address: sheinfej@mskcc.org

Urol Clin N Am 42 (2015) 359–368
http://dx.doi.org/10.1016/j.ucl.2015.04.010
0094-0143/15/$ – see front matter © 2015 Elsevier Inc. All rights reserved.

CLINICAL PRESENTATION AND DETECTION OF LATE RELAPSE

Detection of Late Relapse

LR is most commonly detected during routine follow-up of patients with GCT by detection of increased serum α-fetoprotein (AFP) or human chorionic gonadotropin (HCG) levels, radiographic findings, or clinical symptoms. In the 3 largest series of patients with LR, serum AFP is more commonly increased than HCG (**Table 1**).[7,12,14] In the pooled analysis by Oldenburg and colleagues,[10] this trend holds true: of 426 patients with LR, 207 (49%) had increased serum AFP and 100 (24%) had increased serum HCG levels.

Clinical symptoms including back pain or palpable abdominal mass may indicate LR in patients with GCT, although many patients present without symptoms. Dieckmann and colleagues[7] reported on 122 patients with LR, of whom 30% were symptomatic and 61% were detected incidentally at routine follow-up. In the Indiana and Memorial Sloan Kettering Cancer Center (MSKCC) series, more than 60% of patients were symptomatic at time of LR.[12,14] Early detection of LR before the onset of clinical symptoms may be critical to outcomes, because the presence of clinical symptoms at LR was associated with poorer cancer-specific survival (CSS) (hazard ratio [HR] = 4.9; 95% confidence interval [CI], 1.6–15.2)[14] and overall survival (HR = 3.74; 95% CI, 1.3–11.3)[12] in the MSKCC and Indiana series, although this was not confirmed in 2 other series.[7,9]

Time to Late Relapse

The median time to LR from CR to primary treatment is approximately 4 to 7 years.[7,12,14] Approximately 40% to 50% of LRs occur within 2 to 5 years of initial therapy and 50% to 60% present after more than 5 years.[3,14] More than 30% of LRs may present more than 10 years after CR, with the longest reported time to relapse 37.7 years.[14] The recognition that many LRs can present more than a decade after initial treatment underscores the critical importance of lifelong follow-up in patients with GCTs. Guidelines for follow-up are provided by the National Comprehensive Cancer Network, which recommends follow-up, including physical examination, serum tumor markers (STMs), and imaging, with decreased frequency over time corresponding with a decreased risk of relapse and annual follow-up starting at year 5.[15] Computed tomography (CT) is the standard for surveillance imaging, although there is some concern that radiation exposure from surveillance CT scans may increase the risk of secondary malignancy.[16] Use of magnetic resonance imaging[17] and low-dose CT[18] has been considered to lower the risks of radiation exposure; however, these techniques are unproved in surveillance of GCT. Risk-stratified surveillance has been suggested as a means to minimize radiation exposure, because the risk of recurrence decreases over time.[19]

Patterns of Late Relapse

The retroperitoneum is the most common site of LR, accounting for approximately 45% to 70% of the LRs, regardless of initial histology, treatment of primary, or clinical presentation (**Table 2**).[3,5,7,12,14] Other sites of LR can include the lungs, mediastinum, retrocrural space, neck/supraclavicular nodes, liver, brain, and pelvis. Multiple sites of LR have been reported in 36% to 52% patients.[5,12,14] Factors associated with development of LR include increased tumor burden at the time of primary therapy, absence of primary RPLND, and the presence of teratoma after primary therapy.[3,5,20]

CLINICAL OUTCOMES AND PREDICTORS OF SURVIVAL IN LATE RELAPSE

Disease recurrences more than 24 months after CR to primary treatment in chemotherapy-naive patients tend to show similar outcomes to patients presenting de novo with metastatic GCT.[14] LR after CR to treatment including chemotherapy portends a worse prognosis.[14] Because of the

Table 1
Clinical presentation of patients with LR of GCT

| Series | Total Number of Patients | Clinical Symptoms (%) | Number of Patients with | |
			Increased AFP Levels (%)	Increased HCG Levels (%)
George et al,[12] 2003	83	55 (66)	43 (52)	8 (10)
Sharp et al,[14] 2008	75	45 (60)	36 (48)	18 (24)
Dieckmann et al,[7] 2005	122	36 (30)	48/92 (52)	23/78 (29)

Table 2
Sites of disease in patients with LR of GCT

Series	Total Number of Patients	Number of Patients with Late Relapse in			
		Retroperitoneum (%)	Lungs (%)	Mediastinum (%)	Neck (%)
George et al,[12] 2003	83	39 (47)	21 (25)	8 (10)	7 (8)
Sharp et al,[14] 2008	75	54 (72)	15 (20)	9 (12)	8 (11)
Dieckmann et al,[7] 2005	122	71 (58)	8 (7)	14 (11)	10 (8)
Gerl et al,[5] 1997	25	12 (48)	2 (8)	8 (32)	1 (4)

disparate clinical outcomes based on primary treatment, we have advocated for defining LR only in the postchemotherapy setting. For the purposes of this review, we consider LR based on initial management of GCT and disease stage at presentation.

Late Relapse in Patients Initially Managed with Surveillance

Surveillance is a recognized management strategy for patients with clinical stage (CS) I GCT, and despite a low risk of relapse, most patients are salvaged. In a recent analysis by Kollmannsberger and colleagues,[21] 173 of 1344 (13%) patients with CSI seminoma relapsed overall, with 43 (3.2%) relapsing after 2 years, with all LRs either radiosensitive or chemosensitive. In a separate analysis of 638 patients followed with surveillance for CSI seminoma from 4 centers,[22] there were 38 relapses after 2 years (6% LR rate), with the latest relapse at 12 years. Risk factors for relapse included size of primary tumor, rete testis invasion, and lymphovascular invasion (LVI), although these risk factors have not been validated in other studies.[22] In a single-institution series at Princess Margaret Hospital,[23] 203 men with CSI seminoma were managed by surveillance, and the risk of relapse at 5 years was 4%.

The rate of LR after surveillance for CSI NSGCT is low, with some series having no cases of LR.[24,25] In the recent report by Kollmannsberger and colleagues,[21] of 1139 patients with CSI nonseminoma, 221 (19%) relapsed on surveillance, including 18 (1.6%) after 2 years. Seventeen of the 18 LRs were cured with standard therapy.[21] In another study of 233 patients who underwent surveillance for CSI NSGCT, 3% (7 patients) had LR and all patients were successfully salvaged with chemotherapy with or without RPLND for disease-specific survival of 100% at median follow-up 52 months (range 3–136 months).[26] With appropriate surveillance and early detection, it is possible to salvage most cases of LR.

Rice and colleagues[27] recently reported on a series of patients with LR after surveillance for CSI NSGCT referred to Indiana University. The median time to diagnosis of LR in 28 patients was 48.5 months but occurred as late as 27 years. Thirteen of 28 patients presented with increased STMs, with increased HCG levels in 9 of them. In contrast, AFP level is more commonly increased in all patients with LR.[7,12,14] The retroperitoneum was the dominant site of relapse in these patients, with 26 of 28 patients (94%) experiencing retroperitoneal relapse. The rate of LR in patients with CSI GCT is unknown, because these patients were largely referred from other institutions. Eight of 9 patients who had primary RPLND for LR in this series had viable malignancy, including 2 with secondary somatic malignancy and 1 with teratoma. Of the 19 patients who had postchemotherapy RPLND for LR of CSI GCT, 5 had viable malignancy, 4 had teratoma, and 10 had fibrosis in the RPLND specimen. Of the 13 patients with viable malignancy at RPLND (primary and postchemotherapy), there were 3 with secondary somatic malignancy and 4 died of their disease at median follow-up 21 months (range 1–237 months). Although 86% had no evidence of disease (NED) at last follow-up, these results highlight the potential of even CSI GCT to be lethal and underscores the need for diligent surveillance protocols.

Late Relapse After Adjuvant Radiotherapy or Chemotherapy for Clinical Stage I Seminoma

The LR rate after adjuvant therapy for CSI seminoma is very low. Only 4 of 2466 (0.2%) of patients had relapses after 3 years in results from 3 pooled randomized trials[28] of 20 versus 30 Gy radiotherapy,[29] para-aortic versus dogleg radiotherapy,[30] or radiotherapy versus single-dose carboplatin.[31] However, median follow-up of these studies is short, potentially limiting conclusions about LR.

In studies with longer follow-up, the overall relapse rate after adjuvant radiotherapy for CSI seminoma is reported to be 1.4% to 6.9%.[30,32] In a series of 194 patients treated with adjuvant radiotherapy for CSI seminoma at Princess Margaret Hospital, 11 experienced relapse with 2 relapses after more than 4 years.[33] In a recent study from Mayo Clinic,[34] in patients who received adjuvant radiotherapy for CSI seminoma, only 3 of 199 patients relapsed (1.5%) with 1 LR (median follow-up 13.7 years; range 0.1–37 years).

Powles and colleagues[35] reported an analysis of patients who received adjuvant single-agent chemotherapy for CSI seminoma. In this study of 199 patients with median follow-up of 9 years (range 0.1–20.1 years), 4 patients (2%) had LR. All patients with LR were successfully salvaged with cisplatin chemotherapy.

Late Relapse in Patients Initially Presenting with Low-Stage Nonseminomatous Germ Cell Tumors Managed with Retroperitoneal Lymph Node Dissection or Chemotherapy

A standard option for treatment of CSI/IIa NSGCT is bilateral infrahilar RPLND, and infield recurrences are rare after properly performed RPLND.[3,36,37] However, the retroperitoneum is the most common site of LR in patients with low-stage NSGCT primarily managed with RPLND, suggesting that an inadequately controlled retroperitoneum is a contributing factor and may be caused by inadequate initial management of the retroperitoneum with incomplete removal of lymphatic tissue as a result of surgical technique or modification of surgical templates. Of 19 patients initially treated with primary RPLND and referred to MSKCC for LR from 1990 to 2004, 11 (58%) had received chemotherapy (either adjuvant or for early relapse) before LR. Twelve of the 19 (63%) patients relapsed in the retroperitoneum, including 8 in the primary landing zone, suggesting that LR could have been prevented by proper management of the retroperitoneum at initial treatment. Five-year CSS after LR in patients treated with primary RPLND was 58% (95% CI, 31%–68%) in these patients.[14] In a series of 35 patients with LR reported by Indiana University, primary RPLND was performed in 31 (89%), including 19 (61%) who relapsed in the retroperitoneum despite having received adjuvant chemotherapy for pathologic stage II disease.[3] These results impress the importance of proper surgical management of the retroperitoneum and imply that 2 cycles of chemotherapy cannot compensate for inadequate RPLND.

Eggener and colleagues[38] reported that the use of modified RPLND templates would result in residual extratemplate retroperitoneal disease in 3% to 23% of patients depending on the template used. Carver and colleagues[39] showed that for men undergoing postchemotherapy RPLND for NSGCT, extratemplate disease is found in 4% to 32% of patients, depending on which modified template was used. In a series of 369 patients who had resection of postchemotherapy masses only (not full template),[40] there were 37 (10%) with retroperitoneal relapse.

A single cycle of bleomycin plus etoposide plus cisplatin (BEP) chemotherapy for patients with CSI NSGCT has been advocated by some,[17] with a reduction in relapse risk by approximately 90% compared with surveillance. In a recently published update of this series with median follow-up 7.9 years,[41] there were no LRs in 255 patients with stage CSIa NSGCT without LVI and relapses in 8 of 258 (3.2%) patients with LVI including 3 with LR. Because even 2 cycles of BEP do not eliminate the risk of LR in the adjuvant setting after early relapse, it is likely that as the data from this trial mature, there will also be a predictable increase of LR.

Late Relapse in Patients Initially Presenting with Advanced Stage Germ Cell Tumors

Patients presenting with metastatic GCT (ie, CSIIb or higher) are typically managed with cisplatin-based chemotherapy alone or combined with surgery, although some have advocated treating low stage II patients with surgery alone.[42,43] In the Indiana series there was a relapse rate of 35% in patients with low stage II disease treated with surgery alone but no relapses in patients with stage II disease who received 2 cycles of adjuvant cisplatin-based chemotherapy.[43] In patients with pathologic stage II NSGCT who received primary RPLND and 2 cycles of adjuvant chemotherapy, there were no LRs in 87 patients with median follow-up of 8 years in the MSKCC series.[44]

Ehrlich and colleagues[45] reported a series of 141 patients with metastatic disease who had CR to induction chemotherapy alone, with an overall 9% rate of relapse, including 5 patients (3.5%) with LR (from 3 to 13 years) at median follow-up time 15.5 years, including 2 in the retroperitoneum. As mentioned earlier, the most common site of LR in patients treated with induction chemotherapy is the retroperitoneum. Sharp and colleagues[14] analyzed 75 patients referred to MSKCC from 1990 to 2004 for LR and of the 45 treated with induction chemotherapy, 34 (76%) developed LR in the retroperitoneum, including 17 of 18 who did not have postchemotherapy RPLND. The 5-year CSS rate after LR in the 45 patients with LR after induction chemotherapy was 53% (95% CI, 36%–68%).

Using a combined regimen of induction chemotherapy and postchemotherapy RPLND seems effective at reducing the risk of relapse, with 5-year progression-free survival of 98%.[46] Kondagunta and colleagues[47] reported LR in 3 of 282 (1.1%) International Germ Cell Cancer Collaborative Group (IGCCCG) good-risk patients treated with 4 cycles of etoposide plus cisplatin induction chemotherapy. In a series of 418 patients reported by Gerl and colleagues[5] who received cisplatin-based induction chemotherapy with or without surgery for advanced GCT, the cumulative risk of LR was 1.1% at 5 years and 4.0% at 10 years. Previous early relapse and poor-risk disease (Medical Research Council criteria) were associated with higher risk of LR.

It has proved difficult to predict the presence of fibrosis and necrosis after induction chemotherapy. Even in patients with complete radiographic response to induction chemotherapy, viable malignancy or teratoma can be found in up to 30% of patients.[48,49] Complete resection of teratoma can convey several advantages to the patient. Teratoma is chemoresistant and may grow and invade adjacent structures or become unresectable.[50] Furthermore, there is a risk of malignant transformation to non–germ cell malignancies, including sarcoma or carcinoma. The incidence of malignant transformation in the postchemotherapy setting is 3% to 6%. These tumors do not respond to cisplatin-based chemotherapy regimens like GCTs, and complete surgical resection is the best treatment option for these patients.[51] Because it remains difficult to accurately predict fibrosis/necrosis and eliminate the risk of viable GCT or residual teratoma, a subset of patients who undergo induction chemotherapy alone or undergo incomplete RPLND may remain at risk for LR.

Histopathology of Late Relapse

The histology of the late recurrence is distinct, with more aggressive biology than that found at RPLND for primary GCT (**Table 3**). Whereas teratoma is found in approximately 20% to 30% of node-positive primary RPLND specimens[36] and approximately 40% of postchemotherapy RPLND specimens,[52] teratoma is found in up to 60% of patients with LR.[53] The incidence of somatic malignant transformation of teratoma is around 20% for patients with LR,[14,53] which is significantly increased compared with the rate noted in the MSKCC primary RPLND series (0.4%; 2 of 550 patients) and postchemotherapy series (18 of 532 patients; 3%).[52] The incidence of viable GCT in LR is approximately 60% to 70%[14,53] and significantly higher than the 10% found at postchemotherapy RPLND.[52] Yolk sac tumor is the most common nonteratomatous germ cell element in LR, but all other types can be found.[53] Because of the high rate of teratoma, somatic malignant transformation and chemoresistant viable GCT, late recurrence is not likely to respond to chemotherapy and is best treated with surgical excision. Attempts to define the molecular basis for chemoresistance have been unsuccessful.[12]

PROGNOSIS AND MULTIDISCIPLINARY TREATMENT OF LATE RELAPSE
Prognosis

The overall prognosis for patients with LR is poor, with survival rates of approximately 30% to 60% (**Table 4**).[3,7,12,14] Sharp and colleagues[14] found that LR in patients who had received previous chemotherapy as part of their initial management is associated with significantly worse 5-year CSS compared with chemotherapy-naive patients with LR (**Fig. 1**; 5-year CSS 49% [95% CI, 34%–62%] vs 93% [95% CI, 61%–99%]; HR = 4.0; 95% CI, 1.2–13.6; P = .03). Chemotherapy-naive patients have disease that is clinically and biologically distinct from those who have received chemotherapy and can generally be managed according to CS and IGCCCG risk criteria with comparable outcomes with patients not presenting with LR.

Several investigators have found that the presence of teratoma or necrosis in the late recurrence

		Histology at Late Relapse of GCT		
Series	Total Number of Patients	Number with Any Teratoma (%)	Number with Somatic Malignant Transformation of Teratoma (%)	Number with Viable GCT (%)
Sharp et al,[14] 2008	69	41 (59)	14 (20)	54 (78)
Michael et al,[53] 2000	91	55 (60)	21 (23)	55 (60)

Table 3
Distribution of histologic findings in men undergoing surgical resection for LR of GCT

Table 4
Outcomes after therapy for LR of GCT

Series	Total Number of Patients	Number of Patients with NED (%)	Median Follow-up (mo)
Baniel et al,[3] 1995	81	21 (26)	56
George et al,[12] 2003	83	38 (46)	24
Sharp et al,[14] 2008	75	40 (53)	54
Dieckmann et al,[7] 2005	120	77 (64)	—

is associated with favorable outcomes.[9,14,53] Sharp and colleagues[14] found that teratoma or fibrosis at LR compared with viable GCT was associated with improved CSS (5-year CSS 88% [95% CI, 49%–98%] vs 41% [95% CI, 25%–57%], P = .03). Michael and colleagues[53] reported that 79% of patients with teratoma or necrosis were NED at 4.8 years average follow-up after treatment of LR in contrast to only 36% of patients with malignant histology. In a series of 25 patients with median follow-up of 74 months described by Oldenburg and colleagues,[9] the presence of teratoma or necrosis was associated with 100% CSS, whereas the presence of viable cancer resulted in 50% CSS (**Fig. 2**; 95% CI, 14%–79%, P = .009).[9]

In addition to the presence of teratoma or fibrosis at LR, Sharp and colleagues[14] identified additional risk factors associated with improved CSS, including complete surgical resection (5-year CSS 73% [95% CI, 49%–87%] vs 28% [95% CI, 12%–46%], P = .0003), single site of relapse (5-year CSS 75% [95% CI, 50%–89%] vs 28% [95% CI, 12%–46%], P = .0001), and asymptomatic presentation (5-year CSS 81% [95% CI, 51%–93%] vs 33% [95% CI, 18%–49%], P = .003). On multivariable analysis, patients with symptomatic presentation (HR = 4.9; 95% CI, 1.6–15.2) and multifocal sites of disease (HR = 3.0; 95% CI, 1.3–6.8) were predictive of poorer 5-year CSS. George and colleagues[12] also found that symptoms at LR were associated with worse overall survival (HR = 3.76; 95% CI, 1.25–11.34).

Surgical Management

Complete surgical resection is paramount to the successful management of LR, because of the high rate of chemoresistant elements. Data from MSKCC report 5-year CSS of 79% in patients who had complete surgical resection at time of LR compared with 36% for patients without complete resection (n = 45 and 30; P<.0001).[14] George and colleagues[12] reported on 49 patients treated with primary surgery for LR of GCT, and 64% of the patients with teratoma and 44% of patients with viable GCT remained continuously free of disease. In contrast, only 6 of 32 (19%) had a complete clinical response to primary chemotherapy, including 4 who were chemotherapy naive. Twenty-four (75%) of the 32 patients who received

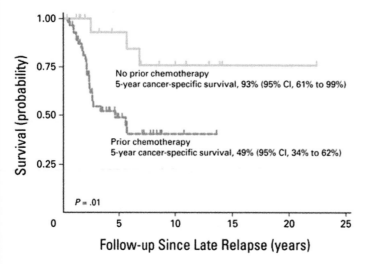

Fig. 1. CSS from time of LR according to previous chemotherapy. (*From* Sharp DS, Carver BS, Eggener SE, et al. Clinical outcome and predictors of survival in late relapse of germ cell tumor. J Clin Oncol 2008;26:5527; with permission.)

No prior chemotherapy
5-year cancer-specific survival, 93% (95% CI, 61% to 99%)

Prior chemotherapy
5-year cancer-specific survival, 49% (95% CI, 34% to 62%)

P = .01

Follow-up Since Late Relapse (years)

Survival (probability)

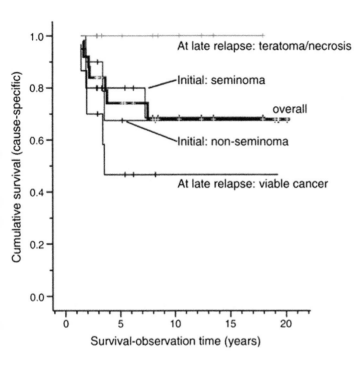

Fig. 2. Histology of LR is associated with CSS. (*From* Oldenburg J, Alfsen GC, Waehre, et al. Late recurrence of germ cell malignancies: a population-based experience over three decades. Br J Cancer 2006;94:826.)

chemotherapy were rendered free of disease with surgical resection. Diekmann and colleagues[7] also reported that treatment of LR with surgery increased the cure rate, although the effect of this factor did not meet statistical significance (P = .07; relative risk, 4.0; 95% CI, 0.9–18.5).

Salvage Chemotherapy

Late recurrence of GCT is usually chemorefractory, as a result of the presence of teratoma or previously chemotherapy-treated viable GCT. Data from the Baniel series[3] showed that only 17 of 65 patients (26%) treated with chemotherapy alone had a CR, with only 2 patients maintaining a durable CR consistent with the low rate of CR to salvage chemotherapy in other smaller series.[5,20] However, in the case of multifocal disease, unresectable disease, or increasing markers at time of LR, salvage chemotherapy is indicated. Motzer and colleagues[54] reported a small series in which 4 of 6 patients with late relapse treated with paclitaxel, ifosfamide, and cisplatin chemotherapy (TIP) had a durable CR with or without surgery. A larger study by Ronnen and colleagues[8] of 246 patients treated with various regimens of salvage chemotherapy included 29 with LR, of whom 17 of 29 (58%) had RPLND as part of initial management. At median follow-up of 50.6 months (range 6.6–88.9 months), the only continuous CRs were in 7 of 14 patients who received TIP chemotherapy. Of the 7 complete responders, 3 had

TIP chemotherapy plus resection of necrosis or teratoma, 3 had TIP plus resection of viable GCT, and 1 patient had chemotherapy without additional surgery. No other salvage regimen resulted in a CR. One patient had a partial response to TIP chemotherapy and was rendered NED by desperation surgery. Gerl and Wilmanns[55] also report success in overcoming resistance of LR GCT by using a paclitaxel-based chemotherapy regimen. Cisplatin plus epirubicin has been examined in a phase 2 trial of 30 patients (70% of whom had an LR), in which 29% of patients had a sustained CR.[56] The role of high-dose chemotherapy (HDCT) in LR is unclear. There are 2 reports including small numbers of patients with LR who achieved CR with HDCT. Feldman and colleagues[57] reported that 2 of 7 patients (29%) achieved long-term disease-free survival with the TI-CE (paclitaxel plus ifosfamide followed by high-dose carboplatin plus etoposide with stem cell support) regimen. Lorch and colleagues[58,59] examined a series of 35 patients with unresectable LR who were treated with HDCT as part of a prospective randomized trial of patients receiving single versus sequential HDCT. At median follow-up of 5.6 years, 5 of 25 patients (14%) had NED progression.

SUMMARY

LR affects approximately 1% to 6% of patients with GCT and may develop after more than

30 years, necessitating long-term follow-up of patients with GCT. Detection of LR before the onset of symptoms may portend a better prognosis. Timely detection of LR is critical to proper management and requires understanding of the patterns of relapse, vigilant adherence to surveillance schedules, and education of our patients on the importance of lifelong follow-up. The most common site of LR is the retroperitoneum, possibly related to suboptimal treatment of the retroperitoneum at the time of initial diagnosis and management. Bilateral templates and meticulous surgical technique may prevent many cases of LR. The primary treatment of LR requires an experienced multidisciplinary team, and most often requires surgery. When surgery is not possible, chemotherapy regimens such as TIP may be used followed by postchemotherapy surgery if possible. A better understanding of the genetics of GCT associated with LR and chemoresistance could help identify patients at risk for LR and new therapeutic options.

REFERENCES

1. Sheinfeld J, Herr HW. Role of surgery in management of germ cell tumor. Semin Oncol 1998;25: 203–9.

2. Einhorn LH. Testicular cancer as a model for a curable neoplasm: The Richard and Hinda Rosenthal Foundation Award Lecture. Cancer Res 1981; 41:3275–80.

3. Baniel J, Foster RS, Gonin R, et al. Late relapse of testicular cancer. J Clin Oncol 1995;13:1170–6.

4. Ravi R, Oliver RT, Ong J, et al. A single-centre observational study of surgery and late malignant events after chemotherapy for germ cell cancer. Br J Urol 1997;80:647–52.

5. Gerl A, Clemm C, Schmeller N, et al. Late relapse of germ cell tumors after cisplatin-based chemotherapy. Ann Oncol 1997;8:41–7.

6. Shahidi M, Norman AR, Dearnaley DP, et al. Late recurrence in 1263 men with testicular germ cell tumors. Multivariate analysis of risk factors and implications for management. Cancer 2002;95:520–30.

7. Dieckmann KP, Albers P, Classen J, et al. Late relapse of testicular germ cell neoplasms: a descriptive analysis of 122 cases. J Urol 2005;173:824–9.

8. Ronnen EA, Kondagunta GV, Bacik J, et al. Incidence of late-relapse germ cell tumor and outcome to salvage chemotherapy. J Clin Oncol 2005;23: 6999–7004.

9. Oldenburg J, Alfsen GC, Waehre H, et al. Late recurrences of germ cell malignancies: a population-based experience over three decades. Br J Cancer 2006;94:820–7.

10. Oldenburg J, Martin JM, Fossa SD. Late relapses of germ cell malignancies: incidence, management, and prognosis. J Clin Oncol 2006;24:5503–11.

11. Carver BS, Motzer RJ, Kondagunta GV, et al. Late relapse of testicular germ cell tumors. Urol Oncol 2005;23:441–5.

12. George DW, Foster RS, Hromas RA, et al. Update on late relapse of germ cell tumor: a clinical and molecular analysis. J Clin Oncol 2003;21:113–22.

13. Geldart TR, Gale J, McKendrick J, et al. Late relapse of metastatic testicular nonseminomatous germ cell cancer: surgery is needed for cure. BJU Int 2006; 98:353–8.

14. Sharp DS, Carver BS, Eggener SE, et al. Clinical outcome and predictors of survival in late relapse of germ cell tumor. J Clin Oncol 2008;26:5524–9.

15. Motzer RJ, Agarwal N, Beard C, et al. Testicular cancer. J Natl Compr Canc Netw 2012;10:502–35.

16. Tarin TV, Sonn G, Shinghal R. Estimating the risk of cancer associated with imaging related radiation during surveillance for stage I testicular cancer using computerized tomography. J Urol 2009;181: 627–32 [discussion: 632–3].

17. Tandstad T, Dahl O, Cohn-Cedermark G, et al. Risk-adapted treatment in clinical stage I nonseminomatous germ cell testicular cancer: the SWENOTECA management program. J Clin Oncol 2009;27:2122–8.

18. O'Malley ME, Chung P, Haider M, et al. Comparison of low dose with standard dose abdominal/pelvic multidetector CT in patients with stage 1 testicular cancer under surveillance. Eur Radiol 2010;20: 1624–30.

19. Martin JM, Panzarella T, Zwahlen DR, et al. Evidence-based guidelines for following stage 1 seminoma. Cancer 2007;109:2248–56.

20. DeLeo MJ, Greco FA, Hainsworth JD, et al. Late recurrences in long-term survivors of germ cell neoplasms. Cancer 1988;62:985–8.

21. Kollmannsberger C, Tandstad T, Bedard PL, et al. Patterns of relapse in patients with clinical stage I testicular cancer managed with active surveillance. J Clin Oncol 2015;33:51–7.

22. Warde P, Specht L, Horwich A, et al. Prognostic factors for relapse in stage I seminoma managed by surveillance: a pooled analysis. J Clin Oncol 2002; 20:4448–52.

23. Chung P, Parker C, Panzarella T, et al. Surveillance in stage I testicular seminoma–risk of late relapse. Can J Urol 2002;9:1637–40.

24. Gels ME, Hoekstra HJ, Sleijfer DT, et al. Detection of recurrence in patients with clinical stage I nonseminomatous testicular germ cell tumors and consequences for further follow-up: a single-center 10-year experience. J Clin Oncol 1995;13:1188–94.

25. Sogani PC, Perrotti M, Herr HW, et al. Clinical stage I testis cancer: long-term outcome of patients on surveillance. J Urol 1998;159:855–8.

26. Kollmannsberger C, Moore C, Chi KN, et al. Non-risk-adapted surveillance for patients with stage I nonseminomatous testicular germ-cell tumors: diminishing treatment-related morbidity while maintaining efficacy. Ann Oncol 2010;21:1296–301.

27. Rice KR, Beck SD, Pedrosa JA, et al. Surgical management of late relapse on surveillance in patients presenting with clinical stage I testicular cancer. Urology 2014;84:886–90.

28. Mead GM, Fossa SD, Oliver RT, et al. Randomized trials in 2466 patients with stage I seminoma: patterns of relapse and follow-up. J Natl Cancer Inst 2011;103:241–9.

29. Jones WG, Fossa SD, Mead GM, et al. Randomized trial of 30 versus 20 Gy in the adjuvant treatment of stage I testicular seminoma: a report on Medical Research Council Trial TE18, European Organisation for the Research and Treatment of Cancer Trial 30942 (ISRCTN18525328). J Clin Oncol 2005;23:1200–8.

30. Fossa SD, Horwich A, Russell JM, et al. Optimal planning target volume for stage I testicular seminoma: a Medical Research Council randomized trial. Medical Research Council Testicular Tumor Working Group. J Clin Oncol 1999;17:1146.

31. Oliver RT, Mason MD, Mead GM, et al. Radiotherapy versus single-dose carboplatin in adjuvant treatment of stage I seminoma: a randomised trial. Lancet 2005;366:293–300.

32. Kollmannsberger C, Tyldesley S, Moore C, et al. Evolution in management of testicular seminoma: population-based outcomes with selective utilization of active therapies. Ann Oncol 2011;22:808–14.

33. Warde P, Gospodarowicz MK, Panzarella T, et al. Stage I testicular seminoma: results of adjuvant irradiation and surveillance. J Clin Oncol 1995;13:2255–62.

34. Hallemeier CL, Choo R, Davis BJ, et al. Excellent long-term disease control with modern radiotherapy techniques for stage I testicular seminoma–the Mayo Clinic experience. Urol Oncol 2014;32:24.e1–6.

35. Powles T, Robinson D, Shamash J, et al. The long-term risks of adjuvant carboplatin treatment for stage I seminoma of the testis. Ann Oncol 2008;19:443–7.

36. Stephenson AJ, Bosl GJ, Motzer RJ, et al. Retroperitoneal lymph node dissection for nonseminomatous germ cell testicular cancer: impact of patient selection factors on outcome. J Clin Oncol 2005;23:2781–8.

37. Donohue JP, Thornhill JA, Foster RS, et al. Primary retroperitoneal lymph node dissection in clinical stage A non-seminomatous germ cell testis cancer. Review of the Indiana University experience 1965-1989. Br J Urol 1993;71:326–35.

38. Eggener SE, Carver BS, Sharp DS, et al. Incidence of disease outside modified retroperitoneal lymph node dissection templates in clinical stage I or IIA nonseminomatous germ cell testicular cancer. J Urol 2007;177:937–42 [discussion: 942–3].

39. Carver BS, Shayegan B, Eggener S, et al. Incidence of metastatic nonseminomatous germ cell tumor outside the boundaries of a modified postchemotherapy retroperitoneal lymph node dissection. J Clin Oncol 2007;25:4365–9.

40. Lutke Holzik MF, Hoekstra HJ, Mulder NH, et al. Non-germ cell malignancy in residual or recurrent mass after chemotherapy for nonseminomatous testicular germ cell tumor. Ann Surg Oncol 2003;10:131–5.

41. Tandstad T, Stahl O, Hakansson U, et al. One course of adjuvant BEP in clinical stage I nonseminoma mature and expanded results from the SWENOTECA group. Ann Oncol 2014;25:2167–72.

42. Rabbani F, Sheinfeld J, Farivar-Mohseni H, et al. Low-volume nodal metastases detected at retroperitoneal lymphadenectomy for testicular cancer: pattern and prognostic factors for relapse. J Clin Oncol 2001;19:2020–5.

43. Donohue JP, Thornhill JA, Foster RS, et al. Clinical stage B non-seminomatous germ cell testis cancer: the Indiana University experience (1965-1989) using routine primary retroperitoneal lymph node dissection. Eur J Cancer 1995;31A:1599–604.

44. Kondagunta GV, Sheinfeld J, Mazumdar M, et al. Relapse-free and overall survival in patients with pathologic stage II nonseminomatous germ cell cancer treated with etoposide and cisplatin adjuvant chemotherapy. J Clin Oncol 2004;22:464–7.

45. Ehrlich Y, Brames MJ, Beck SD, et al. Long-term follow-up of cisplatin combination chemotherapy in patients with disseminated nonseminomatous germ cell tumors: is a postchemotherapy retroperitoneal lymph node dissection needed after complete remission? J Clin Oncol 2010;28:531–6.

46. Stephenson AJ, Bosl GJ, Motzer RJ, et al. Nonrandomized comparison of primary chemotherapy and retroperitoneal lymph node dissection for clinical stage IIA and IIB nonseminomatous germ cell testicular cancer. J Clin Oncol 2007;25:5597–602.

47. Kondagunta GV, Bacik J, Bajorin D, et al. Etoposide and cisplatin chemotherapy for metastatic good-risk germ cell tumors. J Clin Oncol 2005;23:9290–4.

48. Fossa SD, Ous S, Lien HH, et al. Post-chemotherapy lymph node histology in radiologically normal patients with metastatic nonseminomatous testicular cancer. J Urol 1989;141:557–9.

49. Toner GC, Panicek DM, Heelan RT, et al. Adjunctive surgery after chemotherapy for nonseminomatous germ cell tumors: recommendations for patient selection. J Clin Oncol 1990;8:1683–94.

50. Logothetis CJ, Samuels ML, Trindade A, et al. The growing teratoma syndrome. Cancer 1982;50:1629–35.

51. Motzer RJ, Amsterdam A, Prieto V, et al. Teratoma with malignant transformation: diverse malignant

histologies arising in men with germ cell tumors. J Urol 1998;159:133–8.

52. Carver BS, Bianco FJ Jr, Shayegan B, et al. Predicting teratoma in the retroperitoneum in men undergoing post-chemotherapy retroperitoneal lymph node dissection. J Urol 2006;176:100–3 [discussion: 103–4].

53. Michael H, Lucia J, Foster RS, et al. The pathology of late recurrence of testicular germ cell tumors. Am J Surg Pathol 2000;24:257–73.

54. Motzer RJ, Sheinfeld J, Mazumdar M, et al. Paclitaxel, ifosfamide, and cisplatin second-line therapy for patients with relapsed testicular germ cell cancer. J Clin Oncol 2000;18:2413–8.

55. Gerl A, Wilmanns W. Antitumor activity of paclitaxel after failure of high-dose chemotherapy in a patient with late relapse of a non-seminomatous germ cell tumor. Anticancer Drugs 1996;7:716–8.

56. Bedano PM, Brames MJ, Williams SD, et al. Phase II study of cisplatin plus epirubicin salvage chemotherapy in refractory germ cell tumors. J Clin Oncol 2006;24:5403–7.

57. Feldman DR, Sheinfeld J, Bajorin DF, et al. TI-CE high-dose chemotherapy for patients with previously treated germ cell tumors: results and prognostic factor analysis. J Clin Oncol 2010;28:1706–13.

58. Lorch A, Kollmannsberger C, Hartmann JT, et al. Single versus sequential high-dose chemotherapy in patients with relapsed or refractory germ cell tumors: a prospective randomized multicenter trial of the German Testicular Cancer Study Group. J Clin Oncol 2007;25:2778–84.

59. Lorch A, Rick O, Wundisch T, et al. High dose chemotherapy as salvage treatment for unresectable late relapse germ cell tumors. J Urol 2010; 184:168–73.

Role of Extraretroperitoneal Surgery in Patients with Metastatic Germ Cell Tumors

 CrossMark

Brian Hu, MD, Siamak Daneshmand, MD*

KEYWORDS

- Testicular cancer • Extraretroperitoneal • Metastasis • Survival • Surgery • Germ cell tumor

KEY POINTS

- Discordance, in varying degrees, exists between retroperitoneal pathology and histology from extraretroperitoneal sites.
- Surgery for extraretroperitoneal disease (especially pulmonary and hepatic) can be morbid, with a mortality risk as high as 2%.
- In patients with known teratoma or viable germ cell tumor metastasis, all visible extraretroperitoneal disease should be resected.
- In patients with necrosis in the retroperitoneum, extraretroperitoneal disease should be excised if feasible, although surveillance represents an alternative strategy for select patients.
- An individualized surgical approach should be made based on metastatic pattern, prior disorders, patient factors, and institutional considerations.

INTRODUCTION

Approximately half of patients with testicular germ cell tumors (GCTs) present with metastasis. Metastatic spread to the retroperitoneum (RP) is most common, although extraretroperitoneal (ERP) sites are involved in approximately 40% of patients with advanced disease.[1,2] Systemic therapy is efficacious in treating ERP disease, although these masses can persist or recur after initial chemotherapy in up to 35% of patients.[3] In the setting of normal serum tumor markers, resection of ERP masses is favored rather than additional chemotherapy because of its efficacy against teratoma, its side effect profile, and its ability to provide a pathologic diagnosis, which can help guide further therapy. In patients who have residual ERP masses despite salvage chemotherapy, resection can represent the best chance (and sometimes the only chance) for durable survival.

Treating patients with ERP disease can be difficult given the diverse clinical, anatomic, and pathologic spectrum. Although some clinicians advocate removing all residual disease, others think that surgery can be tailored based on available pathology. The morbidity of ERP surgery must also be considered, especially in patients with underlying medical disease. Lung and liver resections carry an operative mortality greater than that seen after postchemotherapy (PC) retroperitoneal lymph node dissection (RPLND), which underscores the high-risk nature of ERP surgery. In addition, the optimal timing of surgery and combining ERP with PC-RPLND can vary widely

Conflicts of Interest: The authors declare no conflicts of interest.
Institute of Urology, USC/Norris Comprehensive Cancer Center, Keck School of Medicine University of Southern California, 1441 Eastlake Avenue, Suite 7416, Los Angeles, CA 90089, USA
* Corresponding author. USC Institute of Urology, 1441 Eastlake Avenue, Suite 7416, Los Angeles, CA 90089.
E-mail address: daneshma@usc.edu

Urol Clin N Am 42 (2015) 369–380
http://dx.doi.org/10.1016/j.ucl.2015.04.011
0094-0143/15/$ – see front matter © 2015 Elsevier Inc. All rights reserved.

and requires a multidisciplinary team with experience in treating advanced disease. This article reviews the role of ERP surgery in metastatic testicular cancer, including discussions on the patterns of metastasis, pathology at ERP sites, surgical considerations, and outcomes after surgery.

PATTERNS OF DISEASE

When treating patients with metastatic GCT, an understanding of the typical patterns of disease is required. The lymphatic drainage from the RP plays a major role in determining this pattern, with the para-aortic and paracaval lymphatics draining behind the crura of the diaphragm to the middle mediastinum. The middle mediastinum is therefore the most common mediastinal compartment involved with GCT and is divided into 3 regions (**Fig. 1**A). Spread to the anterior and posterior compartments (see **Fig. 1**B) likely occurs with lymphatic obstruction and retrograde flow. Kesler and colleagues[4] confirmed this finding by reviewing 268 patients with metastatic mediastinal GCT, in whom the anterior and posterior compartments were only involved if concurrent with middle mediastinal disease. Isolated anterior mediastinal disease should raise suspicion for primary mediastinal GCT. After lymphatics drain from the RP to the middle mediastinum, they flow to the left supraclavicular region, where the thoracic duct enters the left subclavian vein.

Wood and colleagues[5] evaluated the pattern of metastases in 31 patients with testicular GCT, providing clinical validation of this drainage pattern. Neck metastases were more often seen with seminomatous compared with nonseminomatous GCT (NSGCT) (91% vs 65%), and most of these metastases (91%) were on the left side. Mediastinal lymphadenopathy was common in both groups, although it was more often combined with neck disease in patients with seminoma (55% vs 10%). This study confirmed the understanding of more predictable lymphatic spread of seminoma. Hematogenous dissemination of NSGCT was more common and was reflected in the higher rates of lung metastases seen in NSGCT (40% vs 9%). The hematogenous nature of metastases in the lung (and also liver) can manifest as more multifocal disease, which can have implications when planning ERP surgery.

Fizazi and colleagues[6] described the distribution of 126 ERP masses resected in patients who relapsed after cisplatin therapy. The lung (52%) was most commonly involved, followed by the mediastinum (28%), cervical nodes (7%), liver (4%), bone (1.6%), and brain (0.8%). Masterson and colleagues reviewed the sites of disease in 130 patients and found a similar distribution (lung in 68%, mediastinum 29%, liver 13%, neck 12%).[3]

PATHOLOGY
Extraretroperitoneal Disease

After chemotherapy, residual ERP disease is generally in one of 3 pathologic groups, as it is in PC-RPLND specimens: necrosis/fibrosis, teratoma, or viable GCT. Ideally, only patients with

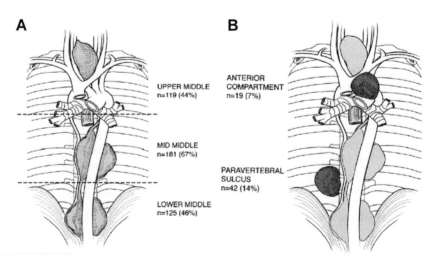

A

UPPER MIDDLE
n=119 (44%)

MID MIDDLE
n=181 (67%)

LOWER MIDDLE
n=125 (46%)

B

ANTERIOR
COMPARTMENT
n=19 (7%)

PARAVERTEBRAL
SULCUS
n=42 (14%)

Fig. 1. (*A*) Middle mediastinum divided into 3 compartments: upper, thoracic inlet to carina; mid, carina to dome of the diaphragm; lower, dome of diaphragm to diaphragmatic crura. The distribution of middle mediastinal metastases in a series from Kesler and colleagues[4] including 268 patients is given for each compartment. (*B*) Metastasis in the paravertebral sulcus and anterior mediastinum occurs much less frequently. In the series by Kesler and colleagues,[4] these lesions always occurred in cases in which middle mediastinal metastases were also present. (*From* Kesler KA. Surgical techniques for testicular nonseminomatous germ cell tumors metastatic to the mediastinum. Chest Surg Clin N Am 2002;12(4):751–52; with permission.)

teratoma or viable GCT would undergo surgery; however, as in the RP, there is currently no reliable method for determining the histology of ERP masses short of surgical resection. However, pathology from the RP or other ERP sites may offer insight. The main reason for studying these relationships is to better predict lesions that represent necrosis, allowing some patients to avoid surgery.

Table 1 presents the histology after ERP surgery for different anatomic sites as well as data on pathologic concordance, if available.[4,7–15] Liu and colleagues[8] and Cagini and colleagues[9] showed high rates of significant disorders (ie, teratoma or viable GCT) in 70% to 77% of patients after lung resections, although not all groups have shown the same distribution of disorders. A review of 19 studies including 996 resection specimens (including both RP and lung) found that necrosis was more common in the lungs compared with RP.[16] Other studies have confirmed that RP disorders had a higher incidence of teratoma or viable GCT than disorders in the lungs.[17,18] Taken together, these data oppose using favorable lung pathology to justify omitting a PC-RPLND.

Concordance Rates

Several studies have described the concordance between pathology at metastatic sites inside and outside the RP. Small series with between 15 and 72 patients have shown pathologic discordance rates of 29% to 47%.[17–21] One study found that metachronously diagnosed ERP disease had a much higher rate of pathologic discordance than synchronous metastases (57% vs 28%).[22] Given these high rates of discordance, many clinicians argue that all residual ERP disease should be resected, regardless of prior pathology.

Although overall discordance rates are useful, stratifying by histology can provide more relevant information, especially if contemplating surveillance in a patient with necrosis in the RP. **Table 2** describes the concordance data stratified by histology from one of the larger ERP surgical series (n = 130).[3] In patients with fibrosis in the RP, there was a 17% incidence of either teratoma or viable GCT. This rate of discordance with necrosis/fibrosis in the RP is similar to the 19% to 20% that have been shown in other studies.[17,18] The discordance rates for necrosis in ERP site–specific studies (see **Table 1**) were 11% in the lungs, 15% in the neck, and 6% in the liver.[7,10,14]

Clinical and primary tumor factors may augment the ability to predict ERP disorders. Tognoni and colleagues[23] reviewed data from patients who underwent a combined PC-RPLND and chest surgery for metastatic GCT (n = 143). RP was concordant with chest disorder in 78% of patients with necrosis, 70% of patients with teratoma, and 69% of patients with cancer. The level of correlation in predicting necrosis increased to 86% when evaluating the uncomplicated subset by Indiana University criteria (ie, normal serum tumor markers, standard first-line chemotherapy, absence of salvage chemotherapy, and no late relapse). In an analysis of 19 studies with data on metastatic disorders, Steyerberg and colleagues[16] correlated teratoma in the primary tumor with lung disorder. The absence of teratoma in the primary tumor was associated with a higher likelihood of cancer in the lung (24%) but a lower rate of teratoma (0%).

SURGICAL CONSIDERATIONS
Lung

The surgical approach to resecting lung disease must be tailored to the patient. In patients with a low number of peripheral lesions, less invasive surgical approaches such as video-assisted thoracoscopic surgery with wedge resection can provide oncologic control and minimize morbidity. With larger or more central lesions, anatomic lung resections may be necessary through a thoracotomy. The presence of synchronous disease must also be assessed, because combining lung surgery with mediastinal or RP surgery is feasible. Circumstances with a large number of lung lesions can also be encountered. Surgery in these patients must be individualized based on the number, location, and size, of the lesions and the response to systemic therapy. Our approach in cases with numerous lung lesions is to resect larger masses, especially those less responsive to chemotherapy. This strategy helps target lesions that are more likely to represent teratoma or viable GCT and allows time to survey smaller lesions that are suspected of harboring necrosis.

Lung resections can be morbid and are associated with a mortality of 1% to 2%.[4,8,24] Many patients have been treated with bleomycin, so there is a level of complexity with 1 series implicating the chemotherapy in 2 of the 3 postoperative mortalities in the series (n = 268). This same group evaluated a subset of patients who underwent pneumonectomy or bilobectomy after bleomycin and found that 4 of 32 (13%) patients died postoperatively secondary to pulmonary complications.[25] The pulmonary morbidity was 18%. In patients who require extensive lung resections, this group limits a patient's total bleomycin dose to 300 units. Alternative regimens with ifosfamide can be considered in those who have significant lung lesions.

Table 1
Distribution of histology after resection of ERP disease by region in patients with metastatic germ cell cancer. Rates of concordance with other metastatic sites are listed, if available

ERP Pathologic Findings by Region

	Lung			Mediastinum	Neck		Liver			
Study	Steyerberg et al,[7] 1997	Liu et al,[8] 1998	Cagini et al,[9] 1998	Kesler et al,[4] 2003	Gupta et al,[10] 2011	Mehra et al,[15] 2012	Rivoire et al,[11] 2001	Hahn et al,[12] 1999	Hartmann et al,[13] 2005	Jacobsen et al,[14] 2010
Number of patients	215	157	141	268	41	34	37	57	43	59
Disorders										
% Necrosis/fibrosis	54	30	23	15	34	29	49	16	67	73
% Teratoma	33	25	45	59	56	56	19	51	12	17
% Viable GCT	13	45	33	16	7	9	32	33	21	10
Other	—	—	—	11% Non-germ cell cancer	3% Benign nodes	6% Benign nodes	—	—	—	—
Notes	Concordance with RP necrosis 89%	—	Overall concordance 76%	—	Overall concordance 77% Concordance with RP necrosis 85%	—	—	—	Overall concordance with second ERP surgery 61%	Overall concordance 49% Concordance with RP necrosis 94%

Table 2 Concordance of the RP and ERP histologic findings reported according to retroperitoneal histology of fibrosis, teratoma, and viable GCT			
	ERP Histology		
RP Histology	Fibrosis	Teratoma	Viable GCT
Fibrosis	83%	12%	5%
Teratoma	52%	42%	6%
Viable GCT	40%	13%	47%

Concordance of metastatic disorder stratified by retroperitoneal histology.

From Masterson TA, Shayegan B, Carver BS, et al. Clinical impact of residual extraretroperitoneal masses in patients with advanced nonseminomatous germ cell testicular cancer. Urology 2012;79(1):158; with permission.

Mediastinum

Given the anatomic diversity of mediastinal lesions, there is a multitude of possible operative options for resecting mediastinal disease, depending on location, disease burden, and presence of synchronous metastases. Access can gained to the mediastinum through multiple techniques, including thoracotomy, median sternotomy, and transpericardial or transabdominal approaches.[26,27] Kesler[27] provided an expert review of these techniques.

The complication rate after mediastinal mass excision was approximately 12%.[4] A unique and serious complication when performing mediastinal surgery is paralysis. For masses that involve circumferential dissection around the descending aorta, ligation of intercostal and spinal arteries can lead to ischemia of spinal cord. The artery of Adamkiewicz, which is the predominant vessel supplying the lower spinal cord, is anatomically variable and cannot be consistently identified on imaging.[28] In one series focusing on mediastinal tumors after resection, 6 patients (2.2%) experienced paralysis.[4] Paralysis was permanent in 2 patients, whereas the other 4 patients had significant improvement in the symptoms. Efforts to spare intercostal or upper spinal arteries in patients undergoing extensive resection are required to reduce the risk of this complication.

Neck

Most lymph node (LN) dissections in the neck are on the left because of the lymphatic drainage into the left subclavian vein. Mehra and colleagues[15] evaluated 34 consecutive patients who underwent excision of a neck metastasis and 15% required right-sided surgery (including 3 patients who had bilateral surgery). The extent of optimal neck

dissection is unknown. **Fig. 2** shows the different LN levels in the neck.[29] Weisberger and colleagues[30] published an early study in which they performed a modified neck dissection routinely including level III to V nodes. Gupta and colleagues[10] described their technique of selective node dissection, removing level IV nodes unless there was known or suspected disease in other regions. A selective neck dissection was also used by See and colleagues,[31] who removed only the lymphatic tissue within the compartment of the residual mass. The complication rates after excising neck masses has been reported to be 0% to 9%.[15,31] Surgery may require sacrificing adjacent structures, such as the spinal accessory nerve, internal jugular vein, or sternocleidomastoid muscle. Chyle leakage has been reported in up to 4% cases.[30]

Liver

The surgical approach to liver lesions depends on the number and location of disease. Smaller, peripheral lesions allow wedge resections, whereas multiple, larger, or central lesions may require an anatomic resection. Intraoperative ultrasonography can be helpful in identifying more central lesions. Hahn and colleagues[12] described the types of resections used from their series of 57 patients and the associated complications (**Table 3**). The complication rate of 30% was high, although this includes most patients who had concurrent surgery. Mortality after liver resections ranges

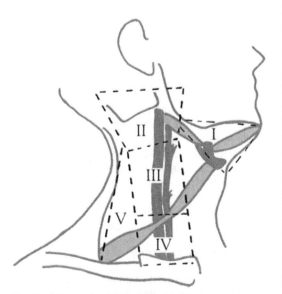

Fig. 2. The anatomic levels of the cervical lymph nodes. (*From* van Vledder MG, van der Hage JA, Kirkels WJ, et al. Cervical lymph node dissection for metastatic testicular cancer. Ann Surg Oncol 2010;17(6):1683; with permission.)

Table 3
Surgical approach to hepatic lesions and complications from hepatic surgery for suspected GCT metastasis

Surgical Procedures for Treatment of Hepatic Lesion (n = 57)	Number
Wedge resection (single or multiple)	22
Right lobectomy	11
Left lobectomy	5
Multiple resections	15
Trisegmentectomy	3
Segmentectomy	4
Complications from Hepatic Surgery	**Number**
Gastrointestinal complications	6
Wound infection/dehiscence	4
Abscess	4
Bile leak	4
Pulmonary complications	4
Deep vein thrombosis	2
Other	2

Adapted from Hahn TL, Jacobson L, Einhorn LH, et al. Hepatic resection of metastatic testicular carcinoma: a further update. Ann Surg Oncol 1999;6(7):641–2.

from 0% to 2.7%.[11,12] This percentage is a reflection of a high-risk surgery in patients with poor-risk disease, underscoring the need for careful consideration of surgery. We do not recommend combining large liver resections with RPLND or other ERP surgery because of this morbidity. In addition, biopsy or ablative techniques (eg, radiofrequency ablation) can have a role when balancing the risks of surgery with oncologic benefit.[32]

Brain

Unlike lung, liver, and neck disease, the role of surgery in patients with brain metastasis is less clear. There is no established standard for treating these patients because stereotactic radiation, whole-brain radiation, chemotherapy, and surgery are efficacious. The optimal timing of surgery is also not known, although it is often dictated by the patient's neurologic symptoms. A study by Fosså and colleagues[33] found that most patients underwent brain surgery within a week of presentation and most of these had a single metastasis.

CONCURRENT SURGERY

Different opinions exist when treating patients with multiple metastatic sites. Some clinicians prefer staging surgery to potentially reduce perioperative complications, allowing patients time for recovery and reassessment of the pathology.[20,34,35] Others think that combining surgery reduces overall

morbidity and streamlines care for patients. These groups argue that because the rates of pathologic discordance can range from 29% to 47%, the decision to remove all residual ERP disease is not influenced by obtaining pathology in a staged fashion.[17–21]

We think that minimizing the burden of treatment to achieve cure is an important aspect of treating ERP disease. In this algorithm, the initial resection of metastatic disease should include the RP unless there is impending compromise to vital ERP structures. One main reason for this is that the RP is the usual first site of metastatic spread and typically produces worse pathology results than ERP sites. Patients with viable GCT in the RP are likely to require salvage systemic therapy regardless of ERP histology. In patients who have received salvage therapy, efforts should be made to limit the number of procedures to achieve complete resection.

During PC-RPLND, if there is concurrent abdominal (eg, liver) or pelvic disease, resection can be combined. Liver resections have been performed concurrently with PC-RPLND in 47% to 65% of cases in published series.[11,12] In situations with a large liver mass and RP disease, our preference is to defer liver resection because RP pathology may dictate further chemotherapy, which can make subsequent surgery easier. If PC-RPLND can be performed with minimal potential for morbidity and without adjuvant surgery (eg, vascular grafting, nephrectomy, liver resection), we think that ERP surgery can safely be combined. Although some clinicians have shown that abdominal, thoracic, and neck surgeries can be performed during 1 anesthetic, we think that limiting dissection to 1 other site represents a better balance of operative efficiency and morbidity.[36]

In our experience, resecting neck disease with the PC-RPLND with 2 operative teams working simultaneously decreases operative time and adds minimal morbidity. Using this approach, disease in the chest, if present, is resected at another time instead of at the same time as concurrent neck and RPLND. In a series of neck dissections, Mehra and colleagues[15] performed an RPLND concurrently in 50% of patients. Neck surgery can also be combined with thoracic surgery for metastatic GCT.[24] Kesler[27] described combining upper mediastinal dissections with neck dissection using a cervicosternotomy approach.

Combining PC-RPLND and chest surgery is feasible. Tognoni and colleagues[23] described this approach with a 35% complication rate, which is higher that of a PC-RPLND alone. Kesler and colleagues[24] described their typical algorithm, which combines a thoracic procedure with the RPLND unless an anatomic pulmonary resection is required or there is bilateral

parenchymal disease.[23] There were 56% of patients in their series who underwent a combined RPLND and thoracic surgery. Skinner and colleagues[37] popularized the thoracoabdominal incision for RPLND, which offers access to the chest and is especially useful for chest disease limited to the lower thorax. Fadel and colleagues[38] described their experience with a transabdominal transdiaphragmatic approach that allows simultaneous resection of RP and mediastinal masses (**Fig. 3**). This technique involves a midline RPLND with incision of the crus of the diaphragm, which provided access the inferior mediastinum on both sides of the aorta. Resection of more superior LNs was performed by partially dividing the sternum. For limited retrocrural disease, we prefer the transabdominal approach with division of the ipsilateral crus. Larger cystic teratomas within the posterior mediastinum can be resected using this technique.

OUTCOMES
All Extraperitoneal Sites

The outcome following ERP surgery depends on various factors. Preoperative variables known to affect survival, such as International Germ Cell

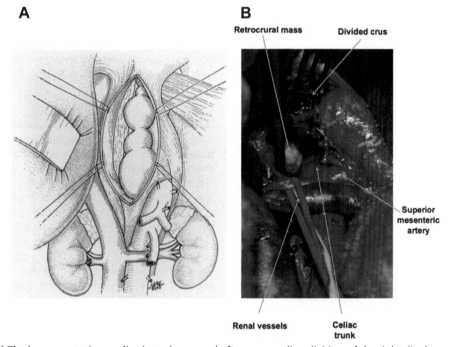

Fig. 3. (*A*) The lower posterior mediastinum is exposed after paramedian division of the right diaphragmatic crus extended anteriorly through the muscular portion, which exposes both sides of the descending aorta. (*B*) Intraoperative view of retrocrural mass after division of crus of diaphragm. ([*A*] *From* Fadel E, Court B, Chapelier AR, et al. One-stage approach for retroperitoneal and mediastinal metastatic testicular tumor resection. Ann Thorac Surg 2000;69(6):1718; with permission.)

Consensus Classification (IGCCC) risk group, salvage chemotherapy, and increase of serum tumor marker levels at time of surgery continue to play a prognostic role after ERP surgery. After surgery has been performed, the histology at the ERP surgery is most prognostic of survival.

Masterson and colleagues[3] evaluated survival in a cohort of 130 patients with a residual ERP mass after chemotherapy and found that 5-year progression-free survival (PFS) was 74% and disease-specific survival (DSS) was 84%. Histology of the ERP site was independently predictive of PFS where patients with necrosis, teratoma, and viable GCT had a 5-year PFS of 93%, 50%, and 8%, respectively (**Fig. 4**). The prognostic ability of ERP histology (hazard ratio [HR] of 7.7 in teratoma and HR 25.0 in viable GCT) for disease progression was independent of a patient's RP pathology.

Fizazi and colleagues[6] evaluated outcomes in 238 patients with resected ERP masses that all had residual GCT following first-line cisplatin therapy. Three factors were independently associated with worse overall survival (OS) and PFS: incomplete ERP resection, greater than or equal to 10% viable GCT at the ERP site, and intermediate-risk or poor-risk IGCCC criteria. When stratifying patients into 3 groups (no risk

factors, 1 risk factor, and >1 risk factor), OS significantly differed (100%, 83%, and 51%).

Survival in a high-risk cohort after salvage chemotherapy with increased serum tumor markers was examined by Albers and colleagues.[39] There were 54% of patients with lung metastases and 40% of patients with visceral metastases who remained disease free after surgical resection. The most important factor in remaining disease free was undergoing a complete resection. Therefore, ERP surgery, especially if fully resected, represents a therapeutic option for some patients after salvage chemotherapy with persistently increased serum tumor markers.

Lung

Two large studies have examined outcomes after resection of metastatic lung lesions. Liu and colleagues[8] evaluated outcomes from 157 patients with testicular GCT who underwent lung resections for suspected metastases. In the entire cohort, 37% of patients experienced a recurrence, with most of them being pulmonary. The 5-year OS was 68% and few deaths were seen after 5 years. The OS increased to 82% in the modern era. Predictors of poor survival included visceral metastases and viable GCT at the time of lung resection. A poor predictor of survival was an early recurrence, because 74% of patients who recurred within a year of the lung resection died. Cagini and colleagues[9] evaluated a similar cohort (n = 141) and OS was 77% at 5 years and was significantly worse in patients who had an incomplete resection (HR, 4.0), viable GCT (HR, 5.7), or multiple sites of lung disease (HR, 4.1).

Mediastinum

Kesler and colleagues[4] presented a review of 268 patients with metastatic mediastinal GCT all treated with surgical resection, with 47% of patients undergoing more than 1 surgery. This group was a high-risk cohort, with 35% of patients who underwent second-line chemotherapy and 32% who had increased serum tumor markers. Five-year and 10-year OS in this cohort was 86% and 74%, respectively. Mediastinal disorder was significantly associated with survival. The presence of necrosis and teratoma had improved survival compared with viable GCT or non–germ cell cancer (**Fig. 5**). Other independent factors predicting poor survival were increased beta human chorionic gonadotropin and advanced age. This group also compared outcomes between patients who underwent excision of lung or mediastinal disease after chemotherapy and found no differences in survival.[24] Therefore, the type of

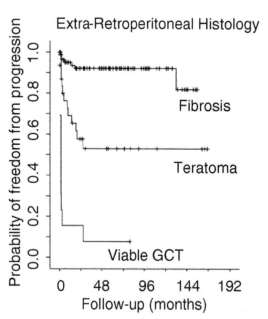

Fig. 4. Kaplan-Meier curve showing the probability of freedom from recurrence after resection of ERP disease stratified according to histology. (*From* Masterson TA, Shayegan B, Carver BS, et al. Clinical impact of residual extraretroperitoneal masses in patients with advanced nonseminomatous germ cell testicular cancer. Urology 2012;79(1):158; with permission.)

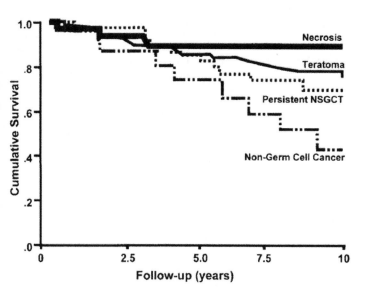

Fig. 5. Long-term survival in metastatic GCT to the mediastinum according to worst postchemotherapy pathologic category. Met, metastasis. (*From* Kesler KA, Brooks JA, Rieger KM, et al. Mediastinal metastases from testicular nonseminomatous germ cell tumors: patterns of dissemination and predictors of long-term survival with surgery. J Thorac Cardiovasc Surg 2003;125(4):918; with permission.)

metastatic spread in the chest (hematogenous [lung] or lymphatic [mediastinal]) did not impact outcomes after chemotherapy and ERP surgery.

Neck

Mehra and colleagues[15] evaluated outcomes after neck dissection in 34 patients. Five-year and 10-year DSS were both 82.3% and viable GCT in the neck predicted DSS. Neck dissection provides excellent local control because no patients in this series experienced local recurrence. Gupta and colleagues[10] had similar findings in their series, with 71% of patients with viable GCT dying of disease, compared with only 8.7% in patients with teratoma.

Liver

Outcomes in patients with liver disease, given that this by definition represents a poor-risk IGCCC category, are generally worse than those seen in other ERP sites. Rivoire and colleagues[11] published a series of patients with GCT and suspected liver metastases after chemotherapy. Forty percent of patients had a solitary liver metastasis and 95% underwent complete resection. With a median follow-up of 66 months, 62% of patients were alive with no evidence of disease. The factors associated with poor outcome included incomplete resection, embryonal carcinoma in the primary tumor, a large metastasis (>3 cm), and residual viable disease. In addition, of the 6 lesions less than 1 cm, all represented necrosis and the patients have remained free of disease.[11] Given that the outcomes in patients with larger (>3 cm) tumors was poor, with almost half of the patients

succumbing to disease, the investigators recommended deferring surgery in this group and to offer resection to patients with growing teratomas. Therefore, the investigators thought that resection of residual liver masses was best reserved for masses 1.0 to 2.9 cm in size.

Hahn and colleagues[12] reviewed their institutional data and came to a different conclusion. The disease-free rates for patients with necrosis, teratoma, and active cancer were 89%, 72%, and 26%, respectively. Of the group with active GCT in the liver, outcomes were especially poor in those with increased tumor markers, with 60% dying of disease progression. The investigators thought that, despite the poor outcomes, liver resection represented the best chance for patients who have already had salvage therapy to achieve durable response.

Brain

Survival in patients with brain metastasis is generally poor, although cure can still be achieved. The mean OS in series reporting on ERP surgery for brain metastases ranged from 16 to 23 months.[40,41] An important factor in determining this survival is the timing of the metastasis diagnosis. Fossa and colleagues[33] found drastically worse survival if a metastasis was identified after treatment compared with at initial presentation (**Fig. 6**). The 5-year cancer specific survival (CSS) in these 2 groups was 45% and 12%, respectively. Surgical resection was associated with an improvement in 2-year CSS (80% vs 49%), whereas radiotherapy was not associated with differences in survival. For patients who were

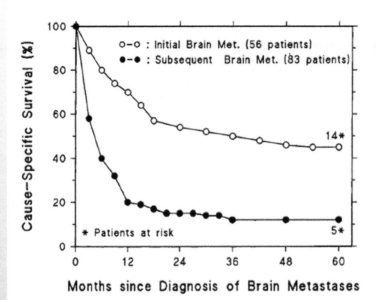

Fig. 6. Cause-specific survival in patients with brain metastases from malignant GCT. (*From* Fosså SD, Bokemeyer C, Gerl A, et al. Treatment outcome of patients with brain metastases from malignant germ cell tumors. Cancer 1999;85(4):993; with permission.)

diagnosed with brain metastases after systemic therapy, improvements in survival were seen in patients who underwent surgery (40% vs 4%) and in those who underwent radiotherapy (18% vs 8%). There was a subset of patients with isolated brain metastases who achieved durable response with a 39% 5-year DSS.

POSTOPERATIVE CHEMOTHERAPY

Two studies provide insight into how to manage patients with residual GCT after ERP surgery. Fox and colleagues[42] retrospectively evaluated the outcomes of patients after PC-RPLND who had 2 courses of cisplatin-based chemotherapy postoperatively. Additional chemotherapy was associated with lower rates of recurrence compared with patients managed expectantly (30% vs 100%). This difference was only seen in patients who underwent primary chemotherapy. Fizazi and colleagues[6] evaluated ERP masses resected showing viable GCT after first-line cisplatin therapy and found that the 5-year PFS rate significantly differed between those who did or did not receive postoperative chemotherapy (69% vs 52%; $P<.001$). Chemotherapy seemed to be most beneficial in intermediate-risk patients (having one of the following variables: incomplete ERP resection, $\geq$10% viable GCT at the ERP site, and intermediate-risk/poor-risk IGCCC criteria). Therefore, 2 additional courses of cisplatin-based chemotherapy may help reduce the risk of relapse after ERP surgery, although its efficacy after salvage chemotherapy seems limited.

SUMMARY

Surgery plays a critical role in treating metastatic GCT outside of the RP. Because surgeries can be safely combined but have potential for significant morbidity, a multidisciplinary team with experience in treating testicular cancer is essential. Pathology from the RP does not always correlate with ERP sites and therefore resection of residual ERP masses after chemotherapy is recommended whenever feasible. However, for patients with favorable pathology (ie, necrosis or fibrosis) in the RP, close surveillance represents an alternative strategy, especially for masses that are difficult to resect or when resection may be associated with significant morbidity.

REFERENCES

1. Carver BS, Sheinfeld J. Management of postchemotherapy extra-retroperitoneal residual masses. World J Urol 2009;27(4):489–92.
2. Daneshmand S, Albers P, Fossa SD, et al. Contemporary management of postchemotherapy testis cancer. Eur Urol 2012;62(5):867–76.
3. Masterson TA, Shayegan B, Carver BS, et al. Clinical impact of residual extraretroperitoneal masses in patients with advanced nonseminomatous germ cell testicular cancer. Urology 2012;79(1):156–9.
4. Kesler KA, Brooks JA, Rieger KM, et al. Mediastinal metastases from testicular nonseminomatous germ cell tumors: patterns of dissemination and predictors of long-term survival with surgery. J Thorac Cardiovasc Surg 2003;125(4):913–23.

5. Wood A, Robson N, Tung K, et al. Patterns of supra-diaphragmatic metastases in testicular germ cell tumours. Clin Radiol 1996;51(4):273–6.

6. Fizazi K, Tjulandin S, Salvioni R, et al. Viable malignant cells after primary chemotherapy for disseminated nonseminomatous germ cell tumors: prognostic factors and role of postsurgery chemotherapy–results from an international study group. J Clin Oncol 2001;19(10):2647–57.

7. Steyerberg EW, Keizer HJ, Messemer JE, et al. Residual pulmonary masses after chemotherapy for metastatic nonseminomatous germ cell tumor. Prediction of histology. ReHiT study group. Cancer 1997;79(2):345–55.

8. Liu D, Abolhoda A, Burt ME, et al. Pulmonary metastasectomy for testicular germ cell tumors: a 28-year experience. Ann Thorac Surg 1998;66(5):1709–14.

9. Cagini L, Nicholson AG, Horwich A, et al. Thoracic metastasectomy for germ cell tumours: long term survival and prognostic factors. Ann Oncol 1998; 9(11):1185–91.

10. Gupta A, Feifer AH, Gotto GT, et al. Outcomes after resection of postchemotherapy residual neck mass in patients with germ cell tumors–an update. Urology 2011;77(3):655–9.

11. Rivoire M, Elias D, De Cian F, et al. Multimodality treatment of patients with liver metastases from germ cell tumors: the role of surgery. Cancer 2001; 92(3):578–87.

12. Hahn TL, Jacobson L, Einhorn LH, et al. Hepatic resection of metastatic testicular carcinoma: a further update. Ann Surg Oncol 1999;6(7):640–4.

13. Hartmann JT, Rick O, Oechsle K, et al. Role of post-chemotherapy surgery in the management of patients with liver metastases from germ cell tumors. Ann Surg 2005;242(2):260–6.

14. Jacobsen NE, Beck SD, Jacobson LE, et al. Is retroperitoneal histology predictive of liver histology at concurrent post-chemotherapy retroperitoneal lymph node dissection and hepatic resection? J Urol 2010;184(3):949–53.

15. Mehra S, Liu J, Gupta A, et al. Cervical metastasis of germ cell tumors: evaluation, management, complications, and outcomes. Laryngoscope 2012; 122(2):286–90.

16. Steyerberg EW, Keizer HJ, Stoter G, et al. Predictors of residual mass histology following chemotherapy for metastatic non-seminomatous testicular cancer: a quantitative overview of 996 resections. Eur J Cancer 1994;30A(9):1231–9.

17. Gerl A, Clemm C, Schmeller N, et al. Sequential resection of residual abdominal and thoracic masses after chemotherapy for metastatic non-seminomatous germ cell tumours. Br J Cancer 1994;70(5):960–5.

18. Hartmann JT, Candelaria M, Kuczyk MA, et al. Comparison of histological results from the resection of residual masses at different sites after chemotherapy for metastatic non-seminomatous germ cell tumours. Eur J Cancer 1997;33(6):843–7.

19. Mandelbaum I, Yaw PB, Einhorn LH, et al. The importance of one-stage median sternotomy and retroperitoneal node dissection in disseminated testicular cancer. Ann Thorac Surg 1983;36(5):524–8.

20. Tiffany P, Morse MJ, Bosl G, et al. Sequential excision of residual thoracic and retroperitoneal masses after chemotherapy for stage III germ cell tumors. Cancer 1986;57(5):978–83.

21. Qvist HL, Fossa SD, Ous S, et al. Post-chemotherapy tumor residuals in patients with advanced nonseminomatous testicular cancer. Is it necessary to resect all residual masses? J Urol 1991;145(2): 300–2 [discussion: 302–3].

22. McGuire MS, Rabbani F, Mohseni H, et al. The role of thoracotomy in managing postchemotherapy residual thoracic masses in patients with nonseminomatous germ cell tumours. BJU Int 2003;91(6):469–73.

23. Tognoni PG, Foster RS, McGraw P, et al. Combined post-chemotherapy retroperitoneal lymph node dissection and resection of chest tumor under the same anesthetic is appropriate based on morbidity and tumor pathology. J Urol 1998;159(6):1833–5.

24. Kesler KA, Kruter LE, Perkins SM, et al. Survival after resection for metastatic testicular nonseminomatous germ cell cancer to the lung or mediastinum. Ann Thorac Surg 2011;91(4):1085–93 [discussion: 1093].

25. Andrade RS, Kesler KA, Wilson JL, et al. Short- and long-term outcomes after large pulmonary resection for germ cell tumors after bleomycin-combination chemotherapy. Ann Thorac Surg 2004;78(4):1224–8 [discussion: 1228–9].

26. de Perrot M, Eaton D, Bedard PL, et al. Anterior transpericardial approach for postchemotherapy residual midvisceral mediastinal mass in metastatic germ cell tumors. J Thorac Cardiovasc Surg 2013; 145(4):1136–8.

27. Kesler KA. Surgical techniques for testicular nonseminomatous germ cell tumors metastatic to the mediastinum. Chest Surg Clin North Am 2002;12(4):749–68.

28. Milen MT, Bloom DA, Culligan J, et al. Albert Adamkiewicz (1850–1921)–his artery and its significance for the retroperitoneal surgeon. World J Urol 1999; 17(3):168–70.

29. van Vledder MG, van der Hage JA, Kirkels WJ, et al. Cervical lymph node dissection for metastatic testicular cancer. Ann Surg Oncol 2010;17(6):1682–7.

30. Weisberger EC, McBride LC. Modified neck dissection for metastatic nonseminomatous testicular carcinoma. Laryngoscope 1999;109(8):1241–4.

31. See WA, Laurenzo JF, Dreicer R, et al. Incidence and management of testicular carcinoma metastatic to the neck. J Urol 1996;155(2):590–2.

32. Kuvshinoff B, Fong Y. Surgical therapy of liver metastases. Semin Oncol 2007;34(3):177–85.

33. Fosså SD, Bokemeyer C, Gerl A, et al. Treatment outcome of patients with brain metastases from malignant germ cell tumors. Cancer 1999;85(4):988–97.

34. Steyerberg EW, Donohue JP, Gerl A, et al. Residual masses after chemotherapy for metastatic testicular cancer: the clinical implications of the association between retroperitoneal and pulmonary histology. Re-analysis of histology in testicular cancer (ReHiT) study group. J Urol 1997;158(2):474–8.

35. Einhorn LH. Do all germ cell tumor patients with residual masses in multiple sites require postchemotherapy resections? J Clin Oncol 1997;15(1):409–10.

36. Brenner PC, Herr HW, Morse MJ, et al. Simultaneous retroperitoneal, thoracic, and cervical resection of postchemotherapy residual masses in patients with metastatic nonseminomatous germ cell tumors of the testis. J Clin Oncol 1996;14(6):1765–9.

37. Skinner DG, Melamud A, Lieskovsky G. Complications of thoracoabdominal retroperitoneal lymph node dissection. J Urol 1982;127(6):1107–10.

38. Fadel E, Court B, Chapelier AR, et al. One-stage approach for retroperitoneal and mediastinal metastatic testicular tumor resection. Ann Thorac Surg 2000;69(6):1717–21.

39. Albers P, Ganz A, Hannig E, et al. Salvage surgery of chemorefractory germ cell tumors with elevated tumor markers. J Urol 2000;164(2):381–4.

40. Oechsle K, Bokemeyer C. Treatment of brain metastases from germ cell tumors. Hematol Oncol Clin North Am 2011;25(3):605–13, ix.

41. Girones R, Aparicio J, Roure P, et al. Synchronous versus metachronous brain metastasis from testicular germ cell tumors (TGCT): an analysis from the Spanish Germ Cell Cancer Group data base. Clin Transl Oncol 2014;16(11):959–65.

42. Fox EP, Weathers TD, Williams SD, et al. Outcome analysis for patients with persistent nonteratomatous germ cell tumor in postchemotherapy retroperitoneal lymph node dissections. J Clin Oncol 1993;11(7):1294–9.

Reoperative Retroperitoneal Surgery
Etiology and Clinical Outcome

Solomon L. Woldu, MD, James M. McKiernan, MD*

KEYWORDS

- Reoperative retroperitoneal lymph node dissection • Redo retroperitoneal lymph node dissection
- Retroperitoneal lymph node dissection • Residual retroperitoneal mass • Testicular cancer

KEY POINTS

- Retroperitoneal recurrences following retroperitoneal lymph node dissection (RPLND) should be viewed as either surgical/technical failures or inappropriate modifications to the original RPLND template.
- Retroperitoneal recurrences in the setting of post-RPLND nonseminomatous germ cell tumors (GCTs) are most commonly found in the para-aortic and periaortic region, owing to the difficulty of dissection within the region of the left renal hilum.
- The most common histology of a retroperitoneal recurrence following RPLND is a teratoma, followed by viable GCT and necrosis/fibrosis.
- Complete resection of all malignant tissue is required, as teratoma is chemoresistant and may undergo malignant transformation, and viable GCT, especially in the postchemotherapy, setting may be chemoresistant.
- In the hands of experienced surgeons at tertiary care centers, reoperative retroperitoneal surgery is associated with long-term survival in a significant proportion of patients, with an acceptable degree of morbidity.

INTRODUCTION

Improvements in the management of germ cell tumors (GCTs), most notably the introduction of highly effective cisplatin-based chemotherapy, has resulted in dramatically improved rates of overall survival, now exceeding 95% for all patients who receive a diagnosis of testicular cancer and 80% for those with metastatic disease.[1] The multimodal approach to the management of GCT with the integration of surgery, chemotherapy, and radiation serves as a model for the successful management of cancer and provides hope for dramatic improvements in the management and prognosis of other malignancies in the future.

Although the advent of effective chemotherapy provides an adjunct to technically challenging surgery, retroperitoneal lymph node dissection (RPLND) remains an essential component of the treatment algorithm for nonseminomatous germ cell tumors (NSGCT)[2,3] and serves as both a therapeutic and a diagnostic and staging procedure (see the article by Masterson and colleagues elsewhere in this issue for further exploration of this topic).

Whether done in the primary or postchemotherapy setting (PC-RPLND), it is apparent that complete resection of all metastatic retroperitoneal disease is the key variable related to long-term relapse-free survival.[4,5] Unfortunately, some

Department of Urology, Columbia University Medical Center, New York Presbyterian Hospital, Herbert Irving Pavilion – 11th Floor, 161 Fort Washington Avenue, New York, NY 10032, USA
* Corresponding author.
E-mail address: jmm23@columbia.edu

Urol Clin N Am 42 (2015) 381–392
http://dx.doi.org/10.1016/j.ucl.2015.05.001

patients will relapse in the retroperitoneum or harbor unresected disease after RPLND, and salvage chemotherapy will rarely adequately compensate for an inadequate initial RPLND, as these late recurrences tend to be chemoresistant malignancies or have chemoresistant teratomatous elements.[6,7] Despite the technical challenges, appropriately selected patients can be effectively managed with reoperative retroperitoneal surgery with an acceptable morbidity rate when performed by experienced surgeons at tertiary care centers.[4,8,9]

This review describes the patterns of metastasis of testicular tumors; incidence, distribution, and histologic findings of retroperitoneal recurrences; indications for reoperative retroperitoneal surgery; and postoperative morbidity/complications and clinical outcomes of patients with GCTs with retroperitoneal recurrences following RPLND.

TESTICULAR TUMORS AND PATTERNS OF METASTASIS

The successful management of testicular GCTs has been facilitated by a predictable pattern of metastatic spread of disease, primarily to the lymph nodes of the retroperitoneum and subsequently to the lung and posterior mediastinum.[10–12] This process holds true for all histologic subtypes of GCTs, with the notable exception of choriocarcinoma, which has a higher reported incidence of hematogenous distribution.[13] The embryologic origin of the testis in the retroperitoneum and, therefore, lymphatic drainage pattern informs the most common location of metastatic disease; tumors of the right testis are first drained by the interaortocaval area, followed by the precaval and preaortic lymph nodes, whereas tumors of the left testis are first drained by the para-aortic and preaortic lymph nodes, followed by the interaortocaval nodes.[11] Right testis tumors are more commonly associated with contralateral spread, and bulky retroperitoneal disease and lymphatic obstruction can result in more caudal deposition of metastatic disease in the retroperitoneum.[14]

Given the predictable patterns of metastatic spread of testicular cancer, RPLND has a well-established role in the management of NSGCT for several reasons. First, because the retroperitoneum is often the first and only site of metastatic disease, patients can be cured with RPLND as long as the initial surgery is thorough enough to removal all sites of gross or micrometastatic disease.[15] Second, although radiologic imaging continues to improve, clinical staging still underestimates the disease burden in the retroperitoneum, with a reported 20% to 30% incidence of pathologic stage II disease (positive retroperitoneal nodes) despite

radiographic suggestion of clinical stage I disease.[16] Third, the uncontrolled retroperitoneum represents a significantly adverse prognostic factor, as untreated retroperitoneal metastases are usually fatal.[7,15,17,18] The management of advanced-stage NSGCT involves the integration of chemotherapy and surgery, and even in the postchemotherapy setting for clinical stage IIA/IIB NSGCT, RPLND reveals a 6% to 8% incidence of viable malignancy and a 31% to 44% incidence of chemoresistant teratoma.[19] Finally, the retroperitoneum is the predominant site of relapse of seminomatous and nonseminomatous GCT for viable malignant tissue, teratoma, or teratoma with malignant transformation.[20,21]

INCIDENCE, DISTRIBUTION, AND HISTOLOGIC FINDINGS OF RETROPERITONEAL RECURRENCES

Tumor recurrence within the retroperitoneum following RPLND is a relatively rare event, with a reported incidence of approximately 1% to 3%, but incidence of as high as 8.2% has been reported (**Table 1**). However, there is reason to believe that residual disease within the retroperitoneum following RPLND may be an underreported phenomenon. The use of effective postoperative cisplatin-based chemotherapy, especially in chemo-naïve patients, may eliminate occult micrometastatic disease that was not resected during initial RPLND.[2,30] In addition, some centers will not perform routine postoperative imaging, and the lack of publications with long-term follow-up likely results in an underreporting of retroperitoneal recurrences.[2,31]

Except in rare cases, a retroperitoneal recurrence following RPLND should be regarded as a technical failure, which may be due to a variety of factors including inappropriate modifications to the original retroperitoneal dissection template or lack of expertise in performing the challenging initial dissection.[2,9,16]

This proposal is supported by the findings of increased retroperitoneal recurrence with left-sided primary testicular tumors, which are associated with a more complex left renal hilar dissection,[4,9,28] and the finding that incomplete lumbar ligation, a prerequisite for clearing the posterior lymphatics behind the great vessels, is a common finding at the time of reoperative retroperitoneal surgery.[9]

RPLND has had a well-established role in the management of NSGCT since 1948, but the surgical template, techniques, and decision to implement this strategy has evolved over the past several decades.[2,14,32] The initial description of

Table 1
Reported incidence of retroperitoneal relapse following RPLND

Authors	No. of Patients	No. of Retroperitoneal Relapses	Notes
Bredael et al,[17] 1982	138	1 (0.7%)	Pathologic stage I NSGCT who underwent RPLND Only 30 received adjuvant chemotherapy CT scans not routinely performed
Lieskovsky et al,[22] 1984	193	1 (0.5%) confirmed 12 unknown sites 2 elevated markers treated with chemotherapy	Clinical stage I, IIA, IIB NSGCT who underwent RPLND and adjuvant chemotherapy
Pizzocaro et al,[23] 1985	202	2 (1.0%)	Clinical stage I NSGCT who underwent RPLND Both recurrences in patients found to have pathologic stage II NSGCT at initial RPLND
Donohue et al,[24] 1990	73	1 (1.4%) 3 additional indeterminate CT scans with elevated serum tumor markers	Clinical stage I NSGCT who underwent nerve-sparing RPLND
Richie,[25] 1990	85	7 (8.2%)	Clinical stage I and IIA NSGCT who underwent RPLND
Weissbach & Hartlapp,[26] 1991	225	3 (1.3%)	Clinical stage IIB NSGCT who underwent RPLND and adjuvant chemotherapy
McLeod et al,[27] 1991	264	7 (2.7%)	Pathologic stage I NSGCT following RPLND
Cespedes & Peretsman,[28] 1990	88	6 (6.8%)	Clinical stage I and II NSGCT who underwent RPLND
Heidenreich et al,[16] 2003	239	3 (1.2%)	Clinical stage I NSGCT who underwent RPLND
Albers et al,[29] 2008	173	7 (4.0%)	Clinical stage I NSGCT

Abbreviations: CT, computed tomography; NSGCT, nonseminomatous germ cell tumor; RPLND, retroperitoneal lymph node dissection.

the RPLND involved an extensive template involving all the nodal tissue between both ureters from the suprahilar region down to the bifurcation of the common iliac arteries.[14,32] Before the advent of cisplatin-based chemotherapy, extensive suprahilar dissection was indicated because of a lack of effective alternative therapy. The discovery of effective systemic chemotherapy, coupled with the relatively low incidence of suprahilar nodal involvement, and significant morbidity associated with suprahilar dissection (including renovascular complications, pancreatic complications, and an increased incidence of chylous ascites), led to one of the first modifications of the RPLND template to exclude the suprahilar region from the standard template.[14,32] Although less morbid, the bilateral infrahilar RPLND was still associated with loss of antegrade ejaculation caused by damage to the paravertebral sympathetic ganglia, postganglionic sympathetic fibers, or the hypogastric plexus, with the incidence of retrograde ejaculation related to the degree of retroperitoneal dissection.[33] Several modified templates has been proposed to preserve antegrade ejaculation (see the article elsewhere in this issue "The Technique and Evolution of Nerve-Sparing Retroperitoneal Lymphadenectomy"). The mainstay of these nerve-sparing templates is to limit the dissection of the contralateral nodal basin, particularly below the level of inferior mesenteric artery, whereas the interaortocaval nodes are variably resected for left-sided primary tumors.[14,32] However, as Jewett and Torbey acknowledge of the limitations of modified templates, "all modified dissections introduce a risk of incomplete resection of involved nodes."[34]

Although modifications to the RPLND template have resulted in reduced morbidity, there is reason to question the adequacy of the anatomic mapping studies of retroperitoneal metastases on which these reduced templates are based. Landmark studies by Ray and colleagues[10] and Donohue and colleagues[11] lack follow-up information, which is a major limitation, as sample error by the surgeon or pathologist cannot be assessed. Without adequate postoperative follow-up the rate of extratemplate recurrence cannot be estimated.[2] Furthermore, it is not possible to accurately determine adequacy of a surgical dissection template, when all patients receive adjuvant chemotherapy. In addition, there is a concern for the potential impact of renal and renovascular anatomic variation on the lymphatic drainage pattern of the testicles, an area of research that has yet to be explored.[2] As such, Eggener and colleagues[35] compared the impact of using 5 modified RPLND templates (Testicular Tumor Study Group [TTSG], Memorial Sloan-Kettering Cancer Center [MSKCC], Indiana, Johns Hopkins University [JHU], Innsbruck) on 500 patients with clinical stage I to IIA NSGCT who underwent primary RPLND at MSKCC. Of the 191 patients with positive nodes, the incidence of extratemplate disease ranged from 3% to 23% depending on the particular node dissection template. For right-sided testicular primary tumors, the most common sites of extratemplate disease were the para-aortic nodes (included in only the MSKCC template) and preaortic nodes (excluded only in the JHU template). Excluding the para-aortic and periaortic nodes would have resulted in unresected disease in 34 (6.8%) patients. For left-sided testicular primary tumors, the most common sites of extratemplate disease were in the interaortocaval regions for those templates which excluded this region (TTSG, Innsbruck). Excluding the interaortocaval nodes for left-sided testicular tumors would have resulted in unresected disease in 23 (4.6%) patients.

Beyond inappropriate reductions in the dissection template, the other main source of retroperitoneal recurrence is lack of expertise or appropriate surgical resolve during the initial RPLND. Recent data suggest that the quality of RPLND is highly correlated with relapse-free survival.[36] Data from Europe, which has largely adopted a model of centralization of health care for complex operations, suggest that patients undergoing RPLND for GCT at higher volume hospitals have significantly improved survival.[37] In the United States, a review of case logs of 8545 urologists certifying between 2003 and 2013 revealed that just 3.4% (290) of urologists logged all the 553 RPLNDs. The median number of RPLNDs logged annually was 1, with just 3 of the 290 urologists performing 23% of all RPLNDs. Three-fourths of urologists logged only a single RPLND.[38] This finding, coupled with data from the American Board of Urology Residency Review Committee, which reports urology residents performed an average of approximately 5 RPLNDs during their 4-year training from 2000 to 2004,[39] and the finding that most recurrences are found within the field of the surgical template, is compelling evidence to suggest that the quality of RPLND may be compromised by inexperienced surgeons.[2,9]

Analysis of reoperative retroperitoneal series further suggests that surgical technique may play a key role in most retroperitoneal recurrences. In their series, Heidenreich and colleagues[40] noted that a significant proportion of retroperitoneal recurrences were located in the para-aortic and interaortocaval regions. The investigators state that complete resection of this area requires mobilization of the pancreas to expose the cranial aspect of the renal vessels and ligation of the lumbar veins entering the left renal vein, both technically challenging maneuvers. This statement is corroborated by the findings of several studies that identified the left renal hilum and left para-aortic regions as the most common sites of relapse following initial RPLND.[4,9,28] Furthermore, Pedrosa and colleagues[9] reported their findings of predictors of retroperitoneal recurrence in 188 patients with unilateral testicular tumors following RPLND. As an indicator of potentially incomplete initial resection, they found incomplete ligation of the lumbar vessels in 56.7% and absent ipsilateral gonadal vein resection in 21.3% of cases at the time of repeat RPLND. Taken together, these studies corroborate the hypothesis that surgical technique during initial RPLND has a significant impact on the rate of retroperitoneal recurrence.

Clearly, the extent of the dissection template will influence the location of possible retroperitoneal recurrences.[35] Pedrosa and colleagues[9] report the Indiana experience of the largest series of reoperative retroperitoneal surgery to date. More than half of their patients had tumors found within the primary landing zone, which should have been resected during the initial RPLND. There were notable differences between the site of recurrence based on the side of the primary testicular tumor. For the 100 patients with primary left-sided testicular tumors who underwent initial RPLND, the most common sites of retroperitoneal recurrence were the periaortic region (53%), followed by the retrocrural (26%), intra-aortocaval (24%), pelvic (19%), suprahilar (17%), and paracaval regions (16%). Of the 88 patients with primary right-sided testicular tumors, the retroperitoneal recurrence site was also most common in the paracaval region (37.5%), followed by the periaortic (35.2%), intra-aortocaval (26.1%), retrocrural (23.8%), pelvic (13.6%), and suprahilar regions (12.5%). These findings correspond with those of the MSKCC series, which found that the left para-aortic and/or hilar region was the most common site of retroperitoneal recurrence (53%).[4] There are 2 reasons for this: as previously noted, this region is often excluded in modified templates for right-sided testicular primary tumors.[35] In addition, the aforementioned technical difficulties of exposure in this region likely contributed to the preponderance of retroperitoneal recurrence within this region. Importantly the investigators from Indiana note that the suprahilar region was the site of recurrence in 12.5% to 17% of cases, a region outside the modern standard RPLND template, and presumably cannot be attributed to surgeon error.[9]

HISTOLOGIC FINDINGS AT REOPERATIVE RETROPERITONEAL SURGERY

The histology of retroperitoneal recurrences is an important consideration, as this affects the required therapies and survival. Just as the surgical template will influence the site of potential recurrence, the previous use of chemotherapy before reoperative retroperitoneal surgery will influence the histopathologic findings afterward. The problem in interpretation of the data is that most patients who undergo reoperative retroperitoneal surgery for recurrence will receive chemotherapy before their resection, either between the initial RPLND and the reoperative surgery, or the

initial RPLND will be performed in the postchemotherapy setting. In the MSKCC series, 86% of patients who underwent reoperation after a primary RPLND received chemotherapy between operations, and 50% of patients who underwent reoperation after a PC-RPLND received additional chemotherapy between operations.[4] In the Indiana series, 97.5% of patients received chemotherapy before reoperative retroperitoneal surgery.[9]

The most common histologic finding in the reoperative setting is teratoma (or teratoma with malignant transformation [TMT]), which makes intuitive sense given that most reoperative retroperitoneal surgeries are performed following chemotherapy, either before the initial RPLND or following it, and teratoma is considered chemotherapy resistant (**Table 2**).[2,4,9,40] Although it is a histologically benign entity, the clinical potential of unresected teratoma is unpredictable; it may grow, obstruct, or invade adjacent structures in what has been called growing teratoma syndrome.[37] In addition, teratoma may undergo malignant/somatic transformation with a change to a non-GCT entity (ie, sarcoma or carcinoma).[4,14] Unresected teratoma is also the main culprit of "late" relapses, defined as occurring after a 2-year disease-free period.[2,7] The clinical implications of residual teratoma are significant, as it necessitates complete surgical extirpation; however, if mature teratoma is the only histology found in the reoperative surgical specimen, the chances of long-term survival are favorable (see the section on clinical outcomes).[4,9]

The MSKCC and Indiana studies differ with regard to the second most common histopathology found on reoperative RPLND: the MSKCC study report fibrosis/necrosis to be the second most common entity found on RPLND, whereas the larger Indiana study reports that viable GCT is the second most common histopathologic finding.[4,9]

Table 2
Histology of masses at reoperative retroperitoneal surgery

Authors	No. of Patients	Viable GCT (%)	Teratoma (%)	TMT/Somatic Type Malignancy (%)	Fibrosis/Necrosis (%)
Sexton et al,[8] 2003	21	24	67	NR	24
McKiernan et al,[4] 2003	56	15	42	17	27
Heidenreich et al,[40] 2005	18	24	39	NR	47
Willis et al,[41] 2007	54	13	35	45	9
Pedrosa et al,[9] 2014	203	37	34	15	15

Abbreviations: GCT, germ cell tumor; NR, not recorded; TMT, teratoma with malignant transformation or somatic type malignancy (ie, sarcoma, carcinoma).
Some patients had tumors of multiple histologies.

Regardless, it is clear that adverse pathologic features are common findings in recurrent retroperitoneal masses, and there is no nonoperative way to determine the histology of these recurrent masses, as positron emission tomography cannot differentiate necrosis/fibrosis from teratoma.[42]

INDICATIONS FOR REOPERATIVE RETROPERITONEAL SURGERY

Reoperative retroperitoneal surgery for GCT recurrence following initial RPLND was initially described by Comisarow and Grabstald in 1976.[43] Although reoperation in this scenario remains a technically challenging operation with increased morbidity, it can result in long-term survival in properly selected patients and may represent the only chance of cure. However, as outcomes are certainly worse than in patients undergoing primary RPLND, reoperative retroperitoneal surgery should not substitute for an inadequate initial RPLND.[4]

Given the significant morbidity associated with reoperative retroperitoneal surgery, proper patient selection is of utmost importance before proceeding with this challenging operation. Several factors should be considered. First, the tumor should be amenable to resection. Even in experienced hands, the Indiana series noted that 27.1% of patients were deemed unresectable after attempting reoperative retroperitoneal surgery.[9] Complete resection is critical given the high rate of viable malignancy and/or teratoma in any unresected mass, so aggressive resection is required to optimize survival. Adjacent organ sacrifice or graft replacement of vessels may be required to perform complete resection.[2,14,44] Second, the patient should be examined carefully to rule out distant disease, as this may be a source of extra-retroperitoneal relapse. Patients with nonretroperitoneal disease should generally be offered resection, as these sites to may harbor chemoresistant teratoma, and extirpative surgery may provide long-term survival (see the article elsewhere in this issue "Role of Extraretroperitoneal Surgery in Patients with Germ Cell Tumors"). Third, the patient should be deemed unlikely to benefit from or tolerate systemic chemotherapy. Most patients in studies reporting on reoperative retroperitoneal surgery have received cisplatin-based chemotherapy before undergoing second surgery. Although more than 50% of recurrent retroperitoneal masses will harbor chemoresistant teratoma, a significant amount of patients with only viable GCT may potentially be cured with chemotherapy or salvage chemotherapy.[4,9] The lack of teratoma in the original RPLND specimen is not an indicator that the residual mass will not contain teratomatous elements; therefore, patients amenable to reoperative retroperitoneal surgery should undergo this salvage operation.[4]

Although elevated serum tumor markers after primary RPLND or PC-RPLND have historically indicated active systemic disease, and have been considered a relative indication for systemic primary or second-/third-line chemotherapy, there is growing evidence to suggest that radiographic recurrences associated with elevated tumor markers may benefit from reoperative retroperitoneal surgery.[45] In addition, although it is often quoted that elevated serum tumor markers indicate active GCT, several studies report finding only teratoma in 20% to 40% of PC-RPLND in the setting of elevated markers.[45–47] Furthermore, the presence of active, and potentially chemosensitive, GCT does not rule out the presence of chemoresistant teratomatous elements within the recurrent retroperitoneal mass. Therefore, the presence of elevated serum tumor markers with a radiographic recurrence after RPLND is not necessarily an indication to proceed with salvage chemotherapy regimens, as this may be consistent with disease limited to the retroperitoneum and these patients may benefit from resection. Both the MSKCC and Indiana studies reported that a significant proportion of patients undergoing reoperative retroperitoneal surgery had elevated serum tumor markers, and although elevated serum tumor markers were associated with increased risk of cancer-related mortality, a significant proportion experienced long-term survival (discussed in the next section).

CLINICAL OUTCOMES

Oncologic outcomes following reoperative retroperitoneal surgery vary according to the status of serum tumor markers, histologic findings at surgery, and the completeness of resection, which is of critical importance for the chance of long-term survival.[8] A review of the literature reveals varied reporting, from 63% to 91.3% survival. This wide variance is explained by differences in inclusion criteria, follow-up, histology found on reoperative surgery, and requirement of salvage chemotherapy (**Table 3**).

In a review of outcomes after reoperative retroperitoneal surgery, it is again important to stress the impact of complete initial resection, as several investigators have consistently demonstrated the negative prognostic significance of incompletely resected disease.[4,5] Stenning and colleagues[49] reported that incomplete resection of all residual masses following chemotherapy was associated with a 4-fold increase in the risk of disease progression.

Table 3
Survival following reoperative retroperitoneal surgery

Authors	No. of Patients	Average Follow-Up (y)	Survival
Waples & Messing,[48] 1993	9	2.7 (mean)	67% overall survival
Sexton et al,[8] 2003	21	4.7 (mean)	71% overall survival
McKiernan et al,[4] 2003	56	3.1 (median)	68% 5-y cancer-specific survival
Heindenreich et al,[40] 2005	18	1.8 (mean)	89% cancer-specific survival
Willis et al,[41] 2007	54	5.8 (median)	91.3% 10-y overall survival
Pedrosa et al,[9] 2014	203	6.1 (median)	65% cancer-specific survival

Furthermore, it is apparent from the MSKCC that reoperative retroperitoneal surgery does not compensate for inadequate initial RPLND (**Fig. 1**). McKiernan and colleagues[4] found a 5-year cancer-specific survival (CSS) after 99.3% survival following primary RPLND not requiring redo RPLND, compared with 86% in those requiring redo RPLND following incomplete primary RPLND ($P = .001$). The postchemotherapy setting exacerbated the discrepancies between complete and incomplete resection; the 5-year CSS after PC-RPLND not requiring redo surgery was 90%, compared with just 56% in those requiring redo PC-RPLND ($P<.0001$).

The investigators also noted that histologic findings and the status of serum tumor markers had a strong association with CSS. Whereas fibrosis or teratoma on resection had a CSS of 80%, viable GCT and TMT on reoperation was associated with 44% and 20% CSS, respectively. Differences in survival depending on status of tumor markers were also significant; those with elevated tumor markers had a 52% 2-year survival in patients with elevated tumor markers, compared with an 80% 2-year survival in patients with normal markers.[4]

Sexton and colleagues,[8] from the MD Anderson Cancer Center (MDACC), reported on outcomes of 21 patients following repeat RPLND, of whom 6 died during the study period, 5 from disease progression and 1 from a postoperative pulmonary embolus. At a mean follow-up of 4.7 years, 71% of patients were alive and 67% remained disease-free. Ten-year actuarial survival was estimated at 63%.

Willis and colleagues,[41] from Charing Cross Hospital, reported on outcomes of 54 patients who underwent repeat RPLND following initial PC-RPLND. With a median follow-up time of 8.5 years, the investigators reported 5- and 10-year CSS of 94.2% and 91.3%, respectively. In addition, unlike the MSKCC report, they found no difference in survival between those patients undergoing reoperative RPLND in comparison with those who underwent PC-RPLND not requiring reoperative surgery ($P = .592$). Also unlike previous studies, the investigators found no difference in survival based on histopathologic findings on reoperative RPLND. The contradictory results from this study in comparison with other reports are likely attributable to differences in the patient

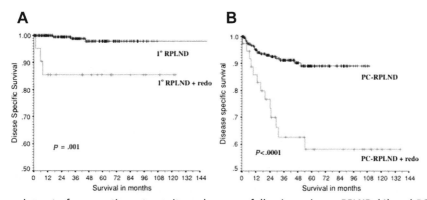

Fig. 1. Adverse impact of reoperative retroperitoneal surgery following primary RPLND (*A*) and PC-RPLND (*B*). (*From* Murphy AM, McKiernan JM. Reoperative retroperitoneal lymph-node dissection for testicular germ cell tumor. World J Urol 2009;27(4):505; with permission.)

populations, as evidenced by finding that only 50% of patients received cisplatin-based chemotherapy before repeat RPLND and 15% of cases were diagnosed with adenocarcinoma on reoperative surgery, at a median time to relapse of 16.9 years.

In a more recent analysis, investigators from Indiana University Medical Center reported the results of 203 patients followed for a median of 73.7 months following reoperative RPLND. At last follow-up, 35% (71 patients) died of disease and 10.3% (21 patients) were alive with disease. The 5- and 10-year CSS rates were 61.2% and 55.4%, respectively. Similarly to the MSKCC study, they found that elevated serum tumor markers (52.8% 5-year CSS, hazard ratio [HR] 2.0), and viable cancer in the resected specimen was associated with worse CSS (44.6% 5-year CSS, HR of death of 4.0 for active GCT and 2.1 for TMT). The most favorable histologic findings at reoperative RPLND were mature teratoma and necrosis, with no difference between the two (log rank $P = .73$). In addition, they found that receiving salvage chemotherapy and nonpulmonary metastatic disease (M1b) were significantly worse

prognostic factors for patients undergoing reoperative RPLND (**Fig. 2**).[9]

Given the larger size of the study, a multivariate analysis could be performed to determine which factors are independently associated with decreased survival. In the preoperative multivariate model, the authors identified 4 factors independently associated with worse CSS: active cancer found on the initial RPLND (HR 1.7), elevated serum tumor markers at the time of reoperative RPLND (HR 1.8), nonpulmonary metastatic disease stage M1b (HR 2.6), and the use of salvage chemotherapy (HR 2.2). Active malignancy in the resected specimen, salvage chemotherapy, and M1b disease were the only predictors to maintain significance in the full multivariate model (including preoperative and postoperative variables), likely attributable to a strong correlation with disease progression and systemic disease.[9]

PERIOPERATIVE MORBIDITY AND COMPLICATIONS

Reoperative retroperitoneal surgery is considered a significantly more challenging operation because

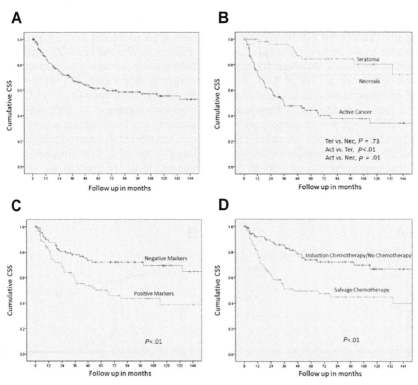

Fig. 2. Cancer-specific survival (CSS): (*A*) in 203 patients undergoing reoperative RPLND at Indiana University Medical Center; (*B*) based on pathology findings in reoperative RPLND specimen; (*C*) based on serum tumor marker status; (*D*) based on salvage chemotherapy history. (*From* Pedrosa JA, Masterson TA, Rice KR, et al. Reoperative retroperitoneal lymph node dissection for metastatic germ cell tumors: analysis of local recurrence and predictors of survival. J Urol 2014;191(6):1780; with permission.)

Table 4
Perioperative complications of reoperative retroperitoneal surgery

Authors	No. of Patients	Average Operative Time (h)	Average EBL (L)	Complication Rate (%)	Summary of Events
Waples & Messing,[48] 1993	9	7.5	5.5	56	1 chylous ascites 1 common bile duct injury 1 aortic injury resulting in lower extremity amputation 1 death from bleomycin toxicity
Sexton et al,[8] 2003	21	8.75	1.6 (median)	48	4 prolonged ileus 3 chylous ascites 2 partial small bowel obstructions 2 reintubation 1 pneumonia 1 abscess 1 chylous thorax 2 deaths
McKiernan et al,[4] 2003	56	NR	NR	30	4 lymphocele 3 Ileus 2 wound infection 2 small bowel obstruction 1 deep venous thrombosis 1 chylous ascites 1 dehiscence 1 pleural effusion 1 postoperative hemorrhage 1 ureteral injury 1 renal infarction 1 death (pulmonary embolus)
Heidenreich et al,[40] 2005	18	2.6	NR	38.8	1 ileus 2 chylous ascites 2 lymphocele 2 deep venous thrombosis
Willis et al,[41] 2007	54	NR	NR	9	1 deep venous thrombosis 1 chest infection 1 lymphocele 1 subphrenic collection 1 right ureteric injury
Pedrosa et al,[9] 2014	203	NR	0.5 (median)	Overall 44.8 Major 9.9 Minor 34.9	1 Clavien V complication 6 Clavien IV complications 14 Clavien III complications 40 Clavien II complications 66 Clavien I complications

Abbreviations: EBL, estimated blood loss; NR, not reported.

of extensive adhesions and a desmoplastic reaction secondary to the prior surgery, prior chemotherapy, and extravasated blood and lymphatic fluid.[2] In addition, identification of operative planes is difficult, which can lead to inadvertent subadventitial vascular dissection and injury to adjacent organs.[8,14,44] Several investigators have published their operative outcomes following reoperative morbidity and complications (**Table 4**).

In 1993, Waples and Messing[48] reported the University of Wisconsin experience of 9 patients who underwent reoperative retroperitoneal surgery and noted a perioperative complication rate of 56% (5 patients), which included chylous ascites requiring peritoneovenous shunting, common bile duct injury requiring pancreatic jejunostomy, and aortic injury resulting in limb loss.

Sexton and colleagues[8] reported the MDACC experience of 21 patients who underwent reoperative retroperitoneal surgery and noted a 29% intraoperative and 48% postoperative complication rate, including 2 cases of subadventitial aortic dissection, 1 of which required aortic grafting. The other most common complications reported were prolonged ileus, partial small bowel obstruction, and chylous ascites. Two patients died within 1 month of hospital discharge, one of pulmonary embolus and the other of failure to thrive and disease progression.

McKiernan and colleagues[4] reported the MSKCC experience of 56 patients who underwent a total of 61 reoperative retroperitoneal surgeries following primary RPLND (23 cases) and PC-RPLND (38 cases). The overall reported perioperative complication rate was 30%, including 1 death from a pulmonary embolus in a patient who underwent reoperative retroperitoneal surgery following a PC-RPLND.

Willis and colleagues[41] reported the Charing Cross Hospital experience of 54 patients who underwent reoperative retroperitoneal surgery following PC-RPLND. The overall reported perioperative complication rate was 9% (5 cases), including a deep venous thrombosis, chest infection, lymphocele, subphrenic collection, and right ureteric injury. In addition, the investigators reported on 2 late complications (4%) of atrophy of the right kidney and a recurrence in the abdominal wall.

Most recently, Pedrosa and colleagues[9] reported the updated experience from Indiana University Medical Center, which represents the largest reported cohort of patients treated with reoperative RPLND, composed of 203 patients treated from 1987 to 2011. This study was the first and only reoperative RPLND study to report complications in a standardized way; although the investigators

reported no perioperative mortalities, the overall complication rate was 44.8%, with a 9.9% classified as major according to the Clavien-Dindo classification scheme, meaning reintervention or intensive care was necessary.

An overall interpretation of the reported morbidity reported for reoperative retroperitoneal surgery by these dedicated tertiary care centers suggests that it can be performed with acceptable, but not minimal, risk. Even more so than with initial RPLND, surgeon expertise is paramount to minimizing patient risks during these challenging cases.[2,3,14] The risks of the operation must be weighed against the benefits of possible cure, especially in the postchemotherapy setting where viable GCT/teratoma may not respond to second-line chemotherapeutics.

SUMMARY

The role for RPLND in the setting of NSGCT is well defined and serves both a diagnostic and therapeutic role. When initial RPLND is not performed completely or accurately, because of either inappropriate modifications of the template or technical errors, the result can be relapse within the retroperitoneum. This uncontrolled retroperitoneum represents a significant adverse prognostic variable in patients with NSGCT and is associated with a significantly decreased overall survival. These recurrences are often found to contain teratoma, viable malignant tissue, or both, which will be unresponsive to cisplatin-based chemotherapy. There is no substitute for a properly performed initial RPLND, and reduced templates or inappropriate attempts to preserve antegrade ejaculation should never compromise oncologic goals. When faced with a retroperitoneal recurrence following RPLND, data from multiple tertiary care centers with experienced surgeons in the modern era of RPLND suggests that reoperative retroperitoneal surgery can be performed, with acceptable morbidity and a significant level of salvage and long-term survival.

REFERENCES

1. Testicular cancer—discoveries and updates. N Engl J Med 2014;371(21):2005–16.
2. Sheinfeld J, Sogani P. Reoperative retroperitoneal surgery. Urol Clin North Am 2007;34(2):227–33 [abstract: x].
3. Murphy AM, McKiernan JM. Reoperative retroperitoneal lymph-node dissection for testicular germ cell tumor. World J Urol 2009;27(4):501–6.
4. McKiernan JM, Motzer RJ, Bajorin DF, et al. Reoperative retroperitoneal surgery for nonseminomatous

germ cell tumor: clinical presentation, patterns of recurrence, and outcome. Urology 2003;62(4):732–6.

5. Donohue JP, Leviovitch I, Foster RS, et al. Integration of surgery and systemic therapy: results and principles of integration. Semin Urol Oncol 1998; 16(2):65–71.

6. Baniel J, Foster RS, Gonin R, et al. Late relapse of testicular cancer. J Clin Oncol 1995;13(5):1170–6.

7. Sheinfeld J. Risks of the uncontrolled retroperitoneum. Ann Surg Oncol 2003;10(2):100–1.

8. Sexton WJ, Wood CG, Kim R, et al. Repeat retroperitoneal lymph node dissection for metastatic testis cancer. J Urol 2003;169(4):1353–6.

9. Pedrosa JA, Masterson TA, Rice KR, et al. Reoperative retroperitoneal lymph node dissection for metastatic germ cell tumors: analysis of local recurrence and predictors of survival. J Urol 2014; 191(6):1777–82.

10. Ray B, Hajdu SI, Whitmore WF Jr. Proceedings: distribution of retroperitoneal lymph node metastases in testicular germinal tumors. Cancer 1974;33(2):340–8.

11. Donohue JP, Zachary JM, Maynard BR. Distribution of nodal metastases in nonseminomatous testis cancer. J Urol 1982;128(2):315–20.

12. Weissbach L, Boedefeld EA. Localization of solitary and multiple metastases in stage II nonseminomatous testis tumor as basis for a modified staging lymph node dissection in stage I. J Urol 1987; 138(1):77–82.

13. Alvarado-Cabrero I, Hernandez-Toriz N, Paner GP. Clinicopathologic analysis of choriocarcinoma as a pure or predominant component of germ cell tumor of the testis. Am J Surg Pathol 2014;38(1):111–8.

14. Sheinfeld J, Bosl GJ. Surgery of testicular tumors. In: Wein AJ, Kavoussi LR, Partin AW, et al, editors. Campbell's urology. Philadelphia: WB Saunders; 2012. p. 871–92.

15. Whitmore WF Jr. Surgical treatment of adult germinal testis tumors. Semin Oncol 1979;6(1):55–68.

16. Heidenreich A, Albers P, Hartmann M, et al. Complications of primary nerve sparing retroperitoneal lymph node dissection for clinical stage I nonseminomatous germ cell tumors of the testis: experience of the German Testicular Cancer Study Group. J Urol 2003;169(5):1710–4.

17. Bredael JJ, Vugrin D, Whitmore WF Jr. Autopsy findings in 154 patients with germ cell tumors of the testis. Cancer 1982;50(3):548–51.

18. Johnson DE, Appelt G, Samuels ML, et al. Metastases from testicular carcinoma. Study of 78 autopsied cases. Urology 1976;8(3):234–9.

19. Stephenson AJ, Bosl GJ, Motzer RJ, et al. Nonrandomized comparison of primary chemotherapy and retroperitoneal lymph node dissection for clinical stage IIA and IIB nonseminomatous germ cell testicular cancer. J Clin Oncol 2007;25(35): 5597–602.

20. Oldenburg J, Wahlqvist R, Fossa SD. Late relapse of germ cell tumors. World J Urol 2009;27(4):493–500.

21. Oldenburg J, Martin JM, Fossa SD. Late relapses of germ cell malignancies: incidence, management, and prognosis. J Clin Oncol 2006;24(35):5503–11.

22. Lieskovsky G, Weinberg AC, Skinner DG. Surgical management of early-stage nonseminomatous germ cell tumors of the testis. Semin Urol 1984; 2(4):208–16.

23. Pizzocaro G, Zanoni F, Salvioni R, et al. Surveillance or lymph node dissection in clinical stage I nonseminomatous germinal testis cancer? Br J Urol 1985;57(6):759–62.

24. Donohue JP, Foster RS, Rowland RG, et al. Nerve-sparing retroperitoneal lymphadenectomy with preservation of ejaculation. J Urol 1990;144(2 Pt 1):287–91 [discussion: 291–2].

25. Richie JP. Clinical stage 1 testicular cancer: the role of modified retroperitoneal lymphadenectomy. J Urol 1990;144(5):1160–3.

26. Weissbach L, Hartlapp JH. Adjuvant chemotherapy of metastatic stage II nonseminomatous testis tumor. J Urol 1991;146(5):1295–8.

27. McLeod DG, Weiss RB, Stablein DM, et al. Staging relationships and outcome in early stage testicular cancer: a report from the Testicular Cancer Intergroup Study. J Urol 1991;145(6):1178–83 [discussion: 1182–3].

28. Cespedes RD, Peretsman SJ. Retroperitoneal recurrences after retroperitoneal lymph node dissection for low-stage nonseminomatous germ cell tumors. Urology 1999;54(3):548–52.

29. Albers P, Siener R, Krege S, et al. Randomized phase III trial comparing retroperitoneal lymph node dissection with one course of bleomycin and etoposide plus cisplatin chemotherapy in the adjuvant treatment of clinical stage I nonseminomatous testicular germ cell tumors: AUO trial AH 01/94 by the German Testicular Cancer Study Group. J Clin Oncol 2008;26(18):2966–72.

30. Fraley EE, Narayan P, Vogelzang NJ, et al. Surgical treatment of patients with stages I and II nonseminomatous testicular cancer. J Urol 1985;134(1):70–3.

31. Yu HY, Madison RA, Setodji CM, et al. Quality of surveillance for stage I testis cancer in the community. J Clin Oncol 2009;27(26):4327–32.

32. Pearce S, Steinberg Z, Eggener S. Critical evaluation of modified templates and current trends in retroperitoneal lymph node dissection. Curr Urol Rep 2013;14(5):511–7.

33. Jewett MA, Kong YS, Goldberg SD, et al. Retroperitoneal lymphadenectomy for testis tumor with nerve sparing for ejaculation. J Urol 1988;139(6):1220–4.

34. Jewett MA, Torbey C. Nerve-sparing techniques in retroperitoneal lymphadenectomy in patients with low-stage testicular cancer. Semin Urol 1988;6(3): 233–7.

35. Eggener SE, Carver BS, Sharp DS, et al. Incidence of disease outside modified retroperitoneal lymph node dissection templates in clinical stage I or IIA nonseminomatous germ cell testicular cancer. J Urol 2007;177(3):937–42 [discussion: 942–3].

36. Carver BS, Cronin AM, Eggener S, et al. The total number of retroperitoneal lymph nodes resected impacts clinical outcome after chemotherapy for metastatic testicular cancer. Urology 2010;75(6):1431–5.

37. Joudi FN, Konety BR. The impact of provider volume on outcomes from urological cancer therapy. J Urol 2005;174(2):432–8.

38. Flum AS, Bachrach L, Jovanovic BD, et al. Patterns of performance of retroperitoneal lymph node dissections by American urologists: most retroperitoneal lymph node dissections in the United States are performed by low-volume surgeons. Urology 2014;84(6):1325–8.

39. Lowrance WT, Cookson MS, Clark PE, et al. Assessing retroperitoneal lymphadenectomy experience in United States urological residency programs. J Urol 2007;178(2):500–3 [discussion: 503].

40. Heidenreich A, Ohlmann C, Hegele A, et al. Repeat retroperitoneal lymphadenectomy in advanced testicular cancer. Eur Urol 2005;47(1):64–71.

41. Willis SF, Winkler M, Savage P, et al. Repeat retroperitoneal lymph-node dissection after chemotherapy for metastatic testicular germ cell tumour. BJU Int 2007;100(4):809–12.

42. Stephens AW, Gonin R, Hutchins GD, et al. Positron emission tomography evaluation of residual radiographic abnormalities in postchemotherapy germ cell tumor patients. J Clin Oncol 1996;14(5):1637–41.

43. Comisarow RH, Grabstald H. Re-exploration for retroperitoneal lymph node metastases from testis tumors. J Urol 1976;115(5):569–71.

44. Nash PA, Leibovitch I, Foster RS, et al. En bloc nephrectomy in patients undergoing postchemotherapy retroperitoneal lymph node dissection for nonseminomatous testis cancer: indications, implications and outcomes. J Urol 1998;159(3):707–10.

45. Beck SD, Foster RS, Bihrle R, et al. Post chemotherapy RPLND in patients with elevated markers: current concepts and clinical outcome. Urol Clin North Am 2007;34(2):219–25 [abstract: ix–x].

46. Albers P, Ganz A, Hannig E, et al. Salvage surgery of chemorefractory germ cell tumors with elevated tumor markers. J Urol 2000;164(2):381–4.

47. Wood DP Jr, Herr HW, Motzer RJ, et al. Surgical resection of solitary metastases after chemotherapy in patients with nonseminomatous germ cell tumors and elevated serum tumor markers. Cancer 1992;70(9):2354–7.

48. Waples MJ, Messing EM. Redo retroperitoneal lymphadenectomy for germ cell tumor. Urology 1993;42(1):31–4.

49. Stenning SP, Parkinson MC, Fisher C, et al. Postchemotherapy residual masses in germ cell tumor patients: content, clinical features, and prognosis. Medical Research Council testicular tumour working party. Cancer 1998;83(7):1409–19.

Long-term Morbidity of Testicular Cancer Treatment

Chunkit Fung, MD, MS[a],*, Sophie D. Fossa, MD, PhD[b],
Annalynn Williams, MS[c], Lois B. Travis, MD, ScD[d]

KEYWORDS

- Testicular cancer • Survivorship • Long-term morbidity • Cardiovascular disease
- Second malignant neoplasms • Neurotoxicity • Hypogonadism • Nephrotoxicity

KEY POINTS

- Potentially long-term life-threatening complications, including second malignant neoplasms, cardiovascular disease, neurotoxicity and ototoxicity, pulmonary complications, hypogonadism, and nephrotoxicity have accompanied the remarkable successes of testicular cancer treatment.
- Testicular cancer survivors should follow applicable national guidelines for cancer screening and management of cardiovascular risk factors.
- Health care providers should capitalize on the time of testicular cancer diagnosis as a teachable moment to introduce and promote lifestyle changes in testicular cancer survivors, including smoking cessation, better nutrition, and participation in a regular exercise regimen.
- Testicular cancer is positioned to become a paradigm in survivorship research for adult-onset cancer and the most comprehensive multi-institutional study to date is currently underway to examine genetic variants associated with long-term toxicities of platinum-based chemotherapy in testicular cancer survivors.

INTRODUCTION

Testicular cancer (TC) is the most common cancer among men age 18 to 39 years.[1] Because of effective cisplatin-based chemotherapy introduced in the 1970s[2] it is also the most curable cancer, with the 10-year relative survival for all patients with TC approaching 95%.[3,4] The incidence of TC has increased steadily in the past 20 years in the United States,[5] likely attributable to genetic and environmental factors.[6] However, potentially life-threatening complications, including second malignant neoplasms (SMN), cardiovascular disease (CVD), neurotoxicity and ototoxicity, pulmonary complications, hypogonadism, and nephrotoxicity,[7–9] have accompanied these remarkable

Conflicts of interest: C. Fung has a consulting or advisory role with Janseen Scientific Affairs, Dendreon, and Bayer HealthCare Pharmaceuticals Inc; receives research funding from Astellas Pharma (ISR000911); and has stock and other ownership interests in GlaxoSmithKline. S.D. Fossa, A. Williams, and L.B. Travis have no conflicts of interest.

[a] Division of Medical Oncology, James P. Wilmot Cancer Institute, University of Rochester Medical Center, 601 Elmwood Avenue, Box 704, Rochester, NY 14642, USA; [b] Departments of Clinical Radiotherapy and Oncology, Norwegian Radium Hospital, Postboks 4959 Nydalen, Oslo 0424, Norway; [c] Department of Public Health Sciences, University of Rochester Medical Center, University of Rochester School of Medicine and Dentistry, Saunders Clinical and Translational Research Building, 265 Crittenden Boulevard, Rochester, NY 14642, USA; [d] Department of Radiation Oncology, Rubin Center for Cancer Survivorship, University of Rochester Medical Center, Saunders Clinical and Translational Research Building, 265 Crittenden Boulevard, CU420318, Rochester, NY 14642, USA
* Corresponding author.
E-mail address: chunkit_fung@urmc.rochester.edu

successes.[3,6] This article focuses on pathogenesis, risks, and management of late effects experienced by long-term TC survivors (TCS), which are defined as individuals who are disease free 5 years or more after primary treatment.[10]

SECOND MALIGNANT NEOPLASMS
Pathogenesis

SMNs can be classified according to their predominant causal factors, including syndromic, cancer treatment, and shared causal exposures.[11] Categories are not mutually exclusive, and reflect the joint contribution of lifestyle factors, genetic susceptibility, environmental exposures, and host effects, including gene-environment interactions (Fig. 1).[12] Age at exposure and attained age are risk modifiers for selected SMNs.[13]

Risks of Leukemia

Radiotherapy for TC is associated with an increased risk of leukemia.[14] An international population-based study of leukemia in 18,567 TCS (n = 36 cases, 106 matched controls) reported a significant 3-fold increased risk of leukemia after abdominal and pelvic radiotherapy (mean dose to active bone marrow = 10.9 Gy).[14] The median latency of the leukemias (22 of 36 occurred after radiotherapy alone) was 5.0 years, with 25% developing after 1 decade. However, the absolute risk of leukemia was low (9 excess cases per 10,000 patients per year followed for 15 years after 25 Gy of abdominal and pelvic radiation).[14]

Both cisplatin and etoposide are also associated with significant excesses of secondary leukemia.[14–17] The cumulative incidences of leukemia 5 years after receiving a cumulative etoposide dose of less than 2000 mg/m^2 and greater than or equal to 2000 mg/m^2 are approximately 0.5% and 2.0%, respectively.[17] In a multivariable model that adjusted for radiation dose, an international nested case-control study of leukemia[14] reported a significant dose-response relationship between

increasing cumulative dose of cisplatin and leukemia (P_{trend} = .001). Although the excess risk was small (16 excess cases among 10,000 patients with TC at 15 years of follow-up), the estimated risk of leukemia after a cumulative cisplatin dose of 650 mg was increased about 3.2-fold.

Risks of Solid Cancers

The overall relative risk (RR) of second solid cancers in TCS compared with the general population is 1.4 to 1.9, with risks increasing 5 years after treatment (Table 1).[13,18,19] In an international population-based investigation of 40,576 TCS, patients with TC who survived at least 10 years (n = 20,984) had significantly increased risks of solid cancers associated with radiotherapy alone (RR = 2.0; 95% confidence interval [CI], 1.9–2.2), chemotherapy alone (RR = 1.8; 95% CI, 1.3–2.5), or both (RR = 2.9; 95% CI, 1.9–4.2).[13] In particular, significantly 1.5-fold to 4.0-fold increased risks for malignant melanoma and cancers of the lung, thyroid, esophagus, pleura, stomach, pancreas, colon, rectum, kidney, bladder, and connective tissue were reported.[13] Compared with population expected risks of 23%, the cumulative risks of solid cancer by 75 years of age among men diagnosed with seminomas or nonseminomas at 35 years of age were 36% and 31%, respectively. In particular, among patients given radiotherapy alone, the risks of SMN at sites included in standard infradiaphragmatic radiotherapy fields were significantly larger than risks at unexposed sites (RR = 2.7 vs 1.6; P<.05), and remained increased for more than 35 years.

Several studies reported significant dose-response relationships between radiotherapy and SMN risks in TCS.[19–22] In a case-control study of 5-year TCS (1959–1987),[22] TCS given radiotherapy had a 5.9-fold increased risk of stomach cancer compared with controls, and risk increased with increasing radiation dose to stomach (P_{trend}<.001). The odds ratios (OR) for developing gastric cancer at radiation doses to the stomach

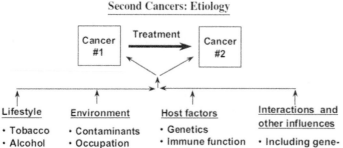

Second Cancers: Etiology

Cancer #1 → Treatment → Cancer #2

Lifestyle
- Tobacco
- Alcohol
- Diet
- Other

Environment
- Contaminants
- Occupation
- Other

Host factors
- Genetics
- Immune function
- Hormonal, other

Interactions and other influences
- Including gene-environment

Fig. 1. Risk factors for second primary cancer (refer to text). Many influences, some of which are shown here, may contribute to the development of multiple primary cancers, including interactions between exposures. (Adapted from Travis LB. Therapy-associated solid tumors. Acta Oncol 2002;41(4):324; with permission.)

of 10.0 to 19.9, 20.0 to 29.9, 30.0 to 39.9, 40 to 40.9, and greater than or equal to 50.0 Gy were 2.0 (95% CI, 0.5–8.7), 2.5 (95% CI, 0.8–7.9), 7.2 (95% CI, 2.1–24.9), 6.7 (95% CI, 1.7–27.1), and 20.5 (95% CI, 3.7–114.3) compared with less than 10 Gy, respectively.[22] In another study,[19] the hazard ratio (HR) for SMN was higher for those who received subdiaphragmatic radiotherapy administered at tumor doses of 40 to 50 Gy (HR = 3.2) and 26 to 35 Gy (HR = 2.3), compared with the surgery-only group. However, radiation tumor doses of greater than 30.0 Gy are no longer commonly used in contemporary radiation treatment of seminoma.[23,24]

Recently, a large population-based series[25] of 12,691 patients with testicular nonseminoma treated in the modern era of cisplatin-based chemotherapy (1980–2008) reported significantly increased 40% excesses of solid tumors after initial chemotherapy (standardized incidence ratio [SIR] = 1.43; 95% CI, 1.2–1.7; n = 111 solid cancers), whereas no increased risk followed surgery alone (SIR = 0.93; 95% CI, 0.8–1.1; n = 99 solid cancers). After chemotherapy, increased risks of solid cancer were reported in most follow-up periods (median latency = 12.5 years), including at more than 20 years after treatment (SIR = 1.54; 95% CI, 0.96–2.3). In particular, the study reported significantly increased 3-fold to 7-fold risks of cancers of the kidney (SIR = 3.4; 95% CI, 1.8–5.8), thyroid (SIR = 4.4; 95% CI, 2.2–7.9), and soft tissue (SIR = 7.5; 95% CI, 3.6–13.8).[25] However, detailed information on cytotoxic drug name and dose were not available.[25]

Management

In general, all survivors of adult-onset cancer, including TCS, should follow applicable national guidelines for cancer screening. Given the increased SMN risk in cancer survivors, screening and early detection strategies have been suggested,[12] particularly in those deemed at high risk because of previous treatment history and/or health habits. Site-specific recommendations regarding screening in cancer survivors were recently summarized by Wood and colleagues[12] (**Table 2**).

CARDIOVASCULAR DISEASE AND RAYNAUD PHENOMENON
Pathogenesis

The pathophysiology of CVD in TCS, including the direct (direct endothelial damage) and indirect hypotheses (increased incidence of cardiovascular risk factors), has been reviewed in detail by Feldman and colleagues.[26]

Risks

The RR of CVD among TCS treated with chemotherapy is significantly increased compared with those in the general population or managed with surveillance (no chemotherapy or radiation), with risks ranging from 1.4 to 7.1.[19,27–30] Among 390 patients treated with chemotherapy in the United Kingdom (1982–1992), a 7% incidence of angina, myocardial infarction (MI), or sudden cardiac death was reported.[28] After a median follow-up of 9.7 years, patients with TC who received chemotherapy had a significantly increased age-adjusted RR of 2.6 (95% CI, 1.2–5.8) for a cardiac event compared with patients with TC treated with surgery alone.[28]

In a retrospective study[30] of a nationwide cohort of 2707 5-year TCS in the Netherlands (1965–1995) with a median follow-up of 18.4 years, an increased incidence of coronary artery disease, defined as MI or angina, was reported compared with age-matched and sex-matched data in the general Dutch population, with an SIR of 1.2 (95% CI, 1.04–1.31). Using multivariate Cox regression analysis, cisplatin, vinblastine, and bleomycin (PVB) chemotherapy was associated with a 1.9-fold (95% CI, 1.7–2.0) increased risk of MI and bleomycin, etoposide, and cisplatin (BEP) chemotherapy was associated with a 1.5-fold (95% CI, 1.0–2.2) increased CVD risk, but not an increased MI risk (HR = 1.2; 95% CI, 0.7–2.1).[30] In a follow-up study[19] using the same cohort (N = 2707 Dutch 5-year TCS with a median follow-up of 17.6 years), chemotherapy (PVB or BEP) increased the risk of CVD by 1.7-fold (95% CI, 1.1–2.5).

Haugnes and colleagues[27] evaluated the incidence of cardiovascular risk factors and long-term incidence of CVD among 990 5-year TCS (median follow-up = 19 years) treated at 5 Norwegian university hospitals (1980–1994). All treatment groups (radiation, chemotherapy, and combined radiation/chemotherapy) had significantly increased prevalence of usage of antihypertensive medications compared with the age-matched male controls in the general population (general population = 13%; surgery = 12%; radiation = 22%; chemotherapy = 26%; and radiation/chemotherapy = 37%). Those in the radiation (10.2%; OR = 2.3; 95% CI, 1.5–3.7) and radiation/chemotherapy groups (15.6%; OR = 3.9; 95% CI, 1.4–10.9) also had higher prevalence of diabetes than the general population (4.3%). Using age-adjusted Cox regression analyses, increased risks of atherosclerotic disease were reported in the radiation (HR = 2.3; 95% CI, 1.04–5.3), chemotherapy (HR = 2.6; 95% CI, 1.1–5.9), and combined radiation/chemotherapy cohorts (HR = 4.8; 95% CI, 1.6–14.4) compared with those

Table 1
RRs of SMNs in TCS

	No. of Patients	Calendar Years of TC Diagnosis	Duration of Follow-up (y)	Treatment	Obs	RR	(95% CI)
Study Populations[a]							
All SMNs							
Norwegian Radium Hospital[98]	2006	1952–1990	Mean = 12.5	Any	153[b]	1.7	1.4–1.9
				RT	130	1.6	1.3–1.9
				CT	4	1.3	0.4–3.4
				RT + CT	15	3.5	2.0–5.8
Fourteen population-based tumor registries in Europe and North America[13]	40,576	1943–2001	Mean = 11.3	Any	1694	1.9	1.8–2.1
				RT	892	2.0	1.9–2.2
				CT	35	1.8	1.3–2.5
				RT + CT	25	2.9	1.9–4.2
Thirteen international cancer registries[99]	29,511	1943–2000	Median = 8.3	Any	1811[c]	1.7	1.6–1.7
Netherlands TCS cohort[19]	2707	1965–1995	Median = 17.6	Any	270[d]	1.7	1.5–1.9
				RT	199	1.7	1.5–2.0
				CT	23	1.4	0.9–2.1
				RT + CT	29	3.0	2.0–4.4
				SDRT	NA	2.6[g]	1.7–4.0
				SDRT + MRT	NA	3.6[g]	2.1–6.0
				PVB/BEP	NA	2.1[g]	1.4–3.1
				SDRT (26–35 Gy)	NA	2.3[g]	1.5–3.6
				SDRT (40–50 Gy)	NA	3.2[g]	2.1–5.1

Swedish Family Cancer Database[100]	5533	1980–2006	NA	Any	274[e]	2.0	1.8–2.2
Second Solid Cancers							
Sixteen population-based registries within the SEER program[25]	12,691	1980–2008	Median = 7.0	Initial surgery only Initial CT (no RT)	99 111[f]	0.9 1.4	0.8–1.1 1.2–1.7
Therapy-associated Leukemia							
Nested case-control study of leukemia in 8 population-based tumor registries in Europe and North America[14]	18,567	1970–1993	NA	No RT/CT RT CT RT + CT	4 22 8 2	1.0 3.1 5.0 5.1	– 0.7–2.2 1.1–40 0.5–28

Abbreviations: BEP, bleomycin, etoposide, cisplatin; CI, confidence interval; CT, chemotherapy; MRT, mediastinal radiation; NA, not available (data not provided); Obs, observed number of cases; PVB, cisplatin, vinblastine, bleomycin; RR, relative risk; RT, any radiation treatment; SDRT, supradiaphragmatic radiation; SEER, Surveillance, Epidemiology, and End Results.

   a There was overlap in the cancer registries included in the cohort studies by Richiardi and colleagues[99] and Travis and colleagues,[13] with Denmark, Finland, Norway, and Sweden contributing patients to both studies.

   b Six cases of leukemia were observed with an RR of 1.9 (95% CI, 0.7–4.1).

   c Thirty-eight cases of myeloid leukemia were observed with an RR of 3.6 (95% CI, 2.6–5.0); 13 cases of lymphoid leukemia were observed with an RR of 1.0 (95% CI, 0.5–1.7); 23 cases of other types of leukemia were observed with an RR of 3.5 (95% CI, 2.2–5.2).

   d Six cases of leukemia were observed with an RR of 1.6 (95% CI, 0.6–3.5).

   e Hazard ratios (HRs) are shown, with the referent group consisting of patients treated with surgery alone (HR = 1.0). Twelve cases of leukemia were observed with an RR of 3.8 (95% CI, 2.0–6.7).

   f Significantly increased risks occurred for cancers of the kidney (standardized incidence ratio [SIR] = 3.4; 95% CI, 1.8–5.7; n = 13); thyroid (SIR = 4.4; 95% CI, 2.2–7.9; n = 11); and soft tissue (SIR = 7.5; 95% CI, 3.6–13.8; n = 10).

   g Hazard ratios (HRs) are shown, with the referent group consisting of patients treated with surgery alone (HR, 1.0).

Adapted from Fung C, Fossa SD, Beard CJ, et al. Second malignant neoplasms in testicular cancer survivors. J Natl Compr Canc Netw 2012;10(4):548. Table 2; with permission.

Table 2
SMN screening and prevention recommendations in cancer survivors at moderate to high risk

SMN Site	Risk Level	Screening Recommendation	Chemoprevention Agents
Colon	Moderate risk: FDR with colon cancer younger than age 60 y or 2 SDRs with colon cancer at any age Radiation in which colon/rectum were included in treatment fields High risk: Family history suggestive of HNPCC	Colonoscopy at age 40 y or 10 y before the earliest case of cancer in the family Colonoscopy at age 35 y or 10 y after radiation Colonoscopy every 1–2 y, starting at age 20–30 y (depending on syndrome)	NSAIDs, COX-2 inhibitors, curcumin, difluoromethyl ornithine, aspirin, isothiocyanates (including sulforaphane), or resveratrol: Not recommended for secondary or tertiary prevention
Skin	High risk: Family history of early melanoma	Annual skin examination and monthly skin self-examination	—
Lung	Increased risk: Prior radiation to chest with or without chemotherapy High risk: Current smokers (>30 pack y); former smokers (>30 pack y and quit <15 y ago)	Smoking cessation Annual low-dose spiral CT	Isotretinoin, etretinate, vitamin E, retinoids, N-acetylcysteine, or aspirin: Not recommended Budesonide, COX-2 inhibitors, 5-LOX inhibitors, and prostacyclin analogs: Not recommended for individuals who have a history of lung cancer
Prostate	High risk: Family history of early prostate cancer (onset younger than age 65 y); personal or family member with mutation in *BRCA1* or *BRCA2*	Serum PSA with or without DRE every 1–2 y, starting at age 45 y	—
Head and neck (upper aerodigestive tract)	—	—	Isotretinoin, β-carotene: Not recommended

Abbreviations: 5-LOX, 5-lipoxygenase; COX-2, cyclooxygenase-2; CT, computed tomography; DRE, digital rectal examination; FDR, first-degree relative; HNPCC, hereditary nonpolyposis colon cancer; NSAID, nonsteroidal antiinflammatory drug; PSA, prostate-specific antigen; SDR, second-degree relative.

Adapted from Wood ME, Vogel V, Ng A, et al. Second malignant neoplasms: assessment and strategies for risk reduction. J Clin Oncol 2012;30:3740–1; with permission.

given surgery only (P_{trend} = .02). In particular, treatment with BEP alone increased the risk of coronary artery disease by 5.7-fold (95% CI, 1.9–17.1) compared with surgery only and increased the risk for MI by 3.1-fold (95% CI, 1.2–7.7) compared with age-matched male controls.[27]

Management

At present, no evidence-based CVD screening recommendations have been developed specifically for TCS. In November 2013, the American College of Cardiology and the American Heart

Associated released guidelines that address the assessment of cardiovascular risk, lifestyle modifications to reduce cardiovascular risk, and management of increased blood cholesterol and body weight in adults.[31] Patients with TC should be advised to adhere to these guidelines for primary prevention of CVD and should also establish care with medical providers who will monitor and modify their CVD risk factors according to currently accepted guidelines.[26]

PULMONARY TOXICITY
Pathogenesis

The proposed primary mechanism for pulmonary toxicity is induction of cytokines and free radicals leading to initial endothelial damage by influx of inflammatory cells and fibroblasts,[32,33] and ultimately causing pulmonary fibrosis.[32,33]

Risks

The long-term prevalence of nonfatal pulmonary toxicity is approximately 7% to 21% in TCS.[34–37] Haugnes and colleagues[38] examined the pulmonary function of 1049 TCS treated (1980–1994) in Norway with a mean observation time of 11.2 years (range = 5–21 years). Compared with the surgery group, cisplatin dose ($P = .007$) and increasing age ($P = .008$) were significantly associated with restrictive lung disease several years after TC treatment in multivariate analyses, including adjustment for doses of bleomycin, etoposide, and vinblastine. In a large population-based study in North America and Europe (1943–2002) of 38,907 1-year TCS (median follow-up = 10 years), Fossa and colleagues[39] reported that men treated with chemotherapy (with or without radiotherapy) in 1975 or later had higher mortality from all respiratory diseases (SMR = 1.58; 95% CI, 1.25–2.01) compared with the general population.

Management

The most effective management for bleomycin-induced pneumonitis is to withhold bleomycin at the earliest signs or symptoms. Corticosteroids are the mainstay of treatment, although there are no data from prospective randomized trials to support this approach.[33] For patients with TC with a history of bleomycin exposure who later undergo surgery, a thorough medical history, physical examination, and conduct of pulmonary function tests, chest radiograph, and cardiac ejection fraction assessments (for those also exposed to cardiotoxic chemotherapy) should be considered preoperatively to identify those at greatest risk

for pulmonary complications.[40] For these patients, intravenous fluids should be administered in the form of colloid and restricted to the lowest volume required to maintain hemodynamic stability and renal output. In addition, supplemental oxygen should be maintained at the minimal concentration (average of 40% fraction of inspired oxygen) necessary for sufficient oxygenation during surgery.[40]

NEPHROTOXICITY
Pathogenesis

Cisplatin causes damage to the proximal and distal tubular epithelium and collecting ducts in animal and human studies.[41,42] At high doses, it also damages the glomerulus.[41,42]

Risks

Long-term studies[43,44] of renal function show persistent changes from baseline values many years after TC treatment. Among 85 patients with malignant germ cell tumor (GCT) surviving more than 10 years after retroperitoneal lymph node dissection (n = 14), radiation treatment (n = 18), or chemotherapy with or without surgery/radiotherapy (n = 53), Fossa and colleagues[44] reported that 25 patients had long-term impaired renal function, with 23 of them in either the radiation or chemotherapy cohort. In particular, renal function decreased by 8% and 14% after radiation and chemotherapy, respectively. The cumulative dose of cisplatin was associated with the degree of renal function damage.[44] In another study, Hansen and colleagues[43] examined long-term effects of cisplatin on renal function in 34 patients with GCT (median follow-up = 65 months [range = 43–97 months]). Cisplatin caused acute nephrotoxicity (median decrease of 18% in glomerular filtration rate [GFR]) with subsequent improvement in 18 of 34 patients (53%) who were observed for 3 to 8 years, suggesting partial reversibility of the renal impairment.[43] Aside from decrease in GFR, increased microalbuminuria in long-term TCS may also be considered a sign of vascular damage within the kidney.[45] Bosl and colleagues[46] reported significant increases in serum renin and aldosterone levels in 24 normotensive patients after cisplatin-based chemotherapy for metastatic GCT (range of follow-up = 9–54 months). The reported increase in incident CV events in long-term TCS[27,28,30] may be partially attributed to nephrotoxicity because various studies report a relationship between decreased GFR and the presence of microalbuminuria leading to increased risks of CV and all-cause mortality in the general population.[47,48]

Management

Hydration is the most effective intervention to limit the severity of renal damage during cisplatin-based chemotherapy.[49] Coadministration of nephrotoxic drugs should also be avoided.[9]

NEUROTOXICITY
Pathogenesis

Mechanisms underlying chemotherapy-induced peripheral neuropathy (CIPN) remain largely unclear and include damage to neuronal cell bodies in the dorsal root ganglion and axonal toxicity through transport deficits or energy failure (reviewed by Travis and colleagues[50]).

Risks

Approximately 7% to 31% of patients with TC undergoing cisplatin-based chemotherapy develop CIPN acutely.[15,51,52] Importantly, 20% to 40% of patients experience persistent long-term symptoms.[53,54] In a Norwegian population-based survey (median = 11 years after TC treatment), 28% and 46% of TCS reported paresthesias after 1 to 4 and greater than or equal to 5 cycles of cisplatin-based chemotherapy, respectively, compared with 10% after orchiectomy alone. Glendenning and colleagues[54] reported a lower incidence of CIPN (20%) as detected by neurophysiologic testing, which was probably attributable to one-third of patients with TC in this study having received carboplatin instead of cisplatin-based chemotherapy.[54]

The incidence of CIPN depends on cumulative cisplatin dose. Compared with a control group of TCS who did not receive chemotherapy, the OR for the development of symptomatic paresthesias of the hands among those treated with 1 to 4 and greater than or equal to 5 cycles of cisplatin-based chemotherapy in Norway (1980–1994) were 2.0 (95% CI, 1.5–2.7) and 3.9 (95% CI, 2.1–7.3), and the OR for symptomatic paresthesias of the feet after 1 to 4 cycles and greater than or equal to 5 cycles of cisplatin-based chemotherapy were 2.2 (95% CI, 1.7–3.0) and 3.1 (95% CI, 1.7–5.7), respectively, compared with those without chemotherapy.[53] In another study, Sprauten and colleagues[55] reported a significant relationship between increasing levels of residual serum platinum levels and CIPN severity after adjusting for initial cisplatin dose.[55] A significant 4-fold to 5-fold association with total Scale for Chemotherapy-Induced Neurotoxicity score emerged for the highest residual platinum quartile.[55]

To understand the large interindividual variations of CIPN after cisplatin-based chemotherapy in TCS, Oldbenburg and colleagues[56] investigated the impact of germline single nucleotide polymorphisms of glutathione S-transferase (GST) P1, M1, and T1 on self-reported paresthesias among long-term TCS. They reported that TCS with the genotype GSTP1-GG had a significantly lower risk of developing paresthesia in the fingers (OR = 0.46; 95% CI, 0.22–0.96) and toes (OR = 0.42; 95% CI, 0.20–0.88) than TCS with the GSTP1-AA and GSTP1-AG genotypes.[56]

Management

No standard treatment has been reported to effectively prevent or reverse CIPN. For symptomatic treatment of CIPN, the recent American Society of Clinical Oncology practice guideline recommends treatment with duloxetine.[57]

OTOTOXICITY
Pathogenesis

Cisplatin causes selective damage to the outer hair cells of the cochlea, resulting in ototoxic symptoms, including tinnitus and hearing loss that impairs high frequencies (4000–8000 Hz) (reviewed by Travis and colleagues[50]).

Risks

After a median follow-up of 58 months (range = 15–159 months) for 86 patients with TC, Bokemeyer and colleagues[58] reported symptomatic ototoxicity in 20% of TCS, with 59%, 18%, and 23% of the 17 affected patients experiencing tinnitus, hearing loss, or both tinnitus and hearing loss, respectively, whereas 10% had reversible ototoxic symptoms between 1 and 18 months after treatment. These symptoms were bilateral in 81% of patients.[58] Among patients with TC who received cumulative doses greater than 400 mg/m^2, 50% of them experienced long-term persistent ototoxicity.[58] In another study (median follow-up = 10.7 years; n = 1409 patients with TC), Brydøy and colleagues[53] reported that patients with TC who received 1 to 4 cycles of cisplatin-based chemotherapy had increased hearing impairment (OR = 1.5; 95% CI, 1.2–2.0) and tinnitus (OR = 1.8; 95% CI, 1.4–2.4) compared with TCS who never received chemotherapy. Similarly, TCS who received 5 or more cycles of chemotherapy also had higher risks of hearing impairment (OR = 3.8; 95% CI, 2.1–6.8) and tinnitus (OR = 3.4; 95% CI, 1.9–5.9) than those not given chemotherapy. In particular, the degree of ototoxicity was most pronounced for TCS after dose-intensive chemotherapy (hearing impairment: OR = 5.3; 95% CI, 3.0–9.2. Tinnitus: OR = 7.1; 95% CI, 4.1–12.4).[53] In addition, older age, high cumulative dose of cisplatin received, and impaired renal and hearing functions seem to be other independent factors associated with more severe ototoxicity.[53,58,59]

A few studies have examined associations of germline genetic polymorphisms in candidate genes with platinum-related ototoxicity. Oldenburg and colleagues[60] reported that both alleles of [105]Val-GSTP1 offered protection against cisplatin-induced hearing impairment as assessed by audiometric testing (up to 4000 dB) in 173 cisplatin-treated TCS. Compared with 105Val/105Val-GSTP1, the risk of having an inferior audiometric result was approximately 4-fold higher in TCS with 105Ile/105Ile-GSTP1 or 105Val/105Ile-GSTP1 (OR = 4.21; 95% CI, 1.99–8.88; P<.001).

In a study of children who received cisplatin as part of cancer treatment, carriers of the minor allele (adenine) of rs12201199 of the TPMT gene and the minor allele (adenine) of rs9332377 of the COMT gene had 17.0-fold (95% CI, 2.3–125.9; P = .00022) and 5.5-fold increased risks (95% CI, 1.9–15.9; P = .00018) of developing cisplatin-induced hearing loss compared with those who were not carriers, respectively.[61] Subsequently, a report[62] of 213 children with medulloblastoma did not replicate the TPMT and COMT results discussed earlier, although Pussegoda and colleagues[63] replicated prior findings for TPMT (rs12201199; OR = 6.1; P = .001) and ABCC3 (rs1051640; OR = 1.8; P = .04) thereafter. In addition, in a recent genomewide association study in 238 children with brain tumors, an inherited genetic variation in ACYP2 (rs1872328) was identified to be associated with cisplatin-related ototoxicity (HR = 4.5; P = 3.9 × 10^{-8}).[64]

Management

There are currently no effective pharmacologic prophylactic interventions or treatments for cisplatin-induced ototoxicity. There is evidence that the degree of ototoxicity may be related to the peak concentration of cisplatin because the risks of developing ototoxicity are lower among TCS who received cisplatin (20 mg/m^2) over 5 days (OR = 5.3) than in those who had cisplatin (50 mg/m2) over 2 days (OR = 7.1).[53] Consequently, the 5-day BEP regimen seems preferable to the shorter regimen with regard to minimizing long-term ototoxicity.[9] For all TCS who work or live in a noisy environment, protective ear equipment is recommended. In addition, TCS should avoid ototoxic agents (eg, aminoglycosides) during or within a few weeks after cisplatin-based chemotherapy.

COGNITIVE IMPAIRMENT
Pathogenesis

The mechanisms behind chemotherapy-related cognitive impairment in patients with cancer are not well characterized. Chemotherapy is hypothesized to affect cognition through several mechanisms, including direct neurotoxicity, systemic inflammation, DNA damage, oxidative stress, and vascular injury.[65]

Risks

Evidence with regard to an association of cisplatin-based chemotherapy with cognitive impairment in TCS is both limited and conflicting. Quality-of-life data were prospectively collected in 666 patients with metastatic TC treated in European Organisation for Research and Treatment of Cancer (EORTC) Trial 30,941/United Kingdom Medical Research Council Trial TE20, using the EORTC Quality-of-Life Questionnaire C30 and a TC module. Approximately 20% of patients reported worsening cognitive function at 2 years of follow-up.[66] Another European cohort of 187 TCS (mean follow-up = 3 years) reported that 32% of patients who received surgery and chemotherapy, or surgery and radiation, reported regular occurrence of cognitive problems compared with 27% in the surgery-only group (P = .85). Importantly, approximately half of the patients who received chemotherapy reported that they were significantly bothered by their cognitive problems. The occurrence of self-report cognitive problems was moderately correlated with measures of anxiety (rho = 0.40) and depression (rho = 0.50).[67] Skoogh and colleagues[68] reported that TCS who received chemotherapy (n = 960; mean follow-up = 11 years) were more than 3 times more likely to say similar but incorrect words compared with TCS who did not receive chemotherapy (OR = 3.3; 95% CI, 1.5–7.1). Similar estimates were reported for saying words in the wrong order (OR = 3.1; 95% CI, 1.7–5.8) and difficulties understanding what other people mean (OR = 3.1; 95% CI, 1.3–7.7). These findings were attenuated after adjustment for anxiety.[68]

Two cross-sectional studies[67,69] used objective neuropsychological assessments and the same definition of cognitive impairment with conflicting results. Schagen and colleagues[67] (n = 187; mean follow-up = 3 years) reported no significant difference in mean scores on individual tests of attention, memory, processing speed, and verbal/motor functioning. However, those survivors who received surgery and chemotherapy or surgery and radiation were at increased risk of cognitive impairment compared with those who only received surgery after adjustment for age and intelligence quotient (chemotherapy: OR = 4.6; 95% CI, 1.1–19.7. Radiation: OR = 3.7; 95% CI, 0.8–15.7).[67] Pedersen and colleagues[69] reported significant differences in tests of verbal recall (chemotherapy mean = 4.6, non-chemotherapy mean = 5.6; P = .03) among TCS who completed treatment 2 to 7 years previously (n = 36 in each group). However, they reported no difference in the proportion of TCS classified as impaired after chemotherapy versus nonchemotherapy (5.6% vs 8.3% respectively; P = .64).[69] In addition, longitudinal studies show that, 1 year after treatment, TCS who received chemotherapy were more likely to experience declines in cognitive function compared with those who received surgery alone.[70,71]

Management

Cognitive complaints among long-term TCS are common[66–69,72] and may be partially attributable to anxiety and depression, which are prevalent in TCS.[67] Addressing specific stressors and advocating effective coping strategies for TCS may therefore be among the initial steps in managing cognitive complaints.

HYPOGONADISM
Pathogenesis

The cause of hypogonadism in TCS is probably multifactorial, attributable to the following 4 primary factors: orchiectomy, underlying testicular dysgenesis syndrome,[73] postorchiectomy chemotherapy or radiation, and the normal aging process.[74] Endocrine (inadequate testosterone production with compensatory increase of luteinizing hormone [LH] level) and exocrine hypogonadism (decreased spermatogenesis with increase of follicle-stimulating hormone [FSH] level) are two of the main long-term adverse effects that TCS may develop.

Risks

Several long-term follow-up studies of TCS[75–77] (range = 244–680 patients with TC) reported that 13% to 15% of patients had subnormal testosterone values (<10 nmol/L) or used androgen replacement therapy. Hypogonadism may not only lead to fertility issues, muscle weakness, depression, loss of energy, and reduced sexual function and well being,[78–82] because it is also associated with increased risk of osteoporosis,[83,84] CVD, and metabolic syndrome.[27,85,86]

Sprauten and colleagues[74] examined 307 Norwegian TCS treated from 1980 to 1994 who had blood samples collected at 3 time points: after orchiectomy but before further treatment, at survey I (SI; 1998–2002), and survey II (SII; 2007–2008). They reported significantly increased risks of lower testosterone and higher LH and FSH levels after radiotherapy or chemotherapy compared with the control group, which included 599 healthy participants in the general Nordic population.[74] Compared with the control group, the risks for lower testosterone were 3.3-fold (95% CI, 2.3–4.7) and 5.2-fold (95% CI, 3.5–7.9) higher in the radiotherapy and chemotherapy cohorts, respectively. The respective risks for increased LH and FSH levels were 3.6-fold (95% CI, 2.4–5.3) and 14.2-fold (95% CI, 8.3–24.4) higher in the chemotherapy cohort and 4.4-fold (95% CI, 3.1–6.5) and 18.9-fold (95% CI, 11.0–32.6) higher after radiotherapy. Cumulative platinum dose was significantly associated with risk of higher LH levels at both surveys and higher FSH at SI (P<.05). Overall, 50% of TCS had at least 1 of 3 sex hormone levels outside the reference range at SII.

Management

Regular assessment of hormonal status (ie, testosterone, FSH, and LH) of TCS should be considered, particularly in symptomatic patients. There is currently no evidence supporting testosterone replacement therapy to prevent late effects related to hypogonadism, such as CVD or metabolic syndrome. Treatment decision regarding optimal timing and/or clinical indication for initiation of testosterone replacement should be guided by clinical symptoms and referral to endocrinologists may be considered for challenging cases.[82]

AVASCULAR NECROSIS
Pathogenesis

Although the exact cause for avascular necrosis in TCS is unknown, it is most likely multifactorial.[9] Avascular necrosis among TCS is likely partially attributable to corticosteroids used as part of the antiemetic regimen during TC chemotherapy.[87–90] The femoral head is most commonly affected and usually bilaterally.[87]

Risks

Among TCS who received cisplatin-based chemotherapy, the incidence of vascular necrosis is approximately 1% to 2%.[87,88] In a cohort of 28 chemotherapy-treated patients with TC with avascular necrosis identified by literature review,[87] all had received chemotherapy with PVB (85%) or BEP (15%). Twenty-seven had received

Box 1
Summary of major research recommendations: late effects of TC and its treatment

1. Overarching recommendation: lifelong follow-up of all TCS

   - Integrate observational and analytical epidemiologic studies with molecular and genetic approaches to ascertain the risk of emerging toxicities and to understand the evolution of known late effects, especially with the aging of TCS

   - Evaluate the influence of race and socioeconomic status on the late effects of TC and its treatment

   - Characterize long-term tissue deposition of platinum (sites, reactivity), serum levels, and correlation with late effects

   - Evaluate the lifelong burden of medical and psychosocial morbidity by treatment

   - Use research findings to establish evidence-based, risk-adapted, long-term follow-up care

2. Specific recommendations

   - SMNs and late relapses

     ○ Determine the effect of reductions in field size and dose of radiotherapy, along with the use of carboplatin as adjuvant therapy in patients with seminoma, on the risk of SMN

     ○ Examine relation between platinum-based chemotherapy and site-specific risk of solid tumors, the associated temporal patterns, and the influence of age at exposure and attained age

     ○ Compare risk of SMN in TCS managed with surgery alone with cancer incidence in the general male population

     ○ Examine delaying influence of platinum-based chemotherapy (and duration and magnitude of effect) on development of contralateral TC

     ○ Characterize the evolution of cured TC; in particular, the molecular underpinnings of late recurrences

   - CVD

     ○ Evaluate the contributions and interactions of subclinical hypogonadism, platinum-based chemotherapy, radiotherapy, lifestyle factors (diet, tobacco use, physical activity), body mass index, family history of CVD, race, socioeconomic status, abnormal laboratory values, and genetic modifiers

     ○ Develop comprehensive risk prediction models, considering the variables listed earlier, to stratify TCS into risk groups in order to customize follow-up strategies and develop evidence-based interventions

   - Neurotoxicity

     ○ Evaluate evolution of neurotoxicity across TCS lifespan, role of genetic modifiers, and extent to which symptoms affect work ability and quality of life

   - Nephrotoxicity

     ○ Determine whether the natural decline in renal function associated with aging is accelerated in TCS, any influence of low-level platinum exposure, and the impact of decreased GFR on CVD and all-cause mortality

     ○ Determine the incidence of hypomagnesemia, together with the role of modifying factors and resultant medical consequences, in long-term TCS

   - Hypogonadism and decreased fertility

     ○ Address the incidence, course, and clinical effects of subclinical hypogonadism

     ○ Evaluate effect of all levels of gonadal dysfunction in TCS on CVD, premature aging, fatigue, osteoporosis, mental health, quality of life, and sexuality

   - Pulmonary function

     ○ Examine role of platinum compounds on long-term pulmonary damage in TCS, and interactions with other influences, including bleomycin, tobacco use and occupational risk factors

   - Psychosocial effects

     ○ Identify prevalence and predictors of depression, cancer-related anxiety, fatigue, infertility-related distress, problems with sexuality and paired relationships, and posttraumatic growth

- ○ Examine the impact of different cultural backgrounds on posttreatment quality of life
- ○ Evaluate TCS work ability throughout life
- ○ Determine whether normal age-related declines in cognitive function are accelerated in TCS

3. Interventions

- Conduct targeted intervention trials to promote smoking cessation, healthy dietary habits, and an increase in physical activity
- Evaluate the role of information and communication technologies in promoting a healthy lifestyle among TCS
- Consider randomized, pharmacologic intervention trials among TCS with biochemical parameters approaching threshold values to avoid accelerated development into treatment-requiring CVD
- Determine optimal schedule of testosterone replacement therapy among TCS with clinical hypogonadism
- Consider screening strategies for selected SMN

4. Genetic and molecular considerations

- Evaluate genetic risk factors (identified in the general male population) as modifiers for all late effects in TCS; in particular, CVD, SMN, neurotoxicity, nephrotoxicity, hypogonadism, and psychosocial effects
- Investigate the role of genomewide association studies, epigenetics, mitochondrial DNA, microRNA, proteomics, and related approaches in identifying genetic variants that contribute to the late effects of treatment
- Develop standardized procedures for biospecimen collection to support genetic and molecular studies, as reviewed previously

5. Risk prediction models

- Develop comprehensive risk prediction models that incorporate genetic modifiers of late sequelae

Adapted from Travis LB, Beard C, Allan JM, et al. Testicular cancer survivorship: research strategies and recommendations. J Natl Cancer Inst 2010;102:1123; with permission.

corticosteroids with the mean equivalent dose of 3730 mg (range = 1890–9010 mg) among 24 patients for whom dose was available. The mean onset of avascular necrosis was 26 months (range = 12–47 months) after completion of chemotherapy.[87]

Management

For any long-term TCS with symptoms suspicious for avascular necrosis, including decreased hip motion and/or limp, prompt investigation with plain radiography or MRI should be considered.[9]

RECOMMENDATIONS FOR FOLLOW-UP
Lifestyle Modifications

In a recent study of TCS from the Pennsylvania State Cancer Registry,[91] smoking (25%), risky drinking (≥2 drinks daily or ≥5 drinks in 1 sitting in the past 30 days) (35%), increased body mass index (83%), poor diet (95% did not meet the guidelines for fruit and vegetable intake), and inadequate exercise (50%) were common. A single-institution study at MD Anderson[92] also reported

that inactivity (46.3%), smoking (17.9%), and problem drinking (≥5 drinks on at least 1 occasion in the past month) (32.7%) were prevalent among TCS. Promotion of smoking cessation, better nutrition, and participation in a regular exercise regimen should be discussed with all TCS.[9,12]

In particular, smoking cessation should be advised in order to lower the risk of CVD and selected SMN. In a large Dutch population of TCS, the risk of developing SMN or CVD was 1.7-fold increased after tobacco use compared with the 1.9-fold increase after cisplatin-based chemotherapy.[19] Health care providers should capitalize on the time of cancer diagnosis as a teachable moment to introduce and promote lifestyle changes.[93]

Testicular Cancer Survivorship Care

The 2005 Institute of Medicine[94] report, *From Cancer Patient to Cancer Survivor: Lost in Transition*, advocated the share-care cancer survivorship model as an approach to facilitate communication and coordination or care between cancer specialists and other health care providers, particularly primary care clinicians. In addition, an integral component in this process is the survivorship care plan, which is a brief synopsis of the cancer, cancer therapy, and plan of care based on the survivor's risks. Integration of the share-care survivorship model and the survivorship care plan document should be considered for all patients with TC.[95]

SUMMARY

For the past 35 years, TC has been the model of a curable cancer[7,96,97] and is now positioned to become a paradigm in survivorship research for adult-onset cancer.[26] TCS comprise an ideal population for survivorship studies, given their young age at diagnosis, long-term survival, and use of largely homogenous therapies.[97] Future research priorities with regard to late effects of TC and its treatment were recently summarized during an international consensus conference (**Box 1**).[97] In particular, development of validated measures to quantify the degree of overall long-term burden of morbidities related to TC and its treatments are necessary because few data exist with regard to the number and severity of long-term toxicities experienced by TCS. The most comprehensive multi-institutional study to date is currently underway to examine genetic variants associated with long-term toxicities of platinum-based chemotherapy in TCS, with an initial focus on ototoxicity and neurotoxicity (NCI 1R01CA157823-01A1).[50] This study also systematically collects clinical data regarding various risk factors for CVD and other morbidities.

REFERENCES

1. Siegel R, Ma J, Zou Z, et al. Cancer statistics, 2014. CA Cancer J Clin 2014;64(1):9–29.
2. Einhorn LH, Donohue J. Cis-diamminedichloroplatinum, vinblastine, and bleomycin combination chemotherapy in disseminated testicular cancer. Ann Intern Med 1977;87(3):293–8.
3. Hanna N, Einhorn LH. Testicular cancer: a reflection on 50 years of discovery. J Clin Oncol 2014; 32(28):3085–92.
4. Verdecchia A, Francisci S, Brenner H, et al. Recent cancer survival in Europe: a 2000–02 period analysis of EUROCARE-4 data. Lancet Oncol 2007; 8(9):784–96.
5. Nigam M, Aschebrook-Kilfoy B, Shikanov S, et al. Increasing incidence of testicular cancer in the United States and Europe between 1992 and 2009. World J Urol 2015;33(5):623–31.
6. Hanna NH, Einhorn LH. Testicular cancer–discoveries and updates. N Engl J Med 2014;371(21): 2005–16.
7. Einhorn LH. Testicular cancer as a model for a curable neoplasm: the Richard and Hinda Rosenthal Foundation Award Lecture. Cancer Res 1981; 41(9 Pt 1):3275–80.
8. Travis LB, Ng AK, Allan JM, et al. Second malignant neoplasms and cardiovascular disease following radiotherapy. J Natl Cancer Inst 2012; 104(5):357–70.
9. Haugnes HS, Bosl GJ, Boer H, et al. Long-term and late effects of germ cell testicular cancer treatment and implications for follow-up. J Clin Oncol 2012; 30(30):3752–63.
10. Aziz NM. Cancer survivorship research: state of knowledge, challenges and opportunities. Acta Oncol 2007;46(4):417–32.
11. Travis LB, Rabkin CS, Brown LM, et al. Cancer survivorship–genetic susceptibility and second primary cancers: research strategies and recommendations. J Natl Cancer Inst 2006;98(1): 15–25.
12. Wood ME, Vogel V, Ng A, et al. Second malignant neoplasms: assessment and strategies for risk reduction. J Clin Oncol 2012;30(30):3734–45.
13. Travis LB, Fossa SD, Schonfeld SJ, et al. Second cancers among 40,576 testicular cancer patients: focus on long-term survivors. J Natl Cancer Inst 2005;97(18):1354–65.
14. Travis LB, Andersson M, Gospodarowicz M, et al. Treatment-associated leukemia following testicular cancer. J Natl Cancer Inst 2000;92(14):1165–71.
15. Bajorin DF, Sarosdy MF, Pfister DG, et al. Randomized trial of etoposide and cisplatin versus etoposide and carboplatin in patients with good-risk germ cell tumors: a multiinstitutional study. J Clin Oncol 1993;11(4):598–606.
16. Kollmannsberger C, Beyer J, Droz JP, et al. Secondary leukemia following high cumulative doses of etoposide in patients treated for advanced germ cell tumors. J Clin Oncol 1998; 16(10):3386–91.
17. Kollmannsberger C, Hartmann JT, Kanz L, et al. Therapy-related malignancies following treatment of germ cell cancer. Int J Cancer 1999;83(6):860–3.
18. Travis LB, Curtis RE, Storm H, et al. Risk of second malignant neoplasms among long-term survivors of testicular cancer. J Natl Cancer Inst 1997;89(19): 1429–39.
19. van den Belt-Dusebout AW, de Wit R, Gietema JA, et al. Treatment-specific risks of second malignancies and cardiovascular disease in 5-year survivors of testicular cancer. J Clin Oncol 2007; 25(28):4370–8.
20. van den Belt-Dusebout AW, Aleman BM, Besseling G, et al. Roles of radiation dose and chemotherapy in the etiology of stomach cancer as a second malignancy. Int J Radiat Oncol Biol Phys 2009;75(5):1420–9.

21. Bachaud JM, Berthier F, Soulie M, et al. Second non-germ cell malignancies in patients treated for stage I-II testicular seminoma. Radiother Oncol 1999;50(2):191–7.

22. Hauptmann M, Fossa SD, Stovall M, et al. Increased stomach cancer risk following radiotherapy for testicular cancer. Br J Cancer 2015; 112(1):44–51.

23. Classen J, Schmidberger H, Meisner C, et al. Radiotherapy for stages IIA/B testicular seminoma: final report of a prospective multicenter clinical trial. J Clin Oncol 2003;21(6):1101–6.

24. Jones WG, Fossa SD, Mead GM, et al. Randomized trial of 30 versus 20 Gy in the adjuvant treatment of stage I testicular seminoma: a report on Medical Research Council Trial TE18, European Organisation for the Research and Treatment of Cancer Trial 30942 (ISRCTN18525328). J Clin Oncol 2005;23(6):1200–8.

25. Fung C, Fossa SD, Milano MT, et al. Solid tumors after chemotherapy or surgery for testicular nonseminoma: a population-based study. J Clin Oncol 2013;31(30):3807–14.

26. Feldman DR, Schaffer WL, Steingart RM. Late cardiovascular toxicity following chemotherapy for germ cell tumors. J Natl Compr Canc Netw 2012; 10(4):537–44.

27. Haugnes HS, Wethal T, Aass N, et al. Cardiovascular risk factors and morbidity in long-term survivors of testicular cancer: a 20-year follow-up study. J Clin Oncol 2010;28(30):4649–57.

28. Huddart RA, Norman A, Shahidi M, et al. Cardiovascular disease as a long-term complication of treatment for testicular cancer. J Clin Oncol 2003; 21(8):1513–23.

29. Meinardi MT, Gietema JA, van der Graaf WT, et al. Cardiovascular morbidity in long-term survivors of metastatic testicular cancer. J Clin Oncol 2000; 18(8):1725–32.

30. van den Belt-Dusebout AW, Nuver J, de Wit R, et al. Long-term risk of cardiovascular disease in 5-year survivors of testicular cancer. J Clin Oncol 2006; 24(3):467–75.

31. Goff DC Jr, Lloyd-Jones DM, Bennett G, et al. 2013 ACC/AHA guideline on the assessment of cardiovascular risk: a report of the American College of Cardiology/American Heart Association Task Force on Practice Guidelines. Circulation 2014;129(25 Suppl 2):S49–73.

32. Nuver J, De Haas EC, Van Zweeden M, et al. Vascular damage in testicular cancer patients: a study on endothelial activation by bleomycin and cisplatin in vitro. Oncol Rep 2010;23(1):247–53.

33. Sleijfer S. Bleomycin-induced pneumonitis. Chest 2001;120(2):617–24.

34. Dearnaley DP, Horwich A, A'Hern R, et al. Combination chemotherapy with bleomycin, etoposide and cisplatin (BEP) for metastatic testicular teratoma: long-term follow-up. Eur J Cancer 1991; 27(6):684–91.

35. Nuver J, Lutke Holzik MF, van Zweeden M, et al. Genetic variation in the bleomycin hydrolase gene and bleomycin-induced pulmonary toxicity in germ cell cancer patients. Pharmacogenet Genomics 2005;15(6):399–405.

36. O'Sullivan JM, Huddart RA, Norman AR, et al. Predicting the risk of bleomycin lung toxicity in patients with germ-cell tumours. Ann Oncol 2003; 14(1):91–6.

37. Van Barneveld PW, van der Mark TW, Sleijfer DT, et al. Predictive factors for bleomycin-induced pneumonitis. Am Rev Respir Dis 1984;130(6): 1078–81.

38. Haugnes HS, Aass N, Fossa SD, et al. Pulmonary function in long-term survivors of testicular cancer. J Clin Oncol 2009;27(17):2779–86.

39. Fossa SD, Gilbert E, Dores GM, et al. Noncancer causes of death in survivors of testicular cancer. J Natl Cancer Inst 2007;99(7):533–44.

40. Donat SM. Peri-operative care in patients treated for testicular cancer. Semin Surg Oncol 1999; 17(4):282–8.

41. Vickers AE, Rose K, Fisher R, et al. Kidney slices of human and rat to characterize cisplatin-induced injury on cellular pathways and morphology. Toxicol Pathol 2004;32(5):577–90.

42. Tanaka H, Ishikawa E, Teshima S, et al. Histopathological study of human cisplatin nephropathy. Toxicol Pathol 1986;14(2):247–57.

43. Hansen SW, Groth S, Daugaard G, et al. Long-term effects on renal function and blood pressure of treatment with cisplatin, vinblastine, and bleomycin in patients with germ cell cancer. J Clin Oncol 1988;6(11):1728–31.

44. Fossa SD, Aass N, Winderen M, et al. Long-term renal function after treatment for malignant germ-cell tumours. Ann Oncol 2002;13(2):222–8.

45. Nuver J, Smit AJ, Sleijfer DT, et al. Microalbuminuria, decreased fibrinolysis, and inflammation as early signs of atherosclerosis in long-term survivors of disseminated testicular cancer. Eur J Cancer 2004;40(5):701–6.

46. Bosl GJ, Leitner SP, Atlas SA, et al. Increased plasma renin and aldosterone in patients treated with cisplatin-based chemotherapy for metastatic germ-cell tumors. J Clin Oncol 1986;4(11):1684–9.

47. Peacock JM, Ohira T, Post W, et al. Serum magnesium and risk of sudden cardiac death in the Atherosclerosis Risk in Communities (ARIC) study. Am Heart J 2010;160(3):464–70.

48. Astor BC, Hallan SI, Miller ER 3rd, et al. Glomerular filtration rate, albuminuria, and risk of cardiovascular and all-cause mortality in the US population. Am J Epidemiol 2008;167(10):1226–34.

49. Hartmann JT, Kollmannsberger C, Kanz L, et al. Platinum organ toxicity and possible prevention in patients with testicular cancer. Int J Cancer 1999; 83(6):866–9.

50. Travis LB, Fossa SD, Sesso HD, et al. Chemotherapy-induced peripheral neurotoxicity and ototoxicity: new paradigms for translational genomics. J Natl Cancer Inst 2014;106(5) [pii:dju044].

51. de Wit R, Roberts JT, Wilkinson PM, et al. Equivalence of three or four cycles of bleomycin, etoposide, and cisplatin chemotherapy and of a 3- or 5-day schedule in good-prognosis germ cell cancer: a randomized study of the European Organization for Research and Treatment of Cancer Genitourinary Tract Cancer Cooperative Group and the Medical Research Council. J Clin Oncol 2001;19(6):1629–40.

52. Williams SD, Birch R, Einhorn LH, et al. Treatment of disseminated germ-cell tumors with cisplatin, bleomycin, and either vinblastine or etoposide. N Engl J Med 1987;316(23):1435–40.

53. Brydoy M, Oldenburg J, Klepp O, et al. Observational study of prevalence of long-term Raynaud-like phenomena and neurological side effects in testicular cancer survivors. J Natl Cancer Inst 2009;101(24):1682–95.

54. Glendenning JL, Barbachano Y, Norman AR, et al. Long-term neurologic and peripheral vascular toxicity after chemotherapy treatment of testicular cancer. Cancer 2010;116(10):2322–31.

55. Sprauten M, Darrah TH, Peterson DR, et al. Impact of long-term serum platinum concentrations on neuro- and ototoxicity in cisplatin-treated survivors of testicular cancer. J Clin Oncol 2012;30(3):300–7.

56. Oldenburg J, Kraggerud SM, Brydoy M, et al. Association between long-term neuro-toxicities in testicular cancer survivors and polymorphisms in glutathione-s-transferase-P1 and -M1, a retrospective cross sectional study. J Transl Med 2007;5:70.

57. Hershman DL, Lacchetti C, Dworkin RH, et al. Prevention and management of chemotherapy-induced peripheral neuropathy in survivors of adult cancers: American Society of Clinical Oncology clinical practice guideline. J Clin Oncol 2014; 32(18):1941–67.

58. Bokemeyer C, Berger CC, Hartmann JT, et al. Analysis of risk factors for cisplatin-induced ototoxicity in patients with testicular cancer. Br J Cancer 1998;77(8):1355–62.

59. Rybak LP. Mechanisms of cisplatin ototoxicity and progress in otoprotection. Curr Opin Otolaryngol Head Neck Surg 2007;15(5):364–9.

60. Oldenburg J, Kraggerud SM, Cvancarova M, et al. Cisplatin-induced long-term hearing impairment is associated with specific glutathione s-transferase genotypes in testicular cancer survivors. J Clin Oncol 2007;25(6):708–14.

61. Ross CJ, Katzov-Eckert H, Dube MP, et al. Genetic variants in TPMT and COMT are associated with hearing loss in children receiving cisplatin chemotherapy. Nat Genet 2009;41(12):1345–9.

62. Yang JJ, Lim JY, Huang J, et al. The role of inherited TPMT and COMT genetic variation in cisplatin-induced ototoxicity in children with cancer. Clin Pharmacol Ther 2013;94(2):252–9.

63. Pussegoda K, Ross CJ, Visscher H, et al. Replication of TPMT and ABCC3 genetic variants highly associated with cisplatin-induced hearing loss in children. Clin Pharmacol Ther 2013;94(2):243–51.

64. Xu H, Robinson GW, Huang J, et al. Common variants in ACYP2 influence susceptibility to cisplatin-induced hearing loss. Nat Genet 2015; 47(3):263–6.

65. Janelsins MC, Kesler SR, Ahles TA, et al. Prevalence, mechanisms, and management of cancer-related cognitive impairment. Int Rev Psychiatry 2014;26(1):102–13.

66. Fossa SD, de Wit R, Roberts JT, et al. Quality of life in good prognosis patients with metastatic germ cell cancer: a prospective study of the European Organization for Research and Treatment of Cancer Genitourinary Group/Medical Research Council Testicular Cancer Study Group (30941/TE20). J Clin Oncol 2003;21(6):1107–18.

67. Schagen SB, Boogerd W, Muller MJ, et al. Cognitive complaints and cognitive impairment following BEP chemotherapy in patients with testicular cancer. Acta Oncol 2008;47(1):63–70.

68. Skoogh J, Steineck G, Stierner U, et al. Testicular-cancer survivors experience compromised language following chemotherapy: findings in a Swedish population-based study 3–26 years after treatment. Acta Oncol 2012;51(2):185–97.

69. Pedersen AD, Rossen P, Mehlsen MY, et al. Long-term cognitive function following chemotherapy in patients with testicular cancer. J Int Neuropsychol Soc 2009;15(2):296–301.

70. Skaali T, Fossa SD, Andersson S, et al. A prospective study of neuropsychological functioning in testicular cancer patients. Ann Oncol 2011;22(5):1062–70.

71. Wefel JS, Vidrine DJ, Marani SK, et al. A prospective study of cognitive function in men with non-seminomatous germ cell tumors. Psychooncology 2014;23(6):626–33.

72. Skaali T, Fossa SD, Andersson S, et al. Self-reported cognitive problems in testicular cancer patients: relation to neuropsychological performance, fatigue, and psychological distress. J Psychosom Res 2011;70(5):403–10.

73. Skakkebaek NE, Rajpert-De Meyts E, Main KM. Testicular dysgenesis syndrome: an increasingly common developmental disorder with environmental aspects. Hum Reprod 2001;16(5):972–8.

74. Sprauten M, Brydoy M, Haugnes HS, et al. Longitudinal serum testosterone, luteinizing hormone, and follicle-stimulating hormone levels in a population-based sample of long-term testicular cancer survivors. J Clin Oncol 2014;32(6):571–8.

75. Huddart RA, Norman A, Moynihan C, et al. Fertility, gonadal and sexual function in survivors of testicular cancer. Br J Cancer 2005;93(2):200–7.

76. Wiechno P, Demkow T, Kubiak K, et al. The quality of life and hormonal disturbances in testicular cancer survivors in Cisplatin era. Eur Urol 2007;52(5):1448–54.

77. Gerl A, Muhlbayer D, Hansmann G, et al. The impact of chemotherapy on Leydig cell function in long term survivors of germ cell tumors. Cancer 2001;91(7):1297–303.

78. Eberhard J, Stahl O, Cohn-Cedermark G, et al. Sexual function in men treated for testicular cancer. J Sex Med 2009;6(7):1979–89.

79. Brydoy M, Fossa SD, Klepp O, et al. Paternity following treatment for testicular cancer. J Natl Cancer Inst 2005;97(21):1580–8.

80. Dahl AA, Bremnes R, Dahl O, et al. Is the sexual function compromised in long-term testicular cancer survivors? Eur Urol 2007;52(5):1438–47.

81. Hintikka J, Niskanen L, Koivumaa-Honkanen H, et al. Hypogonadism, decreased sexual desire, and long-term depression in middle-aged men. J Sex Med 2009;6(7):2049–57.

82. Bhasin S, Cunningham GR, Hayes FJ, et al. Testosterone therapy in men with androgen deficiency syndromes: an Endocrine Society clinical practice guideline. J Clin Endocrinol Metab 2010;95(6):2536–59.

83. Ondrusova M, Ondrus D, Dusek L, et al. Damage of hormonal function and bone metabolism in long-term survivors of testicular cancer. Neoplasma 2009;56(6):473–9.

84. Rochira V, Balestrieri A, Madeo B, et al. Osteoporosis and male age-related hypogonadism: role of sex steroids on bone (patho)physiology. Eur J Endocrinol 2006;154(2):175–85.

85. Haugnes HS, Aass N, Fossa SD, et al. Components of the metabolic syndrome in long-term survivors of testicular cancer. Ann Oncol 2007;18(2):241–8.

86. Nuver J, Smit AJ, Wolffenbuttel BH, et al. The metabolic syndrome and disturbances in hormone levels in long-term survivors of disseminated testicular cancer. J Clin Oncol 2005;23(16):3718–25.

87. Winquist EW, Bauman GS, Balogh J. Nontraumatic osteonecrosis after chemotherapy for testicular cancer: a systematic review. Am J Clin Oncol 2001;24(6):603–6.

88. Cook AM, Dzik-Jurasz AS, Padhani AR, et al. The prevalence of avascular necrosis in patients treated with chemotherapy for testicular tumours. Br J Cancer 2001;85(11):1624–6.

89. Kaila R, Wolman RL. Groin pain in athletes: a consequence of femoral head avascular necrosis after testicular cancer chemotherapy. Clin J Sport Med 2006;16(2):175–6.

90. van den Berkmortel F, de Wit R, de Rooy J, et al. Osteonecrosis in patients with testicular tumours treated with chemotherapy. Neth J Med 2004;62(1):23–7.

91. Reilley MJ, Jacobs LA, Vaughn DJ, et al. Health behaviors among testicular cancer survivors. J Community Support Oncol 2014;12(4):121–8.

92. Shinn EH, Swartz RJ, Thornton BB, et al. Testis cancer survivors' health behaviors: comparison with age-matched relative and demographically matched population controls. J Clin Oncol 2010;28(13):2274–9.

93. Demark-Wahnefried W, Aziz NM, Rowland JH, et al. Riding the crest of the teachable moment: promoting long-term health after the diagnosis of cancer. J Clin Oncol 2005;23(24):5814–30.

94. Hewitt M, Greenfield S, Stovall E, editors. Institute of Medicine. From cancer patient to cancer survivor: lost in transition. Washington, DC: National Academies Press; 2005.

95. Boer H, Nuver J, Lefrandt JD, et al. Easy navigating through the forest of survivorship care. J Clin Oncol 2014;32(1):61–2.

96. Bajorin DF. The graying of testis cancer patients: what have we learned? J Clin Oncol 2007;25(28):4341–3.

97. Travis LB, Beard C, Allan JM, et al. Testicular cancer survivorship: research strategies and recommendations. J Natl Cancer Inst 2010;102(15):1114–30.

98. Wanderas EH, Fossa SD, Tretli S. Risk of subsequent non-germ cell cancer after treatment of germ cell cancer in 2006 Norwegian male patients. Eur J Cancer 1997;33(2):253–62.

99. Richiardi L, Scelo G, Boffetta P, et al. Second malignancies among survivors of germ-cell testicular cancer: a pooled analysis between 13 cancer registries. Int J Cancer 2007;120(3):623–31.

100. Hemminki K, Liu H, Sundquist J. Second cancers after testicular cancer diagnosed after 1980 in Sweden. Ann Oncol 2010;21(7):1546–51.

Infertility with Testicular Cancer

Kevin A. Ostrowski, MD[a],*, Thomas J. Walsh, MD[b]

KEYWORDS

- Testicular cancer • Testicular germ cell tumors • Male infertility • Chemotherapy
- Radiation therapy • Retroperitoneal lymph node dissection (RPLND) • Surveillance

KEY POINTS

- Testicular cancer patients have baseline infertility before treatment due to systemic effects, endocrine changes, possible autoimmune effects, intrinsic testicular damage, and possible congenital abnormalities in testicular maturation.
- Sperm counts are further affected by orchiectomy and radiation and chemotherapy effects.
- There are significant psychological and sexual effects in patients undergoing surveillance or those requiring further treatment after orchiectomy.
- Cryopreservation should be offered to patients and their families before treatment.
- A full discussion of the gonadotoxic effects of cancer treatment and the possibility of sperm or testicular tissue cryopreservation, even in adolescent and prepubertal patients, should become standard of care.

INTRODUCTION

With a survival rate of more than 95%, testicular cancer is one of the most curable cancers worldwide. Although treatment is successful in most cases, the incidence of testicular cancer has doubled over the past 40 years and continues to rise.[1] A majority of patients undergoing treatment are of reproductive age; therefore, the use of gonadotoxic therapies can temporarily or permanently compromise their fertility.

There are many reasons for infertility in the testicular cancer population, including systemic and endocrine effects, autoimmune and intrinsic testicular damage, congenital abnormalities in testicular maturation, and the psychological and treatment effects of testicular cancer. The local and systemic effects of testicular cancer adversely affect spermatogenesis and lower sperm counts before treatment. Sperm counts are further affected by treatment with orchiectomy and the

cytotoxic effects of radiation and chemotherapy. Retroperitoneal lymph node dissection (RPLND) can damage the sympathetic nerve plexus and have negative impacts on ejaculation.

The treatment of testicular cancer is evolving, and there is increased focus on preservation of fertility as well as the psychological and sexual effects of treatment. Patients have more fertility options than ever before with assisted-reproductive technology (ART). This article reviews the reasons for infertility in patients with testicular cancer both before and after treatment and evaluates current options for fertility preservation and infertility treatments.

DISCUSSION: DIAGNOSIS OF MALE INFERTILITY

Infertility is the inability to become pregnant after 1 year of unprotected intercourse and affects approximately 10% to 15% of couples[2]; 20% of cases involve male factors only and another 40%

[a] Department of Urology, Oregon Health and Science University, 3303 Southwest Bond Avenue, CH10U, Portland, OR 97239, USA; [b] Department of Urology, University of Washington School of Medicine, 1959 Northeast Pacific, Box 356510, Seattle, WA 98195, USA
* Corresponding author.
E-mail address: ostrowsk@ohsu.edu

Urol Clin N Am 42 (2015) 409–420
http://dx.doi.org/10.1016/j.ucl.2015.05.003
0094-0143/15/$ – see front matter © 2015 Elsevier Inc. All rights reserved.

involve both male and female factors. Fertility is a couples phenomenon, and therefore all fertility discussions and treatment options should involve both patient and partner.[3] The evaluation for male infertility includes a thorough history and physical examination, semen analyses, and other specialized testing as needed (**Fig. 1**).

RELATIONSHIP BETWEEN INFERTILITY AND TESTICULAR CANCER

The relationship between infertility and testicular cancer has been well established. Multiple studies have shown decreased sperm counts in patients with newly diagnosed testicular cancer prior to cytotoxic treatment. Several studies suggest that testis cancer specifically may portend worse semen quality compared with other cancers.[4–7] In 208 patients evaluated with semen analysis after orchiectomy, only 27% of patients had baseline sperm counts greater than 10 million per mL.[8] Decreased spermatogenesis has been seen

histologically in contralateral testicular biopsies at the time of orchiectomy in more than 2000 patients compared with healthy forensic autopsy controls.[9]

Conversely, multiple studies show that men evaluated for infertility have an increased risk of testicular cancer occurring later in life compared with men from the general population. In 2000, Jacobsen and colleagues[10] studied 32,442 Danish men evaluated for infertility and linked them to the Danish Cancer Registry from 1963 to 1995. They found men evaluated for infertility were 1.6 times more likely than the general population to develop testicular germ cell tumors (TGCTs) (standardized incidence ratio [SIR]; 95% CI, 1.3–1.9) subsequent to their infertility evaluation. Analyses stratified by specific semen characteristics showed that low sperm concentration (SIR 2.3; 95% CI, 1.6–3.2), poor sperm motility (SIR 2.5; 95% CI, 1.0–5.2), and high proportion of morphologically abnormal sperm (SIR 3.0; 95% CI, 0.8–7.6) were associated with an increased risk of testicular cancer. In the United States, Walsh and colleagues[11] studied a

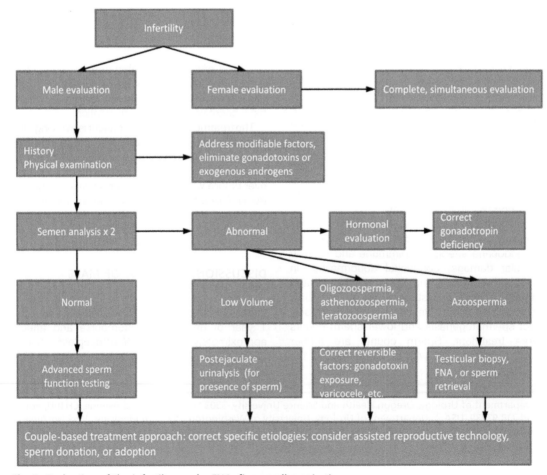

Fig. 1. Evaluation of the infertile couple. FNA, fine-needle aspiration.

cohort of more than 22,000 men from 1968 to 1998 who were evaluated at multiple California infertility clinics. They found 24% of men had male factor infertility based on abnormal semen analysis, and these men were 3 times more likely to be diagnosed with testicular germ cell cancer compared with age-matched men from the general population (SIR 2.8; 95% CI, 1.5–4.8). In multivariate analysis, men with male factor infertility were approximately 3 times more likely to develop testicular cancer (hazard ratio, 2.8; 95% CI, 1.3–6.0) compared with those with normal semen quality.

These studies provide evidence for a common etiology for low semen quality and TGCTs.

Systemic Effects of Testicular Cancer

Several studies have suggested that semen quality at the time of a newly diagnosed testis cancer is abnormal in up to 50% of men.[5,7] In some cases, this may be due to the common etiology between these diseases. In other cases, this may be due to the generalized impact of cancer on the body. Cancer has both systemic and local effects. The systemic effects on the body include temperature changes and hormone and metabolic effects. Fevers greater than 38.5°C have been shown to adversely affect sperm analysis in patients before treatment of their Hodgkin disease.[12]

The body's stress response to cancer has effects on cytokine production (interleukin-1, interleukin-6, tumor necrosis factor α, and interferon-γ). Cytokine effects may be similar to the proposed mechanism of anorexia-cachexia syndrome where cytokines cross the blood-brain barrier, activate central kinase systems, and disturb normal endocrine pathways, especially the hypothalamic-pituitary-gonadal axis (HPGA).[13]

Several cancer types have been shown to decrease sperm counts, with testicular cancer having some of the worst pretreatment sperm counts in multiple studies[7,14] The body's systemic response to cancer is not fully understood, but the systemic effects combined with endocrine regulation as well as local and treatment effects affect spermatogenesis on these young patients.

Endocrine Effects of Testicular Cancer

Spermatogenesis depends on a tightly controlled endocrine system. The effects on the endocrine system from testicular tumors can be due to tumor effects on the HPGA or effects from hormonally active tumors.

Cancer alone can have effects on spermatogenesis and the HPGA. Up to two-thirds of patients with testicular cancer have disrupted gonadotropic hormones or testosterone before orchiectomy.[15] Results from 48 men with hormone levels and semen analysis before and after orchiectomy showed a decrease in median sperm concentration, decrease in total sperm count, decrease in inhibin B, and an increase in luteinizing hormone (LH) and follicle-stimulating hormone (FSH) after orchiectomy. They noted no change in testosterone and sex hormone–binding globulin.[16] Preorchiectomy elevated FSH has been shown to correlate with low post-treatment spermatogenesis.[17,18] In a longitudinal study of 307 testicular cancer patients, half of all patients had at least 1 of 3 hormone levels (testosterone, LH, and FSH) outside the reference range with a median 18 years after diagnosis. The odds of developing low testosterone were 3-fold higher for men with testis cancer who received radiation (odds ratio [OR] 3.3; 95% CI, 2.3–4.7) and 5-fold higher for those who received chemotherapy (OR 5.2; 95% CI, 3.5–7.9) relative to age-matched controls. The cumulative platinum dose was significantly associated with risk of higher LH levels.[19]

In addition, many TGCTs are hormonally active and can produce β–human chorionic gonadotropin (β-hCG) and alpha-fetoprotein (AFP). de Bruin and colleagues[20] evaluated 62 men before orchiectomy with hormone levels and semen analysis. They found that men with β-hCG secreting tumors had lower total motile sperm counts, lower LH and FSH, and higher testosterone, prolactin, and estradiol. Semen quality was negatively correlated with β-hCG, estradiol, and prolactin.

In another study, nonseminomatous germ cell tumors (NSGCTs) that produce AFP were shown on multivariate linear regression analysis to have decreased total sperm counts with almost two-thirds of patients having a low sperm count.[21]

Autoimmune Effects of Testicular Cancer

An intact blood-testis barrier is essential to normal testis function and immune balance. Breakdown of this barrier can affect fertility because sperm that are normally shielded from the host immune system are exposed to immune-competent cells. Approximately 10% of men being evaluated for infertility have antisperm antibodies (ASAs).[22] Studies have shown various correlations between testicular cancer and ASAs (**Table 1**). The effect of ASA on spermatogenesis is not clear both in the infertile population or patients with testicular cancer. The mechanism of infertility with ASA due to tumor invasion is feasible, but further research is needed.

Table 1
Comparison of different studies evaluating antisperm antibodies in testicular cancer treatment patients

Paper	N	Preorchiectomy Antisperm Antibody Positive	N	Postorchiectomy Antisperm Antibody Positive	Type of Assay	Comment
Guazzieri et al,[23] 1985	15	73%	46	28%	ELISA	Stage correlated to ASA
Foster et al,[24] 1991	—	—	52	21%	Immunofluorescence	Low-stage NSGCT
Höbarth et al,[25] 1994	—	—	22	18%	Immunofluorescence	—
Paoli et al,[22] 2009	—	—	190	6%	IBT and GAT[a]	—

[a] Direct immunobead test (IBT) of sperm and serum by the indirect IBT and the gelatin agglutination test (GAT).

Abnormal Testicular Development

The biologic mechanisms linking male infertility and TGCTs are poorly understood. The changes that cause both male infertility and TGCTs have possibly external exposures combined with intrinsic genetic anomalies. The risk of TGCTs is elevated among male relatives of patients with testicular cancer and men with undescended testicles. The elevated risks in these populations may be due to a testicular cancer susceptibility gene and common environmental risk factors that have not been fully elucidated.[26] TGCTs may be linked to undescended testis and hypospadias by way of testicular dysgenesis syndrome (TDS).

TDS has clinical, epidemiologic, biological, and genetic data, which provide evidence for a link between TGCTs, undescended testis, and hypospadias. By TDS theory, alterations in hormones during the masculinization window early in gestation could cause effects linking undescended testis, hypospadias, and TGCTs (**Fig. 2**). There is

an increased risk of carcinoma in situ (CIS) in patients with undescended testis and hypospadias. CIS cells are precursor TGCT cells, and histologic studies show other signs of testicular dysgenesis in these patients, including clusters of undifferentiated seminiferous tubules, microliths, Sertoli cell–only tubules, and Leydig cell micronodules.[27]

Recent studies have advanced understanding of the genetic commonalities between TGCTs and infertility. The human HIWI gene on chromosome 12 acts as a governor for stem cell renewal, gametogenesis, and RNA interference. There has been linkage from this gene to the transformation of CIS to TGCTs. Enhanced HIWI expression was found in 12 of 19 sampled seminomatous TGCTs and 0 of 19 nonseminomatous TGCTs.[28] In addition to HIWI, DNA mismatch repair is crucial to maintaining DNA fidelity. Data from mice suggest that mutations in genes needed for DNA repair (*Pms2* and *Mlh1*) also lead to infertility characterized by meiotic arrest, with a pattern of maturation arrest seen in testis pathology. In mouse studies,

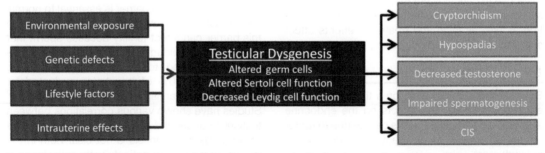

Fig. 2. TDS: multiple types of exposures (*blue boxes*) cause testicular dysgenesis via their effects on Leydig and Sertoli cell function (*purple box*). This has downstream consequences and later symptoms (*green boxes*). (*Adapted from* Juul A, Almstrup K, Andersson AM, et al. Possible fetal determinants of male infertility. Nat Rev Endocrinol 2014;10(9):553–62.)

inactivation of the exonuclease 1 protein, which is critical for the excision step of DNA mismatch repair, has been shown to cause both infertility and cancer. Transcriptional mismatch repair errors in both germline DNA and somatic cell DNA could originate from 1 source, which provides a biologic explanation for infertility and the connection with TGCTs. This is a multifactorial biologic model with intrinsic genetic factors and environmental exposures causing an increased risk for both male infertility and testicular tumors.[29]

CANCER TREATMENT AND FERTILITY

Testicular cancer patients are less fertile for multiple reasons, including disruption of the HPGA; immunologic or cytologic injury to the germinal epithelium; systemic cancer processes, including fever and malnutrition; and psychological issues, such as anxiety and depression.

The types of cancer and treatment affect all these processes and has an effect on pre- and post-treatment fertility. Because spermatogenesis involves rapid cell division, it is extremely sensitive to both chemotherapy and radiotherapy. Orchiectomy decreases spermatogenesis, and an RPLND can effect ejaculation. Finally, there is growing evidence of the psychological and sexual effects of cancer and cancer treatment.

Surveillance

Surveillance is a viable treatment in compliant patients with stage I testicular cancer. Ultimately, approximately 20% to 30% of these patients relapse, requiring gonadotoxic agents. For NSGCTs, approximately 25% progress and require primary chemotherapy and a minority of those require a postchemotherapy RPLND. Therefore, some patients may have worse fertility effects with surveillance than a primary nerve-sparing RPLND.[30]

In men who do not relapse, many studies show semen analysis remains stable or possibly improves. Carroll and colleagues[31] noted 50% of patients with initial oligospermia or azoospermia with stage I NSGCTs on surveillance recovered normal sperm concentrations within 4 to 19 months postorchiectomy. This finding is supported by Jacobsen and colleagues,[32] who evaluated repeat semen analyses of 60 men on surveillance for stage I NSGCTs and found a significant increase in mean sperm concentrations at 1 year postorchiectomy.

In a Norwegian study of fertility after testicular cancer treatment, surveys were sent to 1814 patients; 554 men had attempted post-treatment conception and 71% were successful. This ranged between treatment groups and is shown in **Fig. 3**. Patients who were able to stay on surveillance without need for further treatment had the best fertility. RPLND had the highest fatherhood rate of patients who required treatment after orchiectomy. Assisted reproductive technologies were used by 22% of the couples who attempted conception after treatment. Dry ejaculation, treatment group, pretreatment fatherhood, and marital status were statistically significant independent predictors for post-treatment fatherhood, with dry ejaculation the most important negative factor.[33]

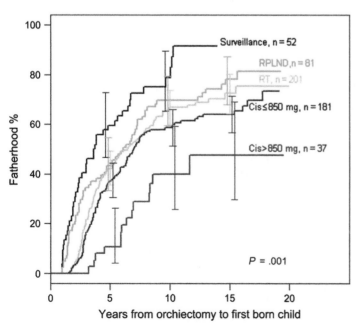

Fig. 3. Comparison of testicular cancer treatment fertility rates. (*From* Brydøy M, Fosså D, Klepp O, et al. Paternity following treatment for testicular cancer. J Natl Cancer Inst 2005;97(21):1583.)

Retroperitoneal Lymph Node Dissection

The removal of retroperitoneal lymph nodes entails a careful dissection around the aorta and inferior vena cava, including the retroperitoneal postganglionic sympathetic nerves. These nerves overlie the aorta and join to form the hypogastric plexus in the pelvis. The ampulla to the vas deferens, seminal vesicles, periurethral glands, internal sphincter, bulbourethral, and periurethral musculature receive innervation from these nerves. Injury to these nerves results in retrograde ejaculation or anejaculation. Improvement in surgical techniques to allow for nerve-sparing RPLNDs, and use of modified templates has improved ejaculatory function significantly.

In a recent review of 176 patients who underwent primary RPLND, 97% had antegrade emission. With bilateral nerve sparing 134 (99%) could ejaculate versus 33 (89%) who underwent template non–nerve-sparing dissection. In those who attempted to have children, 73.4% (47/64 patients) were successful.[34] Postchemotherapy RPLND is a more difficult surgery. In comparing patients with postchemotherapy bilateral template RPLND, antegrade ejaculation was 89% in nerve-sparing patients versus 11% in non–nerve-sparing patients. Anejaculation was also significantly different, 5% versus 75%, respectively. Patients also noted a decreased ejaculatory volume before and after surgery of 4.4 mL to 2.5 mL.[35]

In summary, advances in surgical techniques have allowed for the preservation of ejaculatory function and significantly reduced the risk for infertility associated with RPLND.

Radiotherapy

Radiation can have significant effect on reproductive function because spermatogonia are the most sensitive germ cells to radiation. The loss of germ cells is dose dependent, with doses greater than 2 Gy possibly causing permanent azoospermia. Direct doses to the testicle less than 0.35 Gy are most likely reversible. Leydig cells are less likely to suffer functional impairment than germ cells; however, doses as small as 0.75 Gy can cause a rise in LH. High radiation doses greater than 20 Gy can affect Leydig cell function. The time for recovery is dose dependent, and there is a decline in semen parameters 60 to 70 days after radiation exposure due to the long cycle of spermatogenesis. Testicular cell damage from radiation occurs due to direct radiation or scatter from subdiaphragmatic organs.[36]

In SWOG-8711, 207 patients were treated with orchiectomy and radiotherapy; 50% of patients were subfertile before treatment. The nadir sperm concentration was 4 to 6 months after conclusion of radiotherapy, and changes in FSH mirrored changes in sperm concentration. Return to pretreatment sperm concentration is typically seen 10 to 24 months after completion of radiation therapy; however, the higher the dosage the longer the recovery. The use of shielding devices significantly decreases the radiation dosage received to the testicle. Men receiving infradiaphragmatic radiotherapy for seminoma may experience a transient decrease in sperm counts but can anticipate a recovery of spermatogenesis, which is dose dependent.[37] There are multiple factors that affect recovery of spermatogenesis after radiation (**Box 1**).

Chemotherapy

With the success of chemotherapy regimens, there is increasing focus on spermatogenic side effects because chemotherapy targets rapidly dividing cells. Pubertal status, types of chemotherapy used, and number of cycles all have effect on recovery of spermatogenesis. The chemotherapy agents that can cause or prolong azoospermia are listed in **Table 2**. Recovery of spermatogenesis after chemotherapy is possible, but men who have elevated FSH, receive high-dose cisplatin therapy, and have low pretreatment sperm counts with small testicular volumes are at increased risk for long-term infertility.

Standard chemotherapy for NSGCTs or metastatic seminoma is bleomycin, etoposide, and cisplatin. When administered at conventional doses, bleomycin and etoposide do not seem to affect long-term fertility. The cumulative cisplatin dosage is the most important factor in fertility after treatment. At levels less than 400 mg/m^2 (equivalent to 4 doses of standard cisplatin-based chemotherapy), the effects are most likely transient and affect rapidly proliferating type B spermatogonia with some damage to type A spermatogonia. At doses greater than 400 mg/m^2, there can be partial or complete destruction of

---

Box 1
Factors that affect recovery of spermatogenesis after radiation

Radiation dose[37]

Adjuvant chemotherapy

Pretreatment total motile sperm count

Age (<26 years old more favorable)

Testicular shielding[37]

Fractionated versus single-dose therapy[38]

Table 2
Antineoplastic agents that can cause azoospermia

Effect	Mechanism of Action	Agent
Prolonged azoospermia	Alkylating	Chlorambucil
		Cyclophosphamide
		Procarbazine
		Melphalan
	DNA cross-link	Cisplatin
Azoospermia in adulthood after prepubertal treatment	Alkylating	BCNU
		CCNU
Likely to cause prolonged azoospermia but always given with other highly sterilizing agents	Alkylating	Busulfan
		Ifosfamide
		Nitrogen mustard
	DNA intercalating	Actinomycin D
Reported to be additive with other agents causing prolonged azoospermia, but only temporary reductions in sperm count when not combined	Alkylating	Thiotepa
	DNA intercalating	Adriamycin
	Nucleoside analogue	Cytosine arabinoside
	Microtubule inhibitor	Vinblastine

Abbreviations: BCNU, bis-chloroethylnitrosourea (carmustine); CCNU, 1-(2-chloroethyl)-3-cyclohexyl-1-nitrosourea (lomustine).
Adapted from Meistrich ML. Effects of chemotherapy and radiotherapy on spermatogenesis in humans. Fertil Steril 2013;100(5):1180–6; with permission.

type A spermatogonia, which can cause irreversible loss of spermatogenesis.[39]

Paternity has been found dependent on the number of chemotherapy cycles; 100% of men with 2 cycles (n = 8), 83% with 3 cycles (n = 30), and 76% after 4 cycles (n = 68) were able to achieve pregnancy. There was no differences in LH, testosterone, or sperm counts; however, there was a limited number of patients with semen analysis.[40]

In another large study by Brydoy and colleagues, 554 men treated for testicular cancer were evaluated for paternity. They found that high-dose chemotherapy (>850 mg) had the lowest paternity compared with all other types of treatment. High-dose chemotherapy had a paternity rate of 38% (n = 37) versus 62% in the low-dose chemotherapy group (<850 mg) (n = 183). See **Fig. 3** for a full comparison of testicular cancer treatment and fertility rates.[33]

In summary, there are multiple factors that affect the recovery of germ cells after chemotherapy. Pretreatment factors, pubertal status, pretreatment fertility, and number of cycles and types of chemotherapy drugs all play important roles in determining the recovery of Sertoli and Leydig cell function.

Psychological and Sexual Effects of Cancer

Cancer treatment has significant effects on patient body image and sexual function. Wortel and colleagues[41] prospectively evaluated short-term body image and sexual function with questionnaires on 161 patients with testicular seminoma.

After orchiectomy, 50% expressed fertility concerns and 61% expressed body image concerns. Erectile rigidity was significantly decreased after 6 months of radiotherapy. Body image was directly associated with decreased sexual interest, pleasure, and erectile function, even though 9 out of 10 were sexually active. Arai and colleagues[42] evaluated sexuality and fertility in 85 men after various types of testicular cancer treatment. The rates and nature of sexual dysfunction in the surveillance patients were similar to the chemotherapy, RPLND, and radiotherapy groups except for ejaculatory function. Also, the surveillance group showed the highest incidence of decreased sense of attractiveness. The sexual side effects of patients on surveillance has been reproduced in a longer term study with more than 400 patients.[43]

When comparing testicular cancer treatment with Hodgkin disease, Bloom and colleagues[44] showed worse erectile function (35% vs 26%) and decreased enjoyment of orgasm (46% vs 23%) after testicular cancer treatment, even though both patients are treated during their reproductive years. Both sets of patients had issues with fertility and had significant psychological issues, including depression, anger, and divorce.

When evaluating erectile dysfunction after testicular cancer treatment, up to 84% of patients complained of loss of erection-sustaining capability with mean International Index of Erectile Function domain scores of 16. All patients had normal Doppler ultrasound, with 9 of 10 responding to phosphodiesterase type 5 inhibitors; 1 in 4 had low testosterone (<300 ng/dL).[45]

Overall, there are significant long-term psychological and sexual effects of testicular cancer treatment, regardless of the modality chosen, including surveillance.

FERTILITY PRESERVATION AND INFERTILITY OPTIONS

There has been an increased focus on preservation of fertility and discussion before cancer treatment. Patients with decreased fertility before or after cancer treatment have the ability to conceive with ART. The only guideline currently available, issued by the European Society for Medical Oncology, advocates the deferral of childbearing for at least 12 months after cancer therapy. This is a grade C recommendation based on level IV evidence. Some investigators suggest waiting up to 24 months post-treatment to allow for a decline of aneuploidy rates to baseline frequencies.[46] There is no demonstrated increase in congenital anomalies or disease states in offspring of patients treated for cancer with radiotherapy or chemotherapy (**Box 2**).[47]

Cryopreservation

The best opportunity for sperm preservation is before any cancer treatment has occurred. The sperm retrieval options for cryopreservation are discussed.

- Masturbation
- Postejaculate urinalysis for retrograde ejaculation
- Vibratory stimulation or electroejaculation for anejaculation

Box 2
American Society of Clinical Oncology recommendations for fertility preservation in cancer patients
Discuss the risk of infertility at the earliest possible time
Prompt referral to qualified specialist if the patient is interested
Sperm and embryo cryopreservation are considered standard practice
Promote clinical trials to advance state of knowledge
Adapted from Lee SJ, Schover LR, Partridge AH, et al. American Society of Clinical Oncology. American society of clinical oncology recommendations on fertility preservation in cancer patients. J Clin Oncol 2006;24(18):2917–31.

- Testicular sperm extraction if these measures fail

A proposed outline for a postpubertal patient is shown in **Fig. 4**.

Testicular cancer patients have lower sperm survival (viability) rates with cryopreservation compared with controls. Multivariate analysis shows that testicular cancer has the lowest chance of a post-thaw total motile sperm count greater than 5 million. The goal of cryopreservation is to preserve sperm for future fertility and use the lowest cost option at the time of fertility treatment. If ART is required, intrauterine insemination (IUI) is the cheapest option, but success depends on multiple male and female factors; 5 to 10 million processed total motile count should be used for IUI.[48] Other options include in vitro fertilization and intracytoplasmic sperm injection (ICSI). These are for patients with lower sperm counts who desire fertility after cancer treatment. In the ICSI era, even a few sperm from a single sample can be used for successful fertility treatment.

In a review by Ragni and colleagues[4] of their 15 year experience with cryopreservation, there was an azoospermic rate of 15.3% of men with testicular tumors. One option for these azoospermic men is an oncological testicular sperm extraction (onco-TESE). In a histologic slide review of 77 orchiectomy specimens removed for testicular cancer, 62% had spermatogenesis present. There was a statistically significant inverse relationship between tumor size and spermatogenesis presence; however, a larger tumor size did not preclude the presence of spermatogenesis.[49] Published success rates are up to 40% to 60% for onco-TESE, but it is difficult to generalize due to the low number of patients.[49–51] Also, some surgeons argue that patients with nonobstructive azoospermia should be treated with a microsurgical (micro)-TESE on the side of the testicular tumor. They also recommend having a discussion about a contralateral micro-TESE at the time of orchiectomy.[52]

Hsiao and colleagues published a 37% postchemotherapy success rate with micro-TESE in all cancer types. The mean elapsed time since chemotherapy was 18.6 years. A 57.1% fertilization rate (per injected oocyte) was achieved with ICSI, allowing a 50% clinical pregnancy rate with a live birth rate of 42% overall; 6 of 7 testicular cancer patients had a successful micro-TESE on first attempt, but there was no specific information about number of cycles or type of chemotherapy. There were no differences in age at TESE, FSH, LH, testosterone, time since chemotherapy, and average testis volume between those with successful sperm retrieval versus those without.[53]

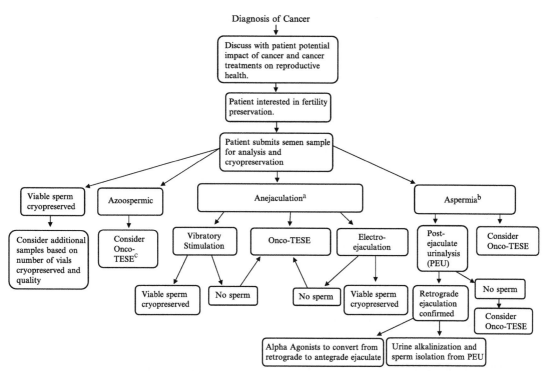

Fig. 4. Postpubertal male fertility preservation algorithm. [a] Patient unable to ejaculate. [b] No semen expelled on ejaculation. [c] onco-TESE. (*From* Brannigan RE. Fertility preservation in adult male cancer patients. Cancer Treat Res 2007;138:41; with permission.)

Postpuberty Adolescent Male Fertility Options

In postpubertal adolescent patients, there should be a careful discussion with the patient and the family members involved about the fertility options. There are multiple barriers to fertility in adolescent patients, including[54]

- Lack of time for complete discussion
- Inadequate knowledge about fertility options and desire
- Perceived awkwardness of discussion
- Lack of adolescent-appropriate educational materials

A team approach with a fertility specialist can help in these difficult discussions. In a questionnaire of 365 parents who had children treated for cancer, only 22% of all parents reported that they knew about the effect of cancer treatment on fertility before they received the questionnaire. However, 64% of parents with boys greater than 12 years of age would agree to masturbation, electroejaculation, or both to collect a semen sample for cryopreservation; 54% of parents with boys less than 12 would agree to a testicular biopsy to store spermatogonial stem cells.[55] This discussion with the patient and family is important, and the options for masturbation and

electroejaculation in adolescent patients are accepted by a significant number of families and should be discussed.

Prepubertal

Sperm banking is not possible for prepubertal males due to the absence of haploid spermatozoa and spermatids in the testis. Spermatogonial stem cells are present in the testis, however, making cryopreservation of testicular tissue a potential option. The tissue must be banked prior to the beginning of gonadotoxic cancer therapy. Several years later, the preserved tissue could be thawed and the stem cells reimplanted into the patient's own testes to continue full maturation there or undergo maturation ex vivo. This approach is experimental in humans, but there has been some success in nonhuman primates.[56]

Testicular biopsy in prepubertal males is experimental, and there are possible harms that should be discussed with families. The concerns are

- Delay in cancer treatment due to biopsy or biopsy-related side effects
- Testicular damage due to removal of testicular tissue causing decreased future fertility
- Surgical risks

- Reintroduction of malignant cells into the testes during spermatogonial stem cell transplantation
- Genetic abnormalities of offspring

Even given all these potential effects, a pilot protocol showed that 76% (n = 21) of prepubertal patients underwent testicular biopsy and cryopreservation after adequate information about the topic.[57]

Although this is an exciting field with significant future upsides, it is still experimental. There have been significant advances over the past 50 years since the discovery of different spermatogonia in the 1960s. The first successful mouse transplantation of spermatonial stem cells was in 1994. Since then, there have been further advances allowing long-term propagation of adult and prepubertal human spermatogonial stem cells.[58] One of the major challenges is that germ cells yield a low number of spermatogonial stem cells. To use prepubertal cryopreserved tissue, the spermatogonial stem cells need to be either matured in vitro or autotransplanted.[57] The use of prepubertal cryopreserved tissue is an exciting area of research, and as techniques develop further, this maybe a possibility in the future.

SUMMARY

Testicular cancer is one of the most curable cancers, affecting mostly young men in their reproductive years, making infertility after treatment important for cancer survivors. Testicular cancer patients have baseline infertility before treatment due to systemic effects, endocrine changes, possible autoimmune effects, intrinsic testicular damage, and possible congenital abnormalities in testicular maturation. Sperm counts are further affected by orchiectomy and radiation and chemotherapy effects. In addition, there are significant psychological and sexual effects in patients undergoing surveillance or those requiring further treatment after orchiectomy. Cryopreservation should be offered to patients and their families before treatment. A full discussion of the gonadotoxic effects of cancer treatment and the possibility of sperm or testicular tissue cryopreservation, even in adolescent and prepubertal patients, should become standard of care.

REFERENCES

1. Huyghe E, Matsuda T, Thonneau P. Increasing incidence of testicular cancer worldwide: a review. J Urol 2003;170:5–11.
2. Spira A. Epidemiology of human reproduction. Hum Reprod 1986;1:111–5.
3. Mosher WD, Pratt WF. Fecundity and infertility in the United States: incidence and trends. Fertil Steril 1991;56:192–3.
4. Ragni G, Somigliana E, Restelli L, et al. Sperm banking and rate of assisted reproduction treatment: insights from a 15-year cryopreservation program for male cancer patients. Cancer 2003;97(7):1624–9.
5. Lass A, Akagbosu F, Abusheikha N, et al. A programme of semen cryopreservation for patients with malignant disease in a tertiary infertility centre: lessons from 8 years' experience. Hum Reprod 1998;13:3256.
6. Bahadur G, Ozturk O, Muneer A, et al. Semen quality before and after gonadotoxic treatment. Hum Reprod 2005;20:774.
7. Williams DH, Karpman E, Sander JC, et al. Pretreatment semen parameters in men with cancer. J Urol 2009;181(2):736–40.
8. Hendry WF, Stedronska J, Jones CR, et al. Semen analysis in testicular cancer and Hodgkin's disease: pre- and post-treatment findings and implications for cryopreservation. Br J Urol 1983;55(6):769–73.
9. Dieckmann KP, Linke J, Pichlmeier U, et al. Spermatogenesis in the contralateral testis of patients with testicular germ cell cancer: histological evaluation of testicular biopsies and comparison with healthy males. BJU Int 2007;99(5):1079–85.
10. Jacobsen R, Bostofte E, Engholm G, et al. Risk of testicular cancer in men with abnormal semen characteristics: cohort study. BMJ 2000;321:789–92.
11. Walsh TJ, Croughan MS, Schembri M, et al. Increased risk of testicular germ cell cancer among infertile men. Arch Intern Med 2009;169:351–6.
12. Marmor D, Elefant E, Dauchez C, et al. Semen analysis in Hodgkin's disease before the onset of treatment. Cancer 1986;57(10):1986–7.
13. Plata-Salamán CR. Central nervous system mechanisms contributing to the cachexia-anorexia syndrome. Nutrition 2000;16(10):1009–12.
14. Hotaling JM, Lopushnyan NA, Davenport M, et al. Raw and test-thaw semen parameters after cryopreservation among men with newly diagnosed cancer. Fertil Steril 2013;99(2):464–9.
15. Carroll PR, Whitmore WF Jr, Herr HW, et al. Endocrine and exocrine profiles of men with testicular tumors before orchiectomy. J Urol 1987;137(3):420–3.
16. Petersen PM, Skakkebaek NE, Rørth M, et al. Semen quality and reproductive hormones before and after orchiectomy in men with testicular cancer. J Urol 1999;161(3):822–6.
17. Fossa SD, Theodorsen L, Norman N, et al. Recovery of impaired pretreatment spermatogenesis in testicular cancer. Fertil Steril 1990;54(3):493–6.
18. Brennemann W, Stoffel-Wagner B, Wichers M, et al. Pretreatment follicle-stimulating hormone: a prognostic serum marker of spermatogenesis status in

patients treated for germ cell cancer. J Urol 1998; 159(6):1942–6.

19. Sprauten M, Brydøy M, Haugnes HS, et al. Longitudinal serum testosterone, luteinizing hormone, and follicle-stimulating hormone levels in a population-based sample of long-term testicular cancer survivors. J Clin Oncol 2014;32(6):571–8.

20. de Bruin D, de Jong IJ, Arts EG, et al. Semen quality in men with disseminated testicular cancer: relation with human chorionic gonadotropin beta-subunit and pituitary gonadal hormones. Fertil Steril 2009; 91(6):2481–6.

21. Hansen PV, Trykker H, Andersen J, et al. Germ cell function and hormonal status in patients with testicular cancer. Cancer 1989;64(4):956–61.

22. Paoli D, Gilio B, Piroli E, et al. Testicular tumors as a possible cause of antisperm autoimmune response. Fertil Steril 2009;91(2):414–9.

23. Guazzieri S, Lembo A, Ferro G, et al. Sperm antibody and infertility in patients with testicular cancer. Urology 1985;26:139–42.

24. Foster RS, Rubin LR, McNulty A, et al. Detection of antisperm- antibodies in patients with primary testicular cancer. Int J Androl 1991;14:179–85.

25. Höbarth K, Klinger HC, Maier U, et al. Incidence of antisperm antibodies in patients with carcinoma of the testis and in subfertile men with normogonadotropic oligoasthenoteratozoospermia. Urol Int 1994; 52:162–5.

26. Garner MJ, Turner MC, Ghadirian P, et al. Epidemiology of testicular cancer: an overview. Int J Cancer 2005;116(3):331–9.

27. Juul A, Almstrup K, Andersson AM, et al. Possible fetal determinants of male infertility. Nat Rev Endocrinol 2014;10(9):553–62.

28. Qiao D, Zeeman AM, Deng W, et al. Molecular characterization of hiwi, a human member of the piwi gene family whose overexpression is correlated to seminomas. Oncogene 2002;21(25):3988–99.

29. Hotaling JM, Walsh TJ. Male infertility: a risk factor for testicular cancer. Nat Rev Urol 2009;6(10): 550–6.

30. Langenstroer P, Rosen MA, Griebling TL, et al. Ejaculatory function in stage T1 nonseminomatous germ cell tumors: retroperitoneal lymph node dissection versus surveillance–a decision analysis. J Urol 2002;168(4 Pt 1):1396–401.

31. Carroll PR, Morse MJ, Whitmore WF Jr, et al. Fertility status of patients with clinical stage I testis tumors on a surveillance protocol. J Urol 1987;138(1):70–2.

32. Jacobsen KD, Theodorsen L, Fossa SD. Spermatogenesis after unilateral orchiectomy for testicular cancer in patients following surveillance policy. J Urol 2001;165(1):93–6.

33. Brydøy M, Fosså SD, Klepp O, et al. Paternity following treatment for testicular cancer. J Natl Cancer Inst 2005;97(21):1580–8.

34. Beck SD, Bey AL, Bihrle R, et al. Ejaculatory status and fertility rates after primary retroperitoneal lymph node dissection. J Urol 2010;184(5):2078–80.

35. Jacobsen KD, Ous S, Waehre H, et al. Ejaculation in testicular cancer patients after post-chemotherapy retroperitoneal lymph node dissection. Br J Cancer 1999;80(1–2):249–55.

36. Shalet SM. Effect of irradiation treatment on gonadal function in men treated for germ cell cancer. Eur Urol 1993;23(1):148–51.

37. Gordon W Jr, Siegmund K, Stanisic TH, et al. A study of reproductive function in patients with seminoma treated with radiotherapy and orchidectomy: (SWOG-8711). Southwest Oncology Group. Int J Radiat Oncol Biol Phys 1997 Apr 1;38(1):83–94.

38. Hansen PV, Trykker H, Svennekjaer IL, et al. Long-term recovery of spermatogenesis after radiotherapy in patients with testicular cancer. Radiother Oncol 1990;18(2):117–25.

39. Pont J, Albrecht W. Fertility after chemotherapy for testicular germ cell cancer. Fertil Steril 1997; 68(1):1–5.

40. Brydøy M, Fosså SD, Klepp O, et al. Norwegian Urology Cancer Group III study group. Paternity and testicular function among testicular cancer survivors treated with two to four cycles of cisplatin-based chemotherapy. Eur Urol 2010;58(1):134–40.

41. Wortel RC, Alemayehu WG, Incrocci L. Orchiectomy and radiotherapy for stage I-II testicular seminoma: a prospective evaluation of short-term effects on body image and sexual function. J Sex Med 2015;12:210–8.

42. Arai Y, Kawakita M, Okada Y, et al. Sexuality and fertility in long-term survivors of testicular cancer. J Clin Oncol 1997;15(4):1444–8.

43. Rossen P, Pedersen AF, Zachariae R, et al. Sexuality and body image in long-term survivors of testicular cancer. Eur J Cancer 2012;48(4):571–8.

44. Bloom JR, Fobair P, Gritz E, et al. Psychosocial outcomes of cancer: a comparative analysis of Hodgkin's disease and testicular cancer. J Clin Oncol 1993;11(5):979–88.

45. Tal R, Stember DS, Logmanieh N, et al. Erectile dysfunction in men treated for testicular cancer. BJU Int 2014;113(6):907–10.

46. Choy JT, Brannigan RE. The determination of reproductive safety in men during and after cancer treatment. Fertil Steril 2013;100(5):1187–91.

47. Hartmann JT, Albrecht C, Schmoll HJ, et al. Long-term effects on sexual function and fertility after treatment of testicular cancer. Br J Cancer 1999; 80(5–6):801–7.

48. Nangia AK, Krieg SA, Kim SS. Clinical guidelines for sperm cryopreservation in cancer patients. Fertil Steril 2013;100(5):1203–9.

49. Choy JT, Wiser HJ, Bell SW, et al. Predictors of spermatogenesis in orchiectomy specimens. Urology 2013;81(2):288–92.

50. Schrader M, Müller M, Sofikitis N, et al. "Onco-tese": testicular sperm extraction in azoospermic cancer patients before chemotherapy-new guidelines? Urology 2003;61(2):421–5.

51. Furuhashi K, Ishikawa T, Hashimoto H, et al. Onco-testicular sperm extraction: testicular sperm extraction in azoospermic and very severely oligozoospermic cancer patients. Andrologia 2013;45(2):107–10.

52. Haddad N, Al-Rabeeah K, Onerheim R, et al. Is ex vivo microdissection testicular sperm extraction indicated for infertile men undergoing radical orchiectomy for testicular cancer? Case report and literature review. Fertil Steril 2014;101(4):956–9.

53. Hsiao W, Stahl PJ, Osterberg EC, et al. Successful treatment of postchemotherapy azoospermia with microsurgical testicular sperm extraction: the weill cornell experience. J Clin Oncol 2011;29(12):1607–11.

54. Nahata L, Cohen LE, Yu RN. Barriers to fertility preservation in male adolescents with cancer: it's time for a multidisciplinary approach that includes urologists. Urology 2012;79(6):1206–9.

55. Sadri-Ardekani H, Akhondi MM, Vossough P, et al. Parental attitudes toward fertility preservation in boys with cancer: context of different risk levels of infertility and success rates of fertility restoration. Fertil Steril 2013;99(3):796–802.

56. Di Pietro ML, Teleman AA. Cryopreservation of testicular tissue in pediatrics: practical and ethical issues. J Matern Fetal Neonatal Med 2013;26(15):1524–7.

57. Ginsberg JP, Carlson CA, Lin K, et al. An experimental protocol for fertility preservation in prepubertalboys recently diagnosed with cancer: a report of acceptability and safety. Hum Reprod 2010;25(1):37–41.

58. Struijk RB, Mulder CL, van der Veen F, et al. Restoring fertility in sterile childhood cancer survivors by autotransplanting spermatogonial stem cells: are we there yet? Biomed Res Int 2013;2013:903142.

Index

Note: Page numbers of article titles are in **boldface** type.

Urol Clin N Am 42 (2015) 421–427
http://dx.doi.org/10.1016/S0094-0143(15)00067-1
0094-0143/15/$ – see front matter © 2015 Elsevier Inc. All rights reserved.

urologic.theclinics.com

Moving?

Make sure your subscription moves with you!

To notify us of your new address, find your **Clinics Account Number** (located on your mailing label above your name), and contact customer service at:

Email: journalscustomerservice-usa@elsevier.com

800-654-2452 (subscribers in the U.S. & Canada)
314-447-8871 (subscribers outside of the U.S. & Canada)

Fax number: 314-447-8029

Elsevier Health Sciences Division
Subscription Customer Service
3251 Riverport Lane
Maryland Heights, MO 63043

*To ensure uninterrupted delivery of your subscription, please notify us at least 4 weeks in advance of move.

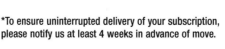

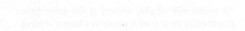

Printed and bound by CPI Group (UK) Ltd, Croydon, CR0 4YY

03/10/2024

01040381-0017